MEDICAL RADIOLOGY

Diagnostic Imaging

Editors:
A. L. Baert, Leuven
M. Knauth, Göttingen
K. Sartor, Heidelberg

T. J. Vogl · T. K. Helmberger · M. G. Mack
M. F. Reiser (Eds.)

Percutaneous Tumor Ablation in Medical Radiology

With Contributions by

A. Boss · D. Dupuy · K. Eichler · R.-T. Hoffmann · N. Hosten · T. F. Jakobs
W. A. Kaiser · G. Kirsch · M. Kirsch · A. Lubienski · A. H. Mahnken · K. Mohnike
H. Müller · M. Nabil · P. L. Pereira · S. O. R. Pfleiderer · D. Proschek · J. Ricke
M. Simon · K. Steinke · C. Trumm · S. Zangos · A. Zinke

Foreword by

A. L. Baert

With 133 Figures in 281 Separate Illustrations, 50 in Color and 33 Tables

Springer

Thomas J. Vogl, MD
Professor, Institute for Diagnostic and
Interventional Radiology
University Hospital
Johann Wolfgang Goethe University
Theodor-Stern-Kai 7
60590 Frankfurt am Main
Germany

Martin G. Mack, MD
PD, Institute for Diagnostic and
Interventional Radiology
University Hospital
Johann Wolfgang Goethe University
Theodor-Stern-Kai 7
60590 Frankfurt am Main
Germany

Thomas K. Helmberger, MD
Professor, Department of Diagnostic and
Interventional Radiology and Nuclear Medicine
Klinikum Bogenhausen, Academic Teaching
Hospital of the Technical University Munich
Engelschalkingerstrasse 77
81925 Munich
Germany

Maximilian F. Reiser, MD
Professor and Chairman
Department of Clinical Radiology
University Hospitals – Grosshadern and Innenstadt
Ludwig-Maximilians-University of Munich
Marchioninistrasse 15
81377 Munich
Germany

Medical Radiology · Diagnostic Imaging and Radiation Oncology
Series Editors:
A. L. Baert · L. W. Brady · H.-P. Heilmann · M. Knauth · M. Molls · C. Nieder · K. Sartor

Continuation of Handbuch der medizinischen Radiologie
Encyclopedia of Medical Radiology

ISBN 978-3-642-06137-0 ISBN 978-3-540-68250-9 (eBook)

Springer is part of Springer Science+Business Media

http//www.springer.com

Softcover reprint of the hardcover 1st edition 2008

Medical Editor: Dr. Ute Heilmann, Heidelberg
Desk Editor: Ursula N. Davis, Heidelberg
Production Editor: Kurt Teichmann, Mauer

Printed on acid-free paper – 21/3180xq – 5 4 3 2 1 0

Foreword

Percutaneous image-guided non-invasive treatment of tumors is now widely regarded as one of the major advances achieved during the past decade in interventional radiology and in medicine.

Over the past years radiologists all over the world have been deeply involved in technological and animal research which has resulted in powerful new clinical tools for tumor ablation.

These include mainly thermal ablative techniques such as laser-induced thermotherapy, radiofrequency and microwave ablation, but also chemoembolization as well as selective internal irradiation therapy.

This volume is one of the most comprehensive books offering a complete overview of our current knowledge in percutaneous tumor ablation. It covers not only all technical aspects of the sophisticated new modalities now available, but also a variety of specific clinical indications for each of these techniques within the framework of a global approach to the oncological patient.

The very well readable text is completed by numerous superb illustrations.

This book should help radiologists not only to improve their skills in percutaneous image-guided ablation techniques, but also to fully assume their role as a key member of the multidisciplinary team that takes responsibility for designing the global treatment strategy and management of oncological patients.

I would like to thank and congratulate most sincerely the editors and authors for preparing this very attractive volume on a highly topical, important though rapidly evolving topic.

This book will be of great interest both to interventional radiologists and to oncologists. I am confident that it will meet with the same success among readers as the previous volumes published in this series.

Leuven — Albert L. Baert

Preface

Technological and oncological advances have provided new methods for the minimally invasive treatment of malignant tumors. A great deal of enthusiasm has developed recently in the use of local oncological treatment options such as thermal ablative therapies and locoregional chemotherapy. The present book features the clinical and practical aspects of thermal ablation as well as the latest advances and applications of this emerging, ground-breaking technology. The editors and authors extensively cover the principles and techniques for the safe usage of local oncological treatment options. Current concepts on the management of hepatic tumors and lung malignancies are presented. The book further stresses applications on primary and secondary bone tumors, primary breast cancer, renal tumors and head and neck cancer. All the technical aspects of locoregional therapies are extensively discussed. Practical guidelines and an evaluation of the results so far obtained are presented. Special focus is also put on the different monitoring technologies such as ultrasound guidance, CT and MRI.

In summary, we have tried to provide a state-of-the-art textbook on the current theoretical and clinical aspects of thermal ablative therapies in order to establish a safe and viable treatment modality for our patients.

Frankfurt	Thomas J. Vogl
Munich	Thomas K. Helmberger
Frankfurt	Martin G. Mack
Munich	Maximilian F. Reiser

Contents

Percutaneous Tumor Ablation

Percutaneous Tumor Ablation

Basic Principles in Oncology

1

Thomas J. Vogl

CONTENTS

1.1 General

The evolving field of interventional oncology can only be considered as a small integrative part in the complex area of oncology. The new field of interventional oncology needs a standardization of the procedures, the terminology, and criteria to facilitate the effective communication of ideas and appropriate comparison between treatments and new integrative technology. In principle, ablative therapy is a part of locoregional oncological therapy and is defined either as chemical ablation using ethanol or acetic acid, or thermotherapies such as radiofrequency, laser, microwave, and cryoablation. All these new evolving therapies have to be exactly evaluated and an adequate terminology has to be used to define imaging findings and pathology. All the different technologies and evaluated therapies have to be compared, and the results have to be analyzed in order to improve the patient outcome.

T. J. Vogl, MD
Professor, Institute for Diagnostic and Interventional Radiology, University Hospital, Johann Wolfgang Goethe University, Theodor-Stern-Kai 7, 60590 Frankfurt am Main, Germany

1.2 Interventional Therapies

"Tumor ablation" is defined as the direct application of thermal or chemical therapies to a specific focal tumor (tumors) in order to achieve either eradication or substantial tumor destruction. The term "direct" is combined with tumor ablation to distinguish these therapies from others that are applied orally or via an intravascular or a peripheral venous route. The area of intravascular tumor therapy, like locoregional chemotherapy or chemoembolization, becomes increasingly important due to newer combined strategies combining thermoablation and locoregional chemotherapy. The expression of image guidance should be added to the term "thermal ablation" because most of these therapies are performed using a host of imaging modalities, such as fluoroscopy, ultrasound, computed tomography (CT), or magnetic resonance imaging (MRI). From a theoretical point nearly all ablation techniques available can be used with more than one modality. The term "minimal invasive procedures" refers to all therapeutic procedures that are less invasive than open conventional surgery. Most of the surgeons refer to these procedures. The term "percutaneous therapies" should only be used when appropriate.

In general, tumor ablation can be divided into two main categories. The first one is *chemical ablation*, the second one is *thermal ablation*. Additionally, other interventional oncological therapeutic approaches have to be defined, such as the percutaneous delivery of radioactive seeds and the transcatheter delivery of chemotherapy and chemoembolization.

"Chemical ablation" is classified based on the used agent, such as ethanol, or acetic acid. By definition, chemical ablation induces coagulation necrosis and tumor ablation. Ethanol ablation is also called "percutaneous ethanol instillation" (PEI), "percutaneous alcohol instillation" (PAI), and others. For all chemical ablations the parameters have to be defined, for example the route (intravenous, intra-arterial, or interstitial), the substances that are injected, the delivery vehicle (size and type of needle or catheter), and the rate of delivery (rapid injection or a defined rate of infusion).

In the category "thermal ablation" all energy sources that destroy a tumor with thermal energy are included, either by heat [radiofrequency (RF), laser, etc.] or by cold (cryoablation). A thermal ablation *procedure* is defined as a single intervention episode which consists of one or more ablations performed on one or more tumors. A *treatment*, on the other hand, consists of one or more "procedures" or "sessions". The energy is normally applied via "applicators". While for RF the applicators are "electrodes", for microwave they are "antennas", and for laser applicators they are "fibers". For cryoablation "cryoprobes" are used to freeze tissue during cryoablation.

In **RF ablation** coagulation is achieved with induction from all electromagnetic energy sources less than 900 kHz. Most of the currently available devices function in their range between 375 and 500 kHz and are either monopolar or bipolar systems. Many electrode variations are currently available, which will be described in more detail in the technical and clinical parts of the book (multi-tined, expandable electrodes, internally cooled electrodes, and perfusion electrodes). For each RF application the algorithm used should be differentiated (ramped energy deposition or impedance regulated and the model number of the generator). Other parameters are the use of monopolar/bipolar systems, the duration of ablation and the amount of energy applied (in current and/or watts). Additional adjuvant therapies are used such as the concomitant percutaneous instillation of sodium chloride solutions to alter the electrical and thermal conductivity during ablation. Hence, the specific details of the adjuvant used (such as drug concentration, rate of administration, route, and timing) should be clearly defined.

"**Laser ablation**" is currently the defined term for all methods of ablation using light energy. Multiple laser technology and application methods are currently in use, such as the superficial therapy contact/noncontact mode or transcutaneous ablation.

The term "interstitial" or "direct" relates to the laser energy that is applied via fibers directly inserted into the tissue.

For the definition of the parameters of laser ablation, laser source (Nd:YAG, Erbium, Holmium, etc.), the precise wavelength, and the device characteristics have to be specified. This includes the type of laser fiber (flexible/glass dome), modifications of the tip (flexible diffuser tip, or scattering dome) with dimensions and materials (length of applicator and diameter of the optic fiber), and the number of laser applicators used. The laser power reported as watts per cm active length, the total duration of energy application, the total amount of energy applied per tumor in the mean and range should be provided as well. In addition to the energy measured before the laser enters the fiber, the actual energy output of the fiber/dome prior to the ablation and/or the end of the procedure should be ideally measured for the applied energy.

For electromagnetic methods for inducing tumor destruction with frequencies greater than or equal to 900 kHz, the term "**microwave ablation (MW)**" is used. Different systems are currently available. Those systems work at 915 MHz and 40 W. The studies showed that microwave and RF ablation zones are similar in pathological appearance and imaging characteristics. Increased length with MW is likely caused by the length of the radiating segment of the antenna. MW ablation offers many of the advantages of RF ablation by possibly overcoming some of the limitations. It does not rely on conduction of electricity into tissue, and it is not limited by charring. Therefore, temperatures greater than 100°C are readily achieved, which potentially results in a larger zone of ablation, faster treatment time and more complete tumor kill. MW ablation has a much broader power field than RF ablation (up to 2 cm in diameter). This allows for larger zones of thermal ablation and a more uniform tumor kill. The cooling effect of blood flow is reduced in comparison to other techniques, thus also enhancing the treatment of perivascular tissue. Other MW systems limit the power at 2450 MHz up to 150 W. The advantage of MW ablation is the proved performance near blood vessels combined with the ability to use multiple simultaneous probes.

For the ultrasound ablation two methods are currently available – extracorporeal (transcutaneous) and direct (or percutaneous) via a needle-like applicator. The term "high intensity focused ultrasound" should be reserved for describing the extracorporeal method. Direct ultrasound ablation means the replacement of an applicator via a percutaneous or laparoscopic insertion.

The destruction of tissue by the application of low temperature freezing is defined as "**cryoablation**". In the past, liquid nitrogen was directly placed on the tissue. In the neck, chest, abdomen, pelvis, and extremities, cryoablation is performed using a closed cryoprobe that is placed on the inside of the tumor. Currently, two main types of systems are used, i.e., either gas/liquid nitrogen, or argon gas. The temperature measurement is either at the tip of the cryoprobe or on the handle. However, the temperature, at which cryoablation is performed, the type of the cryoablation system, the gases used, the probe dimensions, and the number of freeze–thaw cycles should be specified.

For all thermal ablations it is important to be aware of the effects of blood flow because all these methods are negatively influenced by the blood flow as the heat is removed before achieving complete tumor ablation. These cooling effects are described with the term "heat sink effect". The heat sink effect is due to the tumor-adjacent visible (>1 mm diameter) blood vessels when ablated tissues are heated. This results in the shape of thermal lesions altering away from the vessel and the diminishing overall lesion size due to the removal of heat or cold by the flowing blood. It is an advantage that the vessels are protected and bleeding from large vessels is prevented but it can also be a major source of incomplete tumor ablation. Another phenomenon is the term "perfusion mediated tissue cooling (or heating)" which refers to both the effects of the larger heat-sinking vessels and the substantial effects of capillary level microperfusion. This is important because several techniques have been developed or are under consideration to overcome the problem of a pharmacologically induced decrease in blood flow, and temporary vascular balloon occlusion of a specific vessel during ablation (intra-arterial embolization and chemoembolization as well as a Pringle maneuver during surgery). All procedures for thermal ablation are also defined by the expression "**image guidance**", since thermal ablation imaging is used in five separate and distinct ways: (1) planning, (2) ultrasound, (3) CT, (4) MRI, (5) PET.

Ablative Techniques (Percutaneous)

2

Thermal Ablative Techniques

2.1 Radiofrequency Ablation

Thomas K. Helmberger

CONTENTS

The heating effect of alternating radiofrequency (RF) in biological tissue was first described by the French physiologist Jaques D'Arsonval (1851–1940) in the late nineteenth century. From that time on RF gained an important role in many fields of medical treatment. A wide variety of surgical RF instruments were developed, mostly combining tissue dissection and haemostasis by coagulation. In the early 1990s the percutaneous use of needle like probes for interstitial thermal ablation of tumour tissue was reported for the first time (McGahan et al. 1990; Rossi et al. 1990). Since then enormous development of percutaneous RF technology has taken place.

After the initial experience in treatment of hepatic tumours, RF ablation (RFA) was approved as a tissue-sparing, minimally invasive tool for successful tumour eradication resulting in satisfactory survival times in tumours of the kidneys and adrenals, of the lungs, bones, and soft tissue – comparable to surgery even considering the different selection criteria.

2.1.1 Basic Principles of Radiofrequency Ablation

2.1.1.1 Physical Background

In general, the various types of thermoablative techniques differ only by their physical method of generating heat (e.g. radiofrequency, laser, micro wave, focused ultrasound). The fundamental principle of RFA is based upon the biophysical interaction of high-frequency alternating current (typically 450–500 kHz) and biological tissue in terms of resistive (frictional) energy loss. Therefore, the term radiofrequency alludes to the alternating electric current oscillating in a high-frequency range of the alternating current. Between the active and the reference electrode (or two active electrodes in bipolar systems) an electric field is established which oscillates with RF frequency. Ionic oscillatory agitation induced by this oscillating field results in frictional heat followed by "coagulative" necrosis if enough energy is deployed, whereas the field intensity determines directly the frequency of the oscillation.

In consequence, the heat emerges into tissue in the immediate vicinity of the electrode (antenna).

T. K. Helmberger, MD
Professor, Department of Diagnostic and Interventional Radiology and Nuclear Medicine, Klinikum Bogenhausen, Academic Teaching Hospital of the Technical University Munich, Engelschalkinger Str. 77, 81925 Munich, Germany

Further heat dispersion is a result of heat conductivity and convection effects (McGahan et al. 1990).

The generated frictional heat is directly and proportionally dependent on the RF energy delivered, while the total thermal damage caused to the tissue is dependent on both the tissue temperature finally achieved and the duration of heating. An increased temperature of up to 42°C (i.e. hyperthermia) results in an increased susceptibility of the heated tissue to chemotherapy and radiation. A temperature of 45°C for several hours results in irreversible cell damage. The latter cytotoxic effect can be drastically shortened down to a few minutes by increasing the temperature up to 50°–60°C. Almost instant coagulation of tissue is induced at temperatures between 60°C and 100°C and is manifest as irreversible damage to mitochondrial and cytosolic enzymes of the cells and to DNA. At more than 100°–110°C, tissue will vaporize and carbonize (Goldberg 2001; Goldberg and Gazelle 2001).

Due to the specific tissue resistance and the energy dispersion between the needle-like electrode and the dispersive ground pad there is a rapid decay of energy and consequently of heat around the electrode, where the temperature is inversely proportional to the distance from the electrode ($T \approx 1/r^4$; T = temperature, r = radius around the electrode). This means that destructive thermal energy can be deployed sufficiently only within a volume of a maximum diameter of 2.2–2.4 cm around a single, needle-like electrode (Fig. 2.1.1). As a consequence, the energy is delivered quite precisely and focused to the volume around the electrode, making heat-induced damage remote to the source of heat (RFA) rather unlikely.

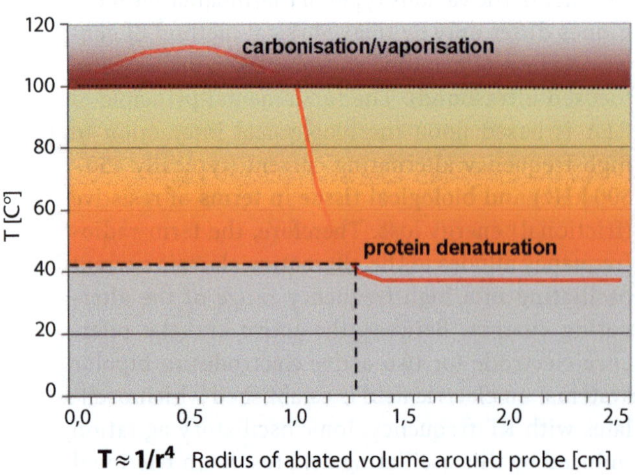

Fig. 2.1.1. The diagram illustrates the interdependency of temperature and radius around a single needle electrode. Note the rapid decay of the temperature over a distance of more than 1 cm from the electrode, which makes the ablation process very focused

Using advanced needle designs volumes of up to 5 cm diameter can be ablated. Accepting an increased time for treatment needle repositioning and creating overlapping volumes may result in even larger volumes (Raman et al. 2000; Scott et al. 2000). Nevertheless, the finally resulting volume of ablation is also considerably dependent on the intrinsic tissue properties such as heat conductivity and convection (Fig. 2.1.2). In this regard two crucial effects must be mentioned: the so-called heat sink effect and the oven effect. The heat sink effect is caused by large vessels – mainly hepatic veins – near to the heat source resulting in heat loss. This effect can be used to increase the ablated volume by temporarily occluding these vessels (e.g. balloon occlusion of a hepatic vein, temporary occlusion of the portal vein, in Pringle's manoeuvre) (de Baere et al. 2002; Elias et al. 2004).

In hepatocellular carcinomas (HCC) within cirrhotic livers in particular, the "oven effect" can be noticed: a well-demarcated ablation, even with volumes larger than expected by the needle design can be achieved because the heat is "trapped" within the (pseudo) encapsulated tumor volume.

In summary the efficacy of the RF energy deposition is determined by the:

- Amount and duration of the energy exposure (watts, time)
- Probe design
- Intrinsic tissue factors (heat connectivity and conversion)
- Heat sink and congestion effects.

In biological tissues, it remains impossible to predict exactly the effect of a specific energy delivery since even in a given biological "system" the system's variables change during the process of energy deployment in a non-linear feed-back mechanism (Fig. 2.1.2). On a theoretical basis for ideal systems, these effects have been calculated in several ways; for example, by Penn's equation or the thermal wave model of bio-heat transfer (Liu et al. 1999). For practical reasons the complex theoretical considerations can be simplified by correlating tissue destruction (i.e. coagulation) to:

- The energy delivered corrected by an (unknown) possibly tissue-specific correction factor (in clinical reality this means that more energy is needed than expected)

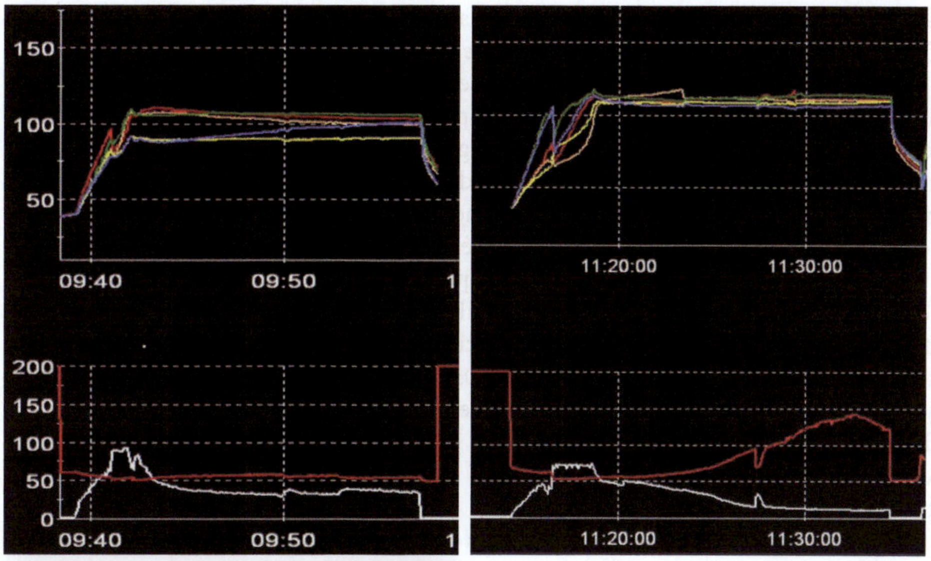

a b

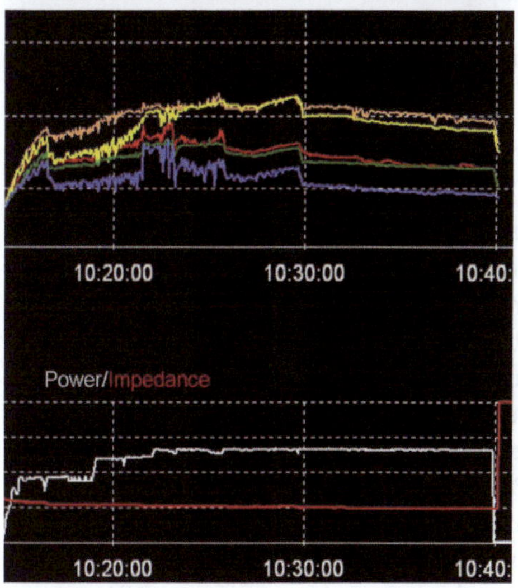

c

Fig. 2.1.2. **a** Intrinsic tissue properties may influence the ablation process as demonstrated in this examples of three different tumor types. In the colorectal metastasis increased power (*white line*, *lower part* of the *diagram*) was necessary only at the beginning of the ablation process to bring the temperature within the tumour to 100°C (*five coloured lines*, *upper part* of the *diagram*) and to maintain it. Tumour impedance remained the same throughout the entire process (*red line*, *lower part* of the *diagram*). **b** While the temperature graphs in a hepatocellular carcinoma (*HCC*) run almost parallel to those for the colorectal carcinoma metastasis, the power and impedance courses are completely different. The impedance rises with progression of the ablation while decreasing power is required to hold the temperature. **c** In contrast, in a sarcoma metastasis maximum power is delivered without reaching the desired temperature of 100°C in all areas of the tumour (*coloured lines*, *upper part* of the *diagram*). Note the spikes of the temperature graphs representing gas blebs. Repositioning of the electrode was necessary in this case to provide complete ablation of the entire tumour volume

- Reduced energy loss resulting from tissue-specific cooling effects (i.e. vascular perfusion, insulation effects, etc.).

In consequence, one has to keep in mind that in clinical practice:

- The energy = definable [$J=W\times t$; J=energy (joule), W=power (watts), t=time (s)]
- The tissue interaction = variable (unpredictable)
- The result = estimation

In consequence, different strategies are conceivable and/or applicable to enhance the ablation process: (1) improving heat conduction, (2) decreasing heat tolerance of the tumour and (3) increasing energy deposition.

Heat conduction can be improved by the injection of saline, which increases the amount of ions with subsequent increased flow of electric current (Goldberg and Gazelle 2001; Kettenbach et al. 2003). The same concept of augmented amplification is applied by injecting iron oxide microparticles into the target tissue (Merkle et al. 1999). Nevertheless, this technique – especially utilizing larger amounts of saline – is not yet common in clinical practice. Potential drawbacks include unpredictable ablation zones following the spreading of the saline and a need for increased energy deposition. Otherwise, there is insufficient energy transfer to the increased number of ions.

According to the theoretical consideration of factors influencing ablation, heat loss by parenchymal perfusion is crucial. Parenchymal perfusion significantly affects the efficacy of a thermal ablation procedure, as shown by Patterson et al.'s (1998) demonstration of ablation with and without Pringle's manoeuvre. Thus, mechanical reduction of local blood flow may enhance the ablation process; however, achieving this can be quite elaborate and can itself be a source for secondary complications. Less invasively lowering perfusion of the tumour pharmacologically, embolizing the tumour's vasculature, and infusing alcohol and acetic acid may also increase the ablation volume, although as yet it is too early to consider these techniques as sufficiently established (Lubienski et al. 2005). Finally, the heat tolerance of tumour cells may be affected by prior chemotherapy and/or radiation therapy. However, the exact effects of "adjuvant" therapeutic regimens to enhance the ablation processes have not yet been systematically evaluated (Goldberg et al. 1999).

2.1.1.2 Monopolar Systems

In the technical setting of monopolar systems the patient is turned into a resistor within a closed-loop circuit consisting of a RF generator, a large dispersive electrode (grounding pads typically placed on the thighs of the patient), and a needle electrode (antenna) in series. Thus, an alternating electric field is created within the tissue of the patient concentrating the electrical energy around the non-insulated tip of the needle-like electrode. Given the relatively high electrical resistance of tissue in comparison with the metal electrodes, there is marked agitation of the ions present in the tissue surrounding the needle-like electrode, concentrating the energy (Ni et al. 2000; Goldberg and Gazelle 2001; Brieger et al. 2003; Lee, Haemmerich et al. 2003; Lee, Han et al. 2003; Pereira et al. 2003).

2.1.1.3 Bipolar Systems

In bipolar systems the two non-insulated electrodes are placed in situ in the same probe. From a physical point of view, bipolar probes seem particularly suitable for avoiding energy dispersion between the dispersive and focusing electrodes. Just recently the first bipolar probes were approved for interstitial tumour ablation. Nevertheless, the same physical properties, i.e. the limited penetration depth of radiofrequency current, apply to both bipolar and monopolar probes. Therefore, the most crucial factor regarding the efficacy of RFA electrodes in terms of reproducible homogenous ablation volumes remains the design of the active electrode tip(s). Recent developments (Olympus-Celon) allow a multiplexed operation of several bipolar electrodes in a cluster-like array where a switch-box controls the electric current between several electrodes (Burdio et al. 2003; Tacke et al. 2004; Frericks et al. 2005; Clasen et al. 2006, 2007).

2.1.1.4 Electrode Designs

In principle, an RF electrode consists of an insulated metallic shaft and a non-insulated, active tip of variable length and/or design. To close the electric circuit of the above-described system of generator, electrodes and patient, the active tip is in contact with the target tissue.

To increase the volume of ablation modifications have been made to the probe design, e.g. extending the length of the antenna (cluster needle, umbrella/inverted umbrella-like design) or internal cooling of the needle to avoid premature carbonization around the probe followed by insulation and energy decay (Fig. 2.1.3). At present, the available electrodes provide ablation volumes with more or less spherical diameters of between 2 and 5 cm.

Pereira et al. compared four different RFA systems in an in vivo animal model: a perfused electrode, an internally cooled electrode, and two different multi-tined electrodes utilizing the vendors' protocols (Pereira et al. 2004). Among the four tested and at that time commercially available systems, larger coagulation volumes could be obtained with the perfusion (at present no longer available) and internally cooled cluster devices. More spherical volumes of ablation were achieved with the 12-tine and cluster electrodes. The cluster and nine-tine electrode produced better reproducibility, which is suggestive of improved predictability of the extent of coagulation with these systems. However, in interpreting these data one has to remember that the unmodified vendors' protocols were used and consequently the deployed power differed significantly (60–250 W).

Beside the specific needle design, and the handling and usability of the different systems, a more

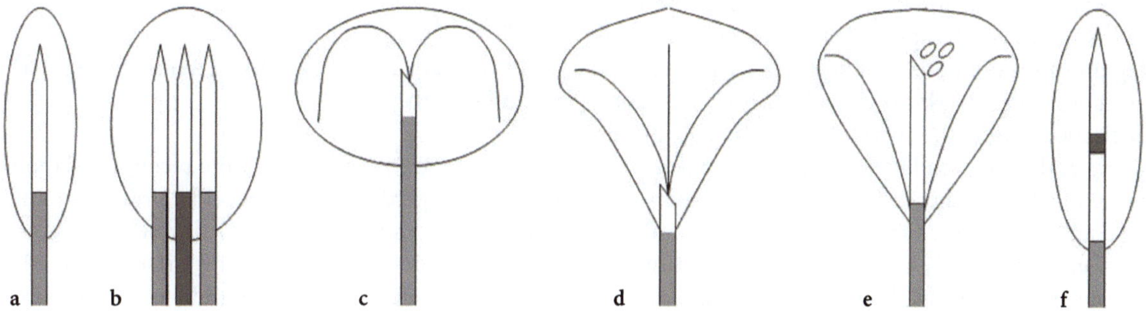

Fig. 2.1.3a–f. Various radiofrequency (*RF*) electrodes: **a** single needle design (Cool Tip, Valleylab System, Tyco), **b** cluster-electrode (Cool Tip Cluster, Valleylab, Tyco); multi-tined electrodes (**c** LeVeen, Radiotherapeutics, Boston Scientific; **d** Starburst XL; **e** perfused Talon needle, AngioDynamics-RITA); **f** internally cooled, bipolar single needle electrode (Olympus Celon)

important role regarding the proper use of a device might be how experienced the user is, as confirmed by Poon et al. (2004b) and Lu et al. (2005). Poon and co-workers could prove in a prospective analysis that the results of percutaneous, laparoscopic and open RFA in terms of morbidity and effectiveness (= complete ablation) increased significantly during the learning period – independently if a single or cluster electrode was used (Poon et al. 2004b). Furthermore the same group could show that there was no significant difference in RFA of hepatocellular carcinomas greater than 3 cm regarding access route (percutaneous, laparoscopic, open), complications, mortality, and success in comparison to tumours smaller than 3 cm in diameter – again independently from the device used (Poon et al. 2004a). These results were confirmed by Lu et al. (2005) since in his work the most important factor influencing the primary success rate was tumour size, independently of electrode design (cluster vs. multi-tined).

2.1.1.5 RF Generators

Different vendors pursue slightly different strategies in terms of generator control and therefore the ablation process. In the internally cooled single and cluster electrode system (Cool-tip, Valleylab, Tyco Healthcare) it are mainly algorithms that are applied, with pulsed delivery of high energy levels over a relatively short period of time (10–15 min) without feedback control. In the multi-tined system with impedance control (Boston Scientific) and the bipolar, single or multi-electrode system (Olympus Celon) a step-wise increased or fixed amount of energy is controlled by the tissue resistance rising with increasing desiccation. In the second multi-tined system (AngioDynamics RITA) the power delivery is controlled by temperature feedback derived from thermistors at the tips of the tines.

As discussed above many different factors influence the process of RFA, which make a vendor's recommendation regarding a specific ablation algorithm only a rough estimate (Goldberg 2001). Therefore, an individual learning curve is necessary to collect enough personal experience to understand and to control the process of ablation sufficiently and to warrant an efficient result in terms of tumour control (Poon et al. 2004b).

2.1.2 Indications and Contraindications

Radiofrequency ablation of primary and secondary hepatic malignancies has been in wide use for more then 10 years. Meanwhile, the continual improvement of generators and probes has led to reproducible and satisfactory results, although the primary local success is often constrained by further progress of the underlying malignant disease. Therefore, there seems almost general agreement that RFA, especially in hepatic metastases (e.g. metastases from colorectal cancer), must be integrated in an interdisciplinary multimodality treatment concept (e.g. adjuvant combination with chemotherapy).

In recent years minimally invasive thermoablative therapy has been applied to almost all kinds of tumours in the human body. Promising initial results were shown for RFA in tumours of the lung, kidney, adrenals, lymph nodes, of the head and neck region, prostate, bone and soft tissue, nerves, and even of the breast (Neeman and Wood 2002; Wood et al. 2002; Lau et al. 2003; Gervais et al. 2005b). Ongoing and future studies will and have to prove the prerequisites for successful treatment in these new fields. Nevertheless, similar basic inclusion and exclusion criteria apply to almost all of these tumours irrespective of their pathological origin or anatomical localization (Table 2.1.1).

Table 2.1.1. Inclusion and exclusion criteria for radiofrequency ablation (*RFA*) of soft-tissue tumours

Prerequisites	Adequate assessment of the overall tumour situation
	Incorporation of thermal therapy into a comprehensive treatment concept
	Balance of advantages and disadvantages of a minimally invasive therapy by an interdisciplinary oncological team
Indications	Exclusion of respectability
	Pre OP in bi-lobar hepatic tumors
	Medical reasons
	Number of lesions <4–5[a]
	Lesion diameter <3.5–5 cm (HCC, kidney and lung tumors)[a]
Contraindications	Progressive systemic disease
	Lesions >5, diameter >5 cm
	Colorectal metastases <3.5 cm[a]
	Thrombosis of portal vein (one branch?)
	Septicemia, coagulopathy
	Tumour volume >50 % organ volume
Relative contraindications	Biliodigestive anastomosis in hepatic tumors
	Pacemaker
	Vicinity to critical structures[b]

[a]Centre dependent, no final agreement. [b]See below "Complications"

2.1.3 Considerations Regarding Lesion Size and Localization

In terms of guidelines no definite recommendations exist yet regarding those specific properties that make a lesion suitable for RFA. Nevertheless, based on the electrophysiological characteristic of the RFA systems, the electrode design and last but not least on oncological considerations, special thought has to be given to the size and localization of a lesion in order to achieve complete ablation (Kuvshinoff and Ota 2002).

To destroy any given tumour completely the ablation volume should envelope the tumour entirely together with a safety margin (5–10 mm) according to surgical rules. The pathophysiological rationale for the safety margin is the high likelihood of scattered tumour cells (invisible to imaging) immediately around the tumour nodule visible by imaging. If only the visible tumour is treated then local recurrence can easily emerge from the tumour cells remaining around the visible tumour. Since the available electrode designs allow more or less spherical ablation volumes with a maximum diameter of about 4–5 cm in a single ablation session lesions with a diameter of 3–4 cm can be treated to achieve an adequate safety margin. Dodd et al. (2001) demonstrated in a computer simulation that tumours of diameters between 1 and 3 cm can be treated sufficiently with a single ablation procedure using 3- to 5-cm electrodes, whereas for diameters up to 4.25 cm and 6.3 cm, respectively, a composite ablation with 6 up to 14 spherical, overlapping ablations is necessary (Dodd et al. 2001). It is easy to understand that in most cases a composite ablation with more than three electrode positions is difficult to operate under clinical conditions.

This considerations are approved by the recent literature, in which local recurrence rates in primary and secondary liver tumours rise with lesion size after a single ablation, or several ablations sessions are necessary to gain compete ablation (Poon et al. 2002, 2004a, 2004b; Gervais et al. 2005a; Lencioni et al. 2005; Lu et al. 2005; Suh et al. 2005; Choi et al. 2007; Yamakado et al. 2007). According to these current references the cut-off lesion diameter for a primary successful RFA is about 3 cm with the RFA systems that are available at present – independent of the anatomical tumour site and histopathological tumour type.

Another independent predictor of a successful ablation is the tumour's vicinity to major vessels causing heat sink effects. Lu et al. (2003) showed that, in 105 tumours with a mean diameter of 2.4 cm treated with two different multi-tined and one cluster RFA system (no difference regarding the RFA system used or whether it was open or percutaneous access!), lesions at least 3 mm from a major vessel presented a primarily incomplete ablation or recurrence only in 7%, while this was true in 48% of tumours that were in the direct vicinity of major vessels (Lu et al. 2003).

In consequence, both these independent predictors of success – lesion size and vascular proximity – have to be incorporated into a RFA treatment concept.

Overall, the primary success rates of RFA in liver, kidney, lung and bone tumours range from 70% to more than 95%, depending on the tumour localization and type – assuming the above-mentioned advice has been considered.

Detailed discussion on the outcome for different tumour and organ entities is provided in several chapters of this volume.

2.1.4 Standard of RFA Procedure

2.1.4.1 Image Guidance and Procedure Monitoring

Radiofrequency ablation can usually be performed as a minimally invasive, percutaneous (outpatient) procedure under conscious sedation. General anaesthesia is usually not necessary. In surgical settings, RFA can be performed laparoscopically or during open surgery. Nevertheless, there are no data supporting the fact that RFA performed during open surgery is superior to a percutaneous approach (Poon et al. 2004a, 2004b).

To direct the RFA probe into the tumour, ultrasound (US), computed tomography (CT), and magnetic resonance imaging (MRI) guidance are applicable, where US is probably the most widely used method for guidance worldwide. As yet there are no ideal imaging and monitoring methods for RFA (or the other thermal ablative techniques) because all imaging methods have both advantages and disadvantages.

Ultrasound is widely available and in many cases allows easy in- and off-plane access to the target and visualization of the probe. However, depending on the given individual's anatomical and pathological characteristics US is not able to tag the target or to follow the probe in all cases. Furthermore, during the process of ablation the target is masked by a cloud of micro gas bubbles (Fig. 2.1.4). This makes it difficult to identify the probe and the target during RFA and to assess the success of the ablation. Recent data suggest that US contrast may help to overcome this problem – nevertheless, the final role for US contrast media in ablation therapy is not yet clear (Solbiati et al. 2004). Furthermore, hybrid systems merging the freedom of US guidance with the superior image information of CT or MRI may overcome the known ultrasound obstacles (Fig. 2.1.5).

Computed tomography guidance is mostly used by interventional radiologists. The advantage of the superior display of anatomical and pathological structures is compromised by the lack of elbowroom within the scanner gantry, the exposure to the

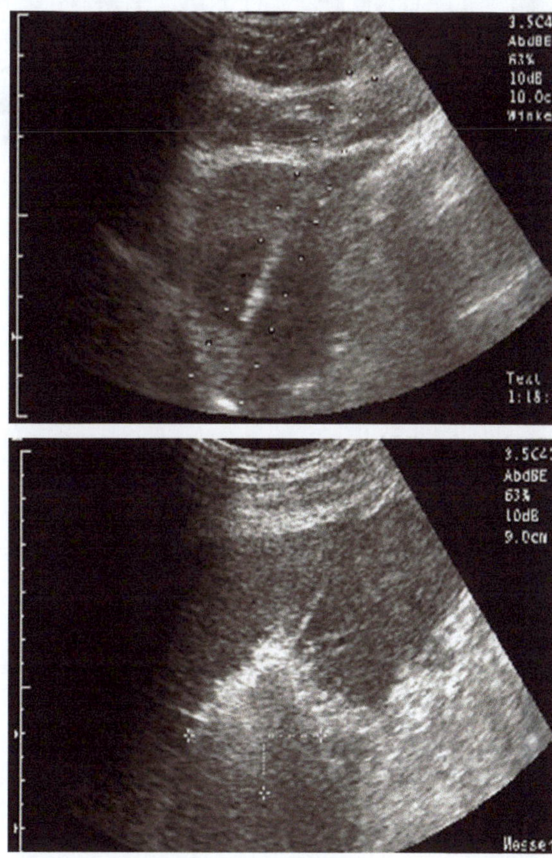

a
b

Fig. 2.1.4. **a** Radiofrequency ablation (*RFA*) of an HCC under ultrasound guidance. Note the bright reflection from the shaft of the electrode; the tumour presents a low echogenicity. **b** Early during the ablation process micro gas bubbles emerge out of the ablation volume masking the tumour. Unfortunately, the volume where the gas bubbles can be appreciated does not correlate very well with ablation volume

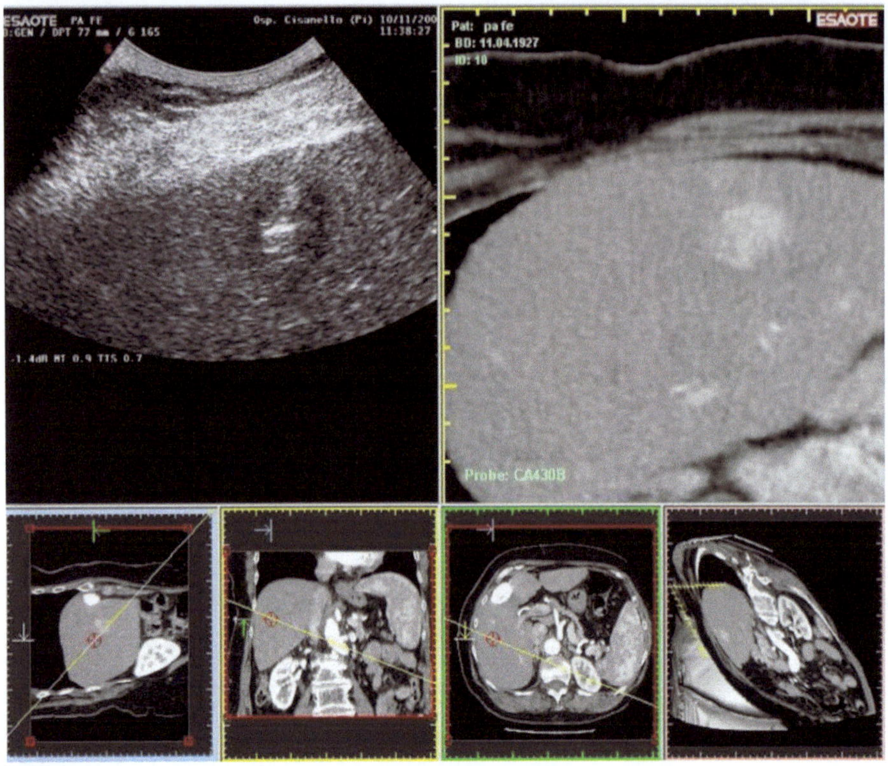

Fig. 2.1.5. Hybrid systems combining the freedom of ultrasound guidance together with the superior image quality of a CT or MRI study (courtesy Laura Crocetti, University of Pisa, Italy) might make an ablation procedure easier and more "comfortable"

radiation dose, and the use of contrast agent for visualization of the potential target lesion.

In contrast to US no significant changes in the treated tissue can be appreciated by CT. A contrast-enhanced CT scan immediately after RFA should display no enhancement within the ablated volume. The full extent of the ablation can be identified only 12–18 h after RFA.

In comparison to US and CT, MRI is the only method that is able to display heat-related intrinsic tissue alterations directly and on-line. Several methods are available for thermal monitoring, e.g. chemical shift imaging and T_1-weighted imaging. Nevertheless, MRI monitoring of thermal ablation is mostly limited to laser applications because MR-compatible RFA probes were only recently presented and are not available for every system. General limitations for performing ablative interventions under MRI guidance are – similar to CT – the restricted freedom of movement, the high technical complexity and costs.

2.1.4.2 Energy Delivery

The control of the process of ablation itself is device-dependent. The heat-related dehydration results in a progressive coagulative necrosis and a loss of conductibility followed by rising tissue impedance (see above). Most RFA systems use the relative increase of impedance as a parameter for controlling the ablative process, while ascending impedance down-regulates the delivered power. At present, only one system is equipped with multiple thermistors at the tips of the antennas, thus offering on-line monitoring of the temperature.

In general, the ablation process takes 10–30 min per needle placement to provide complete tissue necrosis.

2.1.5 Complications

From a procedural and technical point of view, RFA has to be considered a safe and minimally invasive method. The needles used are typically small (14–17.5 G) compared to needles used for biopsy, complemented by the intrinsic capability of cauterization and coagulation (to avoid bleeding from the needle track and tumour seeding along the track cauterization of the track is recommended).

Complications may occur immediately or with a delay after a procedure, and may be related to the puncture, the entire procedure or to the patient's disease and individual situation (DE BAERE et al. 2003).

Immediate complications can be metabolic, vascular and non-vascular, while delayed complications are determined by complex metabolic reactions, infections, biliary obstruction and tumour seeding.

2.1.5.1 Metabolic Complications

This type of complication may represent a permanent risk to the procedure because of the dependency on underlying disease. Changes in blood pressure, sensations of pain, and hormonal reactions (e.g. in RFA of the adrenals or in metastases of neuroendocrine tumours) can affect the patient's condition during the procedure. Therefore, it is mandatory to know the patient's medical condition before the procedure to be able to address any necessary additional medical support ahead of a potential complication.

In treating hormonally active tumours an endocrinologist should be involved. Substitution of corticosteroids and mineralcorticoids may be necessary to minimize the risk of an adrenal crisis due to adrenal insufficiency after partial or complete ablation of the adrenals. In ablation of hormonally active primary or secondary tumours, such as pheochromocytoma, aldosteronomas, insulinomas, or carcinoids, extensive hormone release during the ablation may provoke a hypertensive crisis, or hypoglycemia. Therefore, blood pressure monitoring and blockade of alpha- and beta-receptors are required in pheochromocytomas and glucose infusion in insulinomas (ABRAHAM et al. 2000; PACAK et al. 2001).

2.1.5.2 Vascular Complications

The risk of bleeding depends on the patient's coagulation function and on the type and localization of the lesion that is targeted, the surrounding parenchyma, the pathway to the lesion and the inter-positioned structures. In coagulopathies special attention has to be paid to bleeding from the access route while positioning the probe and special measures should be taken to correct coagulation abnormalities by additional infusion of platelets or fresh frozen plasma and stopping anticoagulative therapies.

Mechanical injuries by the RF probe traversing a vessel and thermal injuries during sustained ablation may cause arterial bleeding, pseudoaneurysm, arterio-venous/arterio-portalvenous fistulae, and hepatic and portal vein thrombosis, with subsequent hepatic infarctions in extremely rare cases. These complications can generally be avoided by applying real-time imaging guidance such as ultrasound or CT-fluoroscopy for placing the probe (Fig. 2.1.6).

Nevertheless, during the ablation process some bleeding – or probably better hemorrhagic diapedesis – can be appreciated, which is usually self-limiting and represents haemorrhage due to thermal damage to the tumour's capillaries.

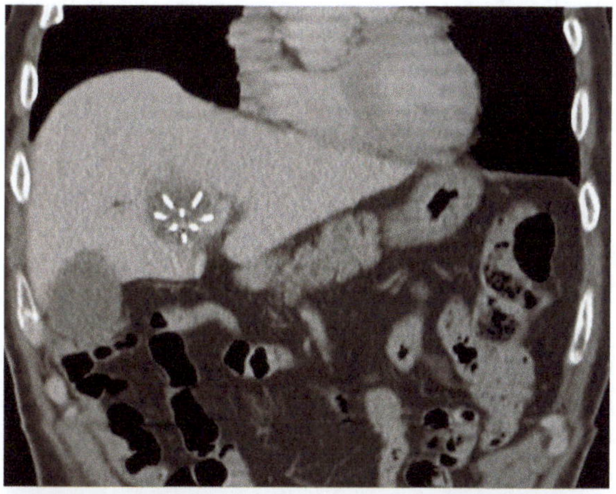
a

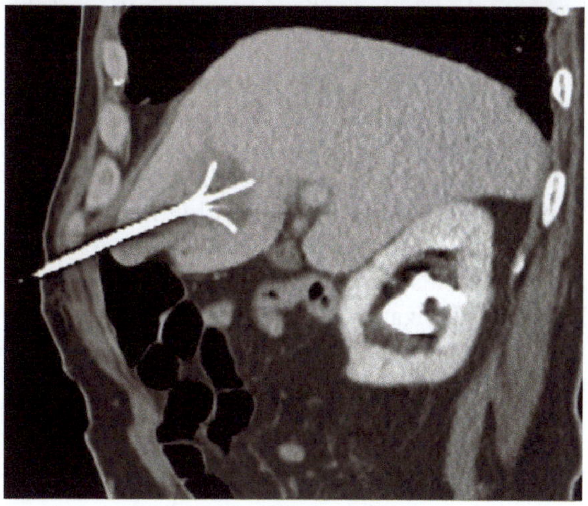
b

Fig. 2.1.6a,b. Multiplanar reformations from 3D CT data sets allow precise assessment of electrode positioning. Note the perfectly centred placement of the multi-tined RFA electrode in the coronal (**a**) and sagittal view (**b**) in a colorectal cancer metastasis (the hooks are not yet fully delpoyed)

If there is suspicion of a vascular complication a base-line follow-up study should be performed within the first 3 h after the procedure, which is absolutely mandatory in cases of intraprocedural bleeding and significant, ongoing pain (Curley et al. 1999; Mulier et al. 2002; de Baere et al. 2003; Chuang et al. 2005).

In suspicious cases, early angiography with interventional stand-by and stabilization of coagulation parameters is crucial to avoid or to minimize bleeding complications.

Nevertheless, based on the principle of cauterization, the coagulative potential of the thermal ablation procedure itself makes the bleeding of a treated lesion quite unusual. To avoid needle track bleeding it is recommended to perform "hot" probe repositioning and removal (i.e. needle track ablation). Therefore, regarding the present literature bleeding in total is a rare, in most cases self-limiting, complication with a frequency of no more than 2%.

2.1.5.3 Infection

Infectious complications are rare; however, they are promoted if the patient is predisposed by an underlying infectious process, a compromised immune system, as in diabetes, or especially in hepatic ablation when biliary enteric communication is present. Patients who underwent a Whipple's procedure, for example, are jeopardized by colonization of the biliary tract by ascending infections and abscess formation within the ablation volume (de Baere et al. 2003; Elias et al. 2006; Kvitting et al. 2006). A delayed onset of infection or abscess formation is typically what makes any persistent or recurrent fever in the 2–3 weeks after RFA highly equivocal. Additionally, there seems to be an increased risk for infection also in patients who have had previous lipiodol embolization for HCC. Overall, the risk of infection is about 1.5% (Shibata et al. 2003; Choi et al. 2005).

2.1.5.3 Tumour Seeding

Tumour seeding by the carrying of tumour cells along the probe's pathway(s) is basically an issue of inappropriate technique and is typically detected 3–12 months after the procedure (Decker et al. 2003; Liu et al. 2003; Espinoza et al. 2005). This risk can be almost eliminated if the probe is properly positioned on the first pass and does not cross the tumour primarily, otherwise tumour cells can be pushed out of the tumour in its periphery. A sufficient safety margin around the tumour and removing the probe by additional ablation of the needle tract will further lower the risk of tumour cell spread. Llovet reported a tumour seeding frequency of 12.5% (4 cases out of 32) while in a large Italian multicentre trial including more than 2000 patients the frequency was only 0.6% (Llovet et al. 2001; Livraghi et al. 2003). In general, multiple or large tumours necessitating several needle passes, subcapsular (hepatic), subpleural (pulmonary) locations, and poor tumour differentiation may favour tumour seeding.

2.1.5.4 Non-Target Thermal Damage

Complications related to the thermal ablation itself include unintentional thermal harm to non-targeted areas including burns at the grounding pads and interference with metallic implants such as pacemaker wires and cardioverter defibrillators.

If the grounding pads are too small or not equidistant from the active electrode in monopolar systems there is an increased risk of grounding pad burns since then the pads can act as another electrode, focusing some energy. The risk of grounding pad burns rises with the amount of energy delivered. In consequence, more or larger grounding pads should be used if more power is applied. If the contact of the grounding pads to the skin surface is not sufficient (e.g. by sweat or hairs under the pad) the RF power is not dispersed efficiently and "spots" of high current flow may be generated, resulting in burns. Defects of the electrode's insulation or metallic coaxial introducers, which may act as secondary antenna by induction, can also create burns at the skin entry site (Fig. 2.1.7).

More critical are unintentional burns to anatomical structures within the vicinity (distance less than 1 cm) of the treated lesion. A thorough planning of the access route and final electrode placement may help to avoid damage of such structures, for example the gallbladder or the renal calices (Ogan et al. 2002; Yamakado et al. 2003). In clinical reality vascular heat sink effects, the peritoneal surfaces and the motility/mobility of some organs such as the stomach and small and large bowel may also have some protective properties. Nevertheless, there are some reports documenting the fatal outcome of secondary thermal damage to the stomach or bowel (Choi et al. 2001; Meloni et al. 2002; Livraghi et al. 2003; Rhim et al. 2003). Dislodgement by air insufflation or injection by glucose injection will protect these structures at risk (Fig. 2.1.8). Therefore, collateral damage to vital structures can be generally avoided if organ-specific anatomical peculiarities are considered.

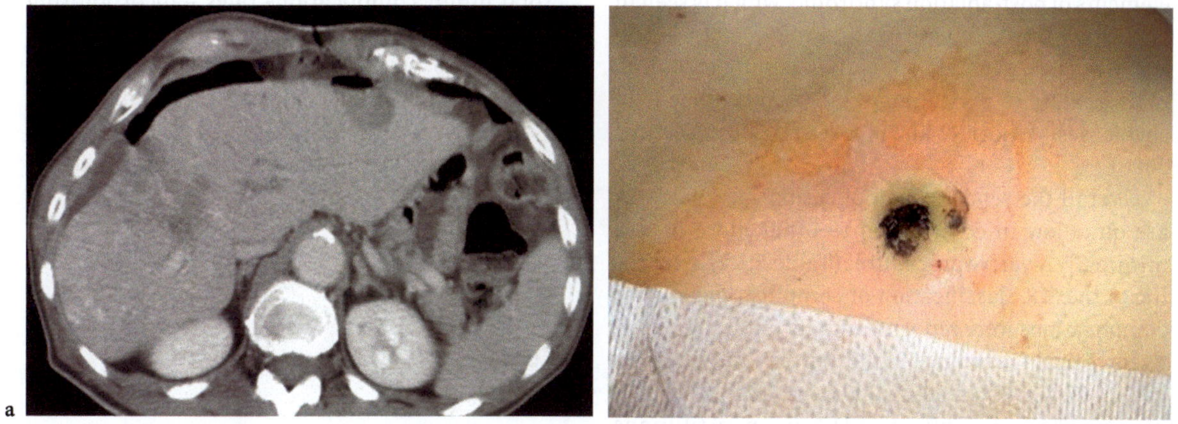

Fig. 2.1.7. a The metastases from a breast cancer, subcapsular located in the left liver lobe, were treated via an oblique access route with the skin entry point at the epigastrium (former selective internal radiation therapy i.e. SIRT caused the parenchymal irregularities in the right liver lobe where active metastases could no longer be appreciated). Note the gas within the treated lesion and gas bubbles along the electrode's pathway. Extensive capsular anaesthesia caused the soft-tissue swelling between peritoneal wall and hepatic surface. **b** Due to an insulation defect, a grade 3 burn occurred at the skin entry point, about 5 cm distant from the electrode's tip. The burn was not appreciated until the end of the procedure because the entry point was draped with a swab and the patient did not feel the burn due to local anaesthesia

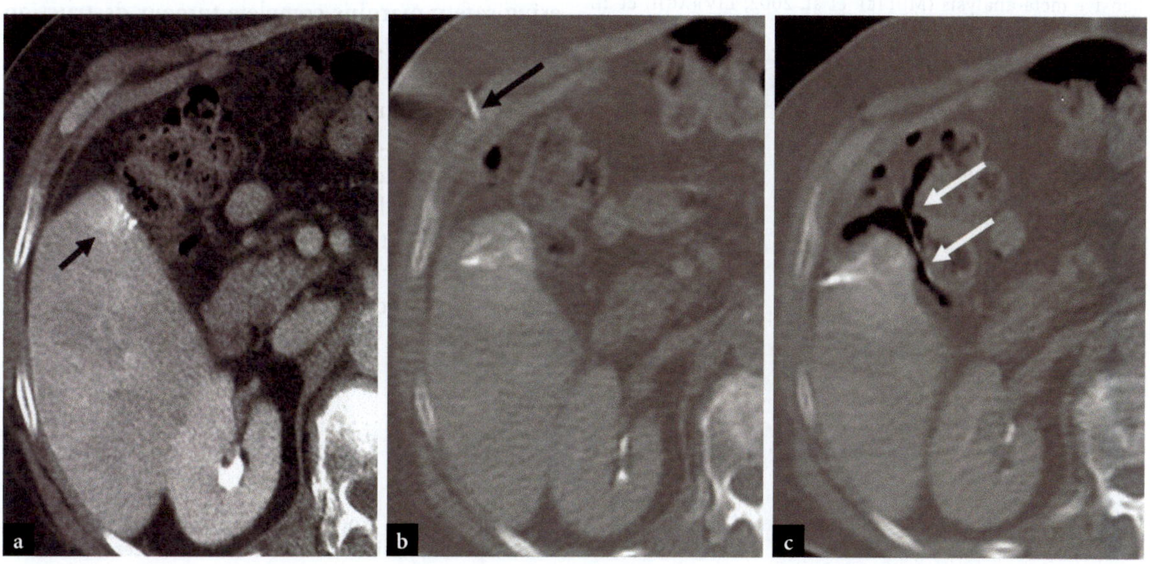

Fig. 2.1.8. a In this patient with recurrent HCC after liver transplantation, colonic adhesions to the hepatic capsule in the area of recurrence (*arrow*) were encountered. On the CT the tumour nodule can be appreciated as faint hypervascularization. Note three tiny clips of the liver capsule resulting from a laparoscopic capsular probe excision. **b** Before starting the process of RFA – the electrode is already in place and the tines are partially deployed – a 21-gauge needle is inserted (*arrow*) to insufflate room air in the space between colon and liver capsule. **c** After the injection of 20 ml room air, the 21-gauge needle is advanced into the space between colon and liver capsule (*arrows*), thus more air can be injected if needed. The ablation can easily be performed down to the capsule, because adjacent structures are insulated by the injected air

2.1.5.5 Minor Complications

Common side-effects in RFA are pain in the area of the puncture site, peritoneal irritation, nausea, vomiting, moderate fever, tiredness and headache. Fever, nausea, tiredness and vomiting are the main elements of post-ablation syndrome, which is seen in about two-thirds of patients and might last for several weeks. In general supportive therapy including mild analgesics and non-steroidals is sufficient in such cases (Ahrar et al. 2005; Rhim 2005; Konety 2006).

Overall the reported complication rates for RFA are quite low in comparison to other more or less minimally invasive procedures (Table 2.1.2). According to the SIR classification of complications, major complications were reported by a recent Italian multicentre trial, including 3554 lesions in 2320 patients, to be 2.4% (Livraghi et al. 2003), paralleled by a figure of 2.43% from a survey of 11 Korean institutions including 1663 lesions in 1139 patients (Rhim et al. 2003, 2004). The total mortality in the studies was 0.3% and 0.09%, respectively, and is similar to the 0.5% mortality rate analysed in a meta-analysis of 82 studies (Mulier et al. 2002). Mulier et al. (2002) also found that the total complication rate in percutaneous RFA of 7.2% is the lowest in comparison to laparoscopic RFA (9.5%), intraoperative RFA (9.5%), and combined procedures with resection and open RFA (31.8%).

Table 2.1.2. Complication rates in RFA of solid organs in the abdomen derived from two multicentre trials and a comprehensive meta-analysis (Mulier et al. 2002; Livraghi et al. 2003; Rhim et al. 2003)

Type of complication	Frequency (%)
Abdominal bleeding	0.5–1.6
Abdominal infection incl. abscess	0.3–1.1
Biliary tract damage incl. bilioma	0.07–1.0
Liver failure	0.07–0.8
Pulmonary complications incl. pneumothorax	0.2–0.8
Dispersive pad skin burn	0.2–0.6
Hepatic vascular damage	0.07–0.6
Visceral damage	0.2–0.5
Cardiac complications incl. vasovagal reflexes	0.13–0.4
Myoglobinaemia or myoglobinuria	0.2
Renal failure	0.07–0.1
Tumour seeding	0.2–0.5
Coagulopathy	0.2
Hormonal complications	0.1

Total minor complications rates – incorporating clinical findings as mentioned above – range between 4.6% and 36%, whereas some of these findings must be considered as expected and inevitable effects and are therefore better classified as side-effects (Mulier et al. 2002; Livraghi et al. 2003; Rhim et al. 2003, 2004).

2.1.6 Conclusion

Over the last 10 years a wide variety of clinical applications for RFA have been developed and RFA has gained clinical acceptance in many centres. Regarding clinical and oncological prerequisites a RF needle can be placed in a target lesion as long as the target can be displayed by US, CT, or MRI. If the RFA is performed in an adequate manner considering safety margins complete tumour destruction can be expected. At present, RFA is still limited by the suboptimal way of monitoring the procedure and the maximum size of the ablation volume that can be achieved. At present, several studies are being conducted to identify the patients that benefit most from local tumour ablation and to identify other adjuvant therapies, such as chemotherapies, that may enhance and stabilize the treatment effects of local tumour control. However, this goal can only be achieved in a multidisciplinary approach.

References

Abraham J, Fojo T, Wood BJ (2000) Radiofrequency ablation of metastatic lesions in adrenocortical cancer. Ann Intern Med 133(4):312–313

Ahrar K, Matin S, Wood CG et al (2005) Percutaneous radiofrequency ablation of renal tumors: technique complications and outcomes. J Vasc Interv Radiol 16(5):679–688

Brieger J, Pereira PL, Trubenbach J et al (2003) In vivo efficiency of four commercial monopolar radiofrequency ablation systems: a comparative experimental study in pig liver. Invest Radiol 38(10):609–616

Burdio F, Guemes A, Burdio JM et al (2003) Bipolar saline-enhanced electrode for radiofrequency ablation: results of experimental study of in vivo porcine liver. Radiology 229(2):447–456

Choi H, Loyer EM, DuBrow RA et al (2001) Radio-frequency ablation of liver tumors: assessment of therapeutic response and complications. Radiographics 21 [Spec No]:S41–S54

Choi D, Lim HK, Kim MJ et al (2005) Liver abscess after percutaneous radiofrequency ablation for hepatocellular carcinomas: frequency and risk factors. AJR Am J Roentgenol 184(6):1860–1867

Choi D, Lim HK, Rhim H et al (2007) Percutaneous radiofrequency ablation for recurrent hepatocellular carcinoma after hepatectomy: long-term results and prognostic factors. Ann Surg Oncol 14(8):2319–2329

Chuang CH, Chen CY, Tsai HM (2005) Hepatic infarction and hepatic artery pseudoaneurysm with peritoneal bleeding after radiofrequency ablation for hepatoma. Clin Gastroenterol Hepatol 3(11):A23

Clasen S, Schmidt D, Boss A et al (2006) Multipolar radiofrequency ablation with internally cooled electrodes: experimental study in ex vivo bovine liver with mathematic modeling. Radiology 238(3):881–890

Clasen S, Schmidt D, Dietz K et al (2007) Bipolar radiofrequency ablation using internally cooled electrodes in ex vivo bovine liver: prediction of coagulation volume from applied energy. Invest Radiol 42(1):29–36

Curley SA, Izzo F, Delrio P et al (1999) Radiofrequency ablation of unresectable primary and metastatic hepatic malignancies: results in 123 patients. Ann Surg 230(1):1–8

de Baere T, Bessoud B, Dromain C et al (2002) Percutaneous radiofrequency ablation of hepatic tumors during temporary venous occlusion. AJR Am J Roentgenol 178(1):53–59

de Baere T, Risse O, Kuoch V et al (2003) Adverse events during radiofrequency treatment of 582 hepatic tumors. AJR Am J Roentgenol 181(3):695–700

Decker GA, Gores GJ, Roberts LR (2003) Tumor seeding complicating radiofrequency ablation of hepatocellular carcinoma. J Hepatol 38(5):692

Dodd GD 3rd, Frank MS, Aribandi M et al (2001) Radiofrequency thermal ablation: computer analysis of the size of the thermal injury created by overlapping ablations. AJR Am J Roentgenol 177(4):777–782

Elias D, Santoro R, Ouellet JF et al (2004) Simultaneous percutaneous right portal vein embolization and left liver tumor radiofrequency ablation prior to a major right hepatic resection for bilateral colorectal metastases. Hepatogastroenterology 51(60):1788–1791

Elias D, Di Pietroantonio D, Gachot B et al (2006) Liver abscess after radiofrequency ablation of tumors in patients with a biliary tract procedure. Gastroenterol Clin Biol 30(6–7):823–827

Espinoza S, Briggs P, Duret JS et al (2005) Radiofrequency ablation of needle tract seeding in hepatocellular carcinoma. J Vasc Interv Radiol 16(5):743–746

Frericks B, Ritz JP, Roggan A et al (2005) Multipolar radiofrequency ablation of hepatic tumors: initial experience. Radiology 237(3):1056–1062

Gervais DA, Arellano RS, McGovern FJ et al (2005a) Radiofrequency ablation of renal cell carcinoma: part 2. Lessons learned with ablation of 100 tumors. AJR Am J Roentgenol 185(1):72–80

Gervais DA, McGovern FJ, Arellano RS et al (2005b) Radiofrequency ablation of renal cell carcinoma: part 1. Indications results and role in patient management over a 6-year period and ablation of 100 tumors. AJR Am J Roentgenol 185(1):64–71

Goldberg SN (2001) Radiofrequency tumor ablation: principles and techniques. Eur J Ultrasound 13(2):129–147

Goldberg SN, Gazelle GS (2001) Radiofrequency tissue ablation: physical principles and techniques for increasing coagulation necrosis. Hepatogastroenterology 48(38):359–367

Goldberg SN, Stein MC, Gazelle GS et al (1999) Percutaneous radiofrequency tissue ablation: optimization of pulsed-radiofrequency technique to increase coagulation necrosis. J Vasc Interv Radiol 10(7):907–916

Kettenbach J, Kostler W, Rucklinger E et al (2003) Percutaneous saline-enhanced radiofrequency ablation of unresectable hepatic tumors: initial experience in 26 patients. AJR Am J Roentgenol 180(6):1537–1545

Konety BR (2006) Percutaneous radiofrequency ablation of renal tumors: technique complications and outcomes. In: Ahrar K, Matin S, Wood CG et al The Department of Diagnostic Radiology. The University of Texas, MD Anderson Cancer Center, Houston, Tex. Urol Oncol 24(1):85–86

Kuvshinoff BW, Ota DM (2002) Radiofrequency ablation of liver tumors: influence of technique and tumor size. Surgery 132(4):605–611; discussion 611–612

Kvitting JP, Sandstrom P, Thorelius L et al (2006) Radiofrequency ablation of a liver metastasis complicated by extensive liver necrosis and sepsis caused by gas gangrene. Surgery 139(1):123–125

Lau WY, Leung TW, Yu SC et al (2003) Percutaneous local ablative therapy for hepatocellular carcinoma: a review and look into the future. Ann Surg 237(2):171–179

Lee FT Jr, Haemmerich D, Wright AS et al (2003) Multiple probe radiofrequency ablation: pilot study in an animal model. J Vasc Interv Radiol 14(11):1437–1442

Lee JM, Han JK, Kim SH et al (2003) A comparative experimental study of the in-vitro efficiency of hypertonic saline-enhanced hepatic bipolar and monopolar radiofrequency ablation. Korean J Radiol 4(3):163–169

Lencioni R, Cioni D, Crocetti L et al (2005) Early-stage hepatocellular carcinoma in patients with cirrhosis: long-term results of percutaneous image-guided radiofrequency ablation. Radiology 234(3):961–967

Liu C, Frilling A, Dereskewitz C et al (2003) Tumor seeding after fine needle aspiration biopsy and percutaneous radiofrequency thermal ablation of hepatocellular carcinoma. Dig Surg 20(5):460–463

Liu J, Chen X, Xu LX (1999) New thermal wave aspects on burn evaluation of skin subjected to instantaneous heating. IEEE Trans Biomed Eng 46(4):420–428

Livraghi T, Solbiati L, Meloni MF et al (2003) Treatment of focal liver tumors with percutaneous radio-frequency ablation: complications encountered in a multicenter study. Radiology 226(2):441–451

Llovet JM, Vilana R, Bru C et al (2001) Increased risk of tumor seeding after percutaneous radiofrequency ablation for single hepatocellular carcinoma. Hepatology 33(5):1124–1129

Lu DS, Raman SS, Limanond P et al (2003) Influence of large peritumoral vessels on outcome of radiofrequency ablation of liver tumors. J Vasc Interv Radiol 14(10):1267–1274

Lu DS, Yu NC, Raman SS et al (2005) Radiofrequency ablation of hepatocellular carcinoma: treatment success as defined by histologic examination of the explanted liver. Radiology 234(3):954–960

Lubienski A, Dux M, Lubienski K et al (2005) Radiofrequency thermal ablation: increase in lesion diameter with continuous acetic acid infusion. Cardiovasc Intervent Radiol 28(6):789–794

McGahan JP, Browning PD, Brock JM et al (1990) Hepatic ablation using radiofrequency electrocautery. Invest Radiol 25(3):267–270

Meloni MF, Goldberg SN, Moser V et al (2002) Colonic perforation and abscess following radiofrequency ablation treatment of hepatoma. Eur J Ultrasound 15(1–2):73–76

Merkle EM, Goldberg SN, Boll DT et al (1999) Effects of superparamagnetic iron oxide on radio-frequency-induced temperature distribution: in vitro measurements in polyacrylamide phantoms and in vivo results in a rabbit liver model. Radiology 212(2):459–466

Mulier S, Mulier P, Ni Y et al (2002) Complications of radiofrequency coagulation of liver tumours. Br J Surg 89(10):1206–1222

Neeman Z, Wood BJ (2002) Radiofrequency ablation beyond the liver. Tech Vasc Interv Radiol 5(3):156–163

Ni Y, Miao Y, Mulier S et al (2000) A novel cooled-wet electrode for radiofrequency ablation. Eur Radiol 10(5):852–854

Ogan K, Jacomides L, Dolmatch BL et al (2002) Percutaneous radiofrequency ablation of renal tumors: technique limitations and morbidity. Urology 60(6):954–958

Pacak K, Fojo T, Goldstein DS et al (2001) Radiofrequency ablation: a novel approach for treatment of metastatic pheochromocytoma. J Natl Cancer Inst 93(8):648–649

Patterson EJ, Scudamore CH, Owen DA et al (1998) Radiofrequency ablation of porcine liver in vivo: effects of blood flow and treatment time on lesion size. Ann Surg 227(4):559–565

Pereira PL, Trubenbach J, Schmidt D (2003) Radiofrequency ablation: basic principles techniques and challenges. Rofo 175(1):20–27

Pereira PL, Trubenbach J, Schenk M et al (2004) Radiofrequency ablation: in vivo comparison of four commercially available devices in pig livers. Radiology 232(2):482–490

Poon RT, Fan ST, Lo CM et al (2002) Long-term survival and pattern of recurrence after resection of small hepatocellular carcinoma in patients with preserved liver function: implications for a strategy of salvage transplantation. Ann Surg 235(3):373–382

Poon RT, Ng KK, Lam CM et al (2004a) Effectiveness of radiofrequency ablation for hepatocellular carcinomas larger than 3 cm in diameter. Arch Surg 139(3):281–287

Poon RT, Ng KK, Lam CM et al (2004b) Learning curve for radiofrequency ablation of liver tumors: prospective analysis of initial 100 patients in a tertiary institution. Ann Surg 239(4):441–449

Raman SS, Lu DS, Vodopich DJ et al (2000) Creation of radiofrequency lesions in a porcine model: correlation with sonography CT and histopathology. AJR Am J Roentgenol 175(5):1253–1258

Rhim H (2005) Complications of radiofrequency ablation in hepatocellular carcinoma. Abdom Imaging 30(4):409–418

Rhim H, Yoon KH, Lee JM et al (2003) Major complications after radio-frequency thermal ablation of hepatic tumors: spectrum of imaging findings. Radiographics 23(1):123–134; discussion 134–136

Rhim H, Dodd GD 3rd, Chintapalli KN et al (2004) Radiofrequency thermal ablation of abdominal tumors: lessons learned from complications. Radiographics 24(1):41–52

Rossi S, Fornari F, Pathies C et al (1990) Thermal lesions induced by 480 KHz localized current field in guinea pig and pig liver. Tumori 76(1):54–57

Scott DM, Young WN, Watumull LM et al (2000) Development of an in vivo tumor-mimic model for learning radiofrequency ablation. J Gastrointest Surg 4(6):620–625

Shibata T, Yamamoto Y, Yamamoto N et al (2003) Cholangitis and liver abscess after percutaneous ablation therapy for liver tumors: incidence and risk factors. J Vasc Interv Radiol 14(12):1535–1542

Solbiati L, Ierace T, Tonolini M et al (2004) Guidance and monitoring of radiofrequency liver tumor ablation with contrast-enhanced ultrasound. Eur J Radiol Suppl 51: S19–S23

Suh R, Reckamp K, Zeidler M et al (2005) Radiofrequency ablation in lung cancer: promising results in safety and efficacy. Oncology (Williston Park) 19 [11 Suppl. 4]:12–21

Tacke J, Mahnken A, Roggan A et al (2004) Multipolar radiofrequency ablation: first clinical results. Rofo 176(3):324–329

Wood BJ, Ramkaransingh JR, Fojo T et al (2002) Percutaneous tumor ablation with radiofrequency. Cancer 94(2):443–451

Yamakado K, Nakatsuka A, Akeboshi M et al (2003) Percutaneous radiofrequency ablation of liver neoplasms adjacent to the gastrointestinal tract after balloon catheter interposition. J Vasc Interv Radiol 14(9 Pt 1):1183–1186

Yamakado K, Hase S, Matsuoka T et al (2007) Radiofrequency ablation for the treatment of unresectable lung metastases in patients with colorectal cancer: a multicenter study in Japan. J Vasc Interv Radiol 18(3):393–398

Ablative Techniques (Percutaneous)

2

Thermal Ablative Techniques

2.2 Microwave Ablation

Andreas Boss, Damian Dupuy, and Philippe L. Pereira

CONTENTS

2.2.1 Overview

Microwave (MW) interstitial thermoablation offers several advantages over the more commonly applied thermal ablative technique of radiofrequency (RF) ablation for targeted tumor destruction, such as higher ablation temperature, faster treatment time, reduced heat-sink effect, effective ablation of cystic lesions, a technologically easier multi-applicator approach, no necessity for grounding pads, and no risk of skin burns. The technique may be used in different treatment approaches, including imaging-guided percutaneous, laparoscopic, and open surgical access. MW ablation constitutes one of the most recent developments in interstitial tumor ablation techniques; however, as yet no FDA-approved commercial device is available. In MW ablation, electromagnetic MW irradiation applied to the tumor tissue causes water molecules to vibrate and rotate, resulting in tissue heating and subsequently cell death via thermal-induced protein denaturation. In first pilot studies, MW ablation has shown immense potential for the treatment of primary and secondary liver tumors, primary and secondary lung cancer, renal cell carcinoma, and bone metastases.

A. Boss, MD; P. L. Pereira, MD
Institute for Diagnostic Radiology, University Clinics, Eberhards-Karls-University, Hoppe-Seyler-Strase 3, 72076 Tübingen, Germany
D. Dupuy, MD
Diagnostic Radiology, Rhode Island Hospital, Warren Alpert Medical School of Brown University, 593 Eddy Street, Providence, RI, USA

2.2.2 Introduction

In tumor ablation techniques, chemical substances or thermal energy is delivered to a targeted tissue leading to cell death and subsequent targeted destruction of the pathological tissue structures. The principle of tissue heating by application of electric energy was first described by Jacques-Arsène d'Arsonval in 1892. In modern tumor treatment, several different modalities for thermal energy deposition have been developed, among which the most commonly applied techniques are: RF ablation (Goldberg and Gazelle 2001), laser interstitial thermotherapy (LITT) (Vogl et al. 2002), high-intensity focused ultrasound (HIFU) (Huber et al. 2001), and MW ablation (Shibata et al. 2002). Many other ablation techniques have been proposed, including ethanol or acetic acid injection, all of which are obsolete now as in clinical trials they were shown to be inferior to the first mentioned techniques in efficiency of tumor destruction. RF ablation has evolved as the most extensively used ablation modality with its ease of applicator positioning, large achievable coagulation diameters, minimally invasive character, and its relative cost efficacy. However, MW ablation has not yet been extensively studied.

MW ablation, which refers to modalities of tissue heating using electromagnetic energy deposition at frequencies in the gigahertz (GHz) order, possibly offers several advantages over RF ablation (Table 2.2.1). The potential benefits are: higher intratumoral temperature, faster treatment times, larger volumes of coagulation necrosis, easier multi-applicator approach, less heat-sink effect, efficient thermal ablation of cystic tumors, no necessity for the placement of grounding pads, and, therefore, no risk of skin burn. In magnetic-resonance- (MR-) guided treatment monitoring, the frequency of MW ablation does not interfere with the receiver frequency of the MR scanner possibly allowing for on-line treatment monitoring, which is currently not possible in MR-guided RF ablation.

By means of thermal ablation devices, target temperatures in excess of 48–50°C are generated within the pathological tissue leading to cellular death and coagulation necrosis. The duration of the treatment, the spatial distribution of the thermal energy as well as the maximal reachable tissue temperature vary among the different treatment modalities. The higher the temperature leading to irreversible damage to critical cell proteins, the shorter the necessary treatment duration for secure cell death and tissue necrosis. The tissue thermal damage at high-temperature exposure may be predicted by means of biophysical relationships such as the Pennes bioheat equation (Pennes 1948), an Arrhenius analysis (Dewey 1994), or the Sapareto-Dewey iso-effect thermal dose relationship (Sapareto and Dewey 1984). These relationships have been tested in several in vivo systems, which demonstrated that within defined temperature ranges the thermal damage in tissue is approximately linearly dependent upon treatment time and exponentially dependent upon the increase in temperature. The sensitivity to heat exposure among different tissue types is variable (Dewey 1994).

In combination with radiological imaging-guidance, tissue ablation may be performed percutaneously as a minimally invasive treatment modality, reducing health-care costs and patient morbidity. Computed tomography (CT) and ultrasound (US) are widely used for positioning of applicators into the tumor, and for treatment monitoring. However, neither CT nor US can confirm complete tumor ablation after energy application. In using US for monitoring, the production of steam bubbles by the heating process disturbs the image acquisition. At native CT scan, the coagulated tissue only shows slight changes (actually the density decreases 0.4 HU per elevation of 1°C) in the imaging pattern compared to the tumor tissue. In MR-guided ablation, a drop in signal intensity is visible in T_2-weighted imaging due to the deprivation of free tissue water, which, therefore, might permit a near-real-time control of the ablation course and therefore allows a higher efficiency in terms of treatment outcome. In the area of lower but still lethal thermal damage at the borders of the coagulation necrosis, the cells typically die within 2–7 days. Surrounding the contour of lethal cell damage, physiological changes take place due to tissue inflammation, with increased blood flow and vascular permeability visible in MR scan and contrast-enhanced CT. For the avoidance of local tumor relapse, the coagulation zone of immediate cell death should encompass at least a 5- to 10-mm layer of peritumoral margin in addition to the complete tumor.

In this manuscript, authors focus on the technique of MW tumor ablation, the physics of the MW heating, and the technique of percutaneous interventional MW ablation. The authors give a literature survey on current clinical applications as well as results of experimental studies.

Table 2.2.1. Microwave ablation compared to radiofrequency ablation

	Microwave ablation	Radiofrequency ablation
Typical frequency	~1 GHz (915 MHz)	365–480 kHz
Physics of energy deposition	Induction of oscillations in water molecules by propagating electromagnetic waves	Resistive heating by electrical alternating current
Generator power control	No feedback used	Temperature and/or impedance
Internally cooled applicators	Not yet available	Available
MR-compatible applicators	Not yet available	Available
Multi-applicator approach	Possible (amplitude, phase)	Limited
Available devices	No FDA-approved devices (Vivant Medical)	FDA approved devices: e.g., ValleyLab, Boston Scientific, RITA

2.2.3 Physics of Microwave Heating

Microwaves belong to the electromagnetic waves with wavelengths in the range of 30 cm (frequency = 1 GHz) to 1 mm (300 GHz), meaning, therefore, that the microwaves have wavelengths longer than those of infrared light, but shorter than those of radio waves. The boundaries are, however, arbitrarily chosen and differ in various fields of science and engineering. Microwaves are used in many areas of modern technology, especially in the field of communication (cellular phones, wireless internet connections, satellite television). For medical uses specific frequencies between 915 mHz and 2.4 GHz have been designated so as not to interfere with communications in the aviation and military frequencies. Common MW ovens operate at approximately 2.45 GHz. As the water molecule exhibits an electric dipole moment, the electric field of the MW excites harmonic oscillations in the water as they try to align themselves with the alternating electric field, resulting in warming. Other molecules are heated by convection due to the fact that macromolecules are not directly affected by microwaves.

The lowest resonance frequency of the water molecule is at 22.2 GHz. However, even at MW frequencies in the range of 1–2 GHz, the electromagnetic energy is effectively absorbed with a typical efficiency factor of 50%–60%. As microwaves are electromagnetic waves, they may be refracted or reflected at boundaries of matter. In metallic conductors, significant reflection occurs at frequencies higher than 1 GHz, and microwaves at frequencies over 1 GHz can hardly be transported in electric cables, but lead instead to notable cable heating. Therefore, newly developed clinically used MW ablation devices work at frequencies below 1 GHz.

2.2.4 Microwave Ablation Compared to Radiofrequency Ablation

Compared to RF ablation, which deposits thermal energy in the tissue by resistive heating using alternating current at 365–480 kHz, MW ablation uses a different principle providing theoretically several advantages. The MW antenna emits electromagnetic radiation into the tissue without the necessity of an electrical current. The resulting coagulation necrosis, however, is similar in histopathological examination in both modalities (Simon et al. 2005; Wright et al. 2005). As no electrical current is applied, carbonization, tissue boiling and steam bubbles surrounding the applicator do not hamper the energy deposition. Much higher tumor temperatures may, therefore, be reached as compared to RF ablation of up to temperatures of 150°C. As there is an exponential dependence between tissue temperature and induced cell death, complete coagulation of malignant tissue may be achieved in much shorter treatment time. As no electric current is passing through the patient's body in MW ablation, there is no necessity for the placement of grounding pads. The danger of tissue heating in unwanted areas is strongly reduced, which may occur in RF ablation especially at transitions of anatomical structures with relatively high electrical resistance, such as vessel walls and the skin-to-grounding pad transition.

Both modalities are reported to show comparable ablation diameters. RF ablation typically creates ablation diameters of 2–4 cm depending on the ablation system applied (multi-tined, internally cooled single or cluster) (Pereira et al. 2004). The clinically used MW devices show varying sizes of coagulation volume depending on their geometry: applicators of straight geometry are reported to achieve coagulation diameters of up to 2.5 cm (Wright et al. 2003), whereas single loop-antenna applicators were reported to result in coagulation diameters of up to 3.5 cm (Shock et al. 2004). To increase the coagulation volume, multi-applicator approaches may be used (multi-polar RF devices, multi-applicator MW). With increasing ablation power, however, the danger of tissue heating in unwanted areas significantly increases in RF ablation, whereas this is not an issue in MW ablation. The pathway of the electrical current through the body in RF ablation is dependent on anatomical structures, and notable distortions of the spherical geometry of the ablation volume have been reported for RF ablation, decreasing the predictability of the ablation outcome. Another drawback of RF ablation is the limited possibility of multi-applicator use in conventional monopolar techniques due to a shielding effect of the electric current among the multiple RF applicators (Goldberg et al. 1995), leading to unpredictable coagulation geometries for arbitrary placement of electrodes. No interference between different electrodes is found in MW ablation (Wright et al.

2003). Three different modalities of energy disposition in a MW multi-applicator approach have been described (Haemmerich and Lee 2005): the coherent application of energy with one generator for each electrode, which is the conventionally applied technique. In the incoherent approach, one generator switches rapidly between the multiple applicators. To further improve uniformity of power deposition, phase modulation between applicators has been proposed. The last two modalities, however, have not as yet been sufficiently investigated.

Vascular flow may cause a significant reduction in the effectiveness of RF ablation due to cooling of the perivascular area, which is called the heat-sink effect (Goldberg et al. 1998). In several recent publications (Deardorff et al. 2001; Wright et al. 2003), the opposite effect was described for MW ablation, where a selective tracking of the ablation zone along blood vessels was discovered. Up to now, no complete explanation has been found for this effect. It was suggested that the presence of a vessel causes a distortion or extension of the energy distribution pattern of the electromagnetic irradiation (Deardorff et al. 2001). The effect was also suggested to possibly be caused by thermally produced vapor traveling though the vessel (Wright et al. 2003). The increased performance of MW ablation close to vessels may reduce the local relapse rate close to liver veins as compared to RF ablation. However, it may carry an increased risk of complications associated with thrombosis of major vessels.

2.2.5 Available Microwave Devices

Two different devices are described in the literature in the Asian region: a Japanese MW generator (Microtaze; Nippon Shoji, Osaka, Japan) (Sato et al. 1996; Matsukawa et al. 1997; Shimada et al. 1998; Ohmoto et al. 1999; Midorikawa et al. 2000; Ido et al. 2001; Shibata et al. 2002), and a Chinese device (UMC-I Ultrasound-Guided Microwave Coagulator, Institute 207 of the Aerospace Industry Company, Beijing, China, and Department of Ultrasound of Chinese PLA General Hospital, Beijing, China) (Lu et al. 2001; Dong et al. 2003), both operating at 2.450 MHz emission frequency with generator power of up to 90 W and 80 W, respectively. Available straight needle electrodes were 1.6 mm in diameter (14 gauge) with a 2-cm active tip (Japanese system), and 1.6 mm in diameter and a 2.7-cm active tip (Chinese system).

Recently, two newly developed systems were reported operating at 915 MHz with up to 60 W generator output (Vivant Medical, Mountain View, Calif., USA) and 2.450 MHz (Microsulis, Bath, England) (Shock et al. 2004; Simon et al. 2005), possibly offering lower loss due to electromagnetic reflection within the cable and improved convection profile. Straight MW antennae are available that are 1.5 mm in diameter (14.5 gauge). Three applicators may be applied in a triangular configuration with applicator distances of between 1.5 and 2.5 cm. Additionally, the development of an expandable 24-gauge (0.5-mm) circular loop antenna was reported with a diameter of 2.7 cm. As yet there are no approved devices for patient treatment commercially available within the USA or Europe.

2.2.6 Treatment Procedure

MW ablation allows for application in different treatment approaches including open surgical access, laparoscopy, and imaging-guided percutaneous treatment. Increasing interest is focused on the indication for percutaneous treatment, as this may be regarded as a minimally invasive approach potentially offering several benefits such as reduced patient recovery time and lower overall health-care costs. For this reason, the typical imaging-guided procedure is described here in greater detail.

The indication for percutaneous interventional thermoablative treatment in oncology has to be given in an interdisciplinary assessment including consultations for internal medicine, oncology, surgery, and interventional radiology. A possible locally curative treatment by thermoablation should be included in a comprehensive treatment strategy for the malignant disease, potentially including surgery, chemotherapy, and radiation therapy. Treatment strategies have to be discussed relying on medical history, physical examination, laboratory parameters, patient compliance, and sufficient radiological assessment of the local extent and generalization of the malignant disease. Imaging guidance may be performed with US or CT. Figure 2.2.1 shows the CT-guided interventional treatment of

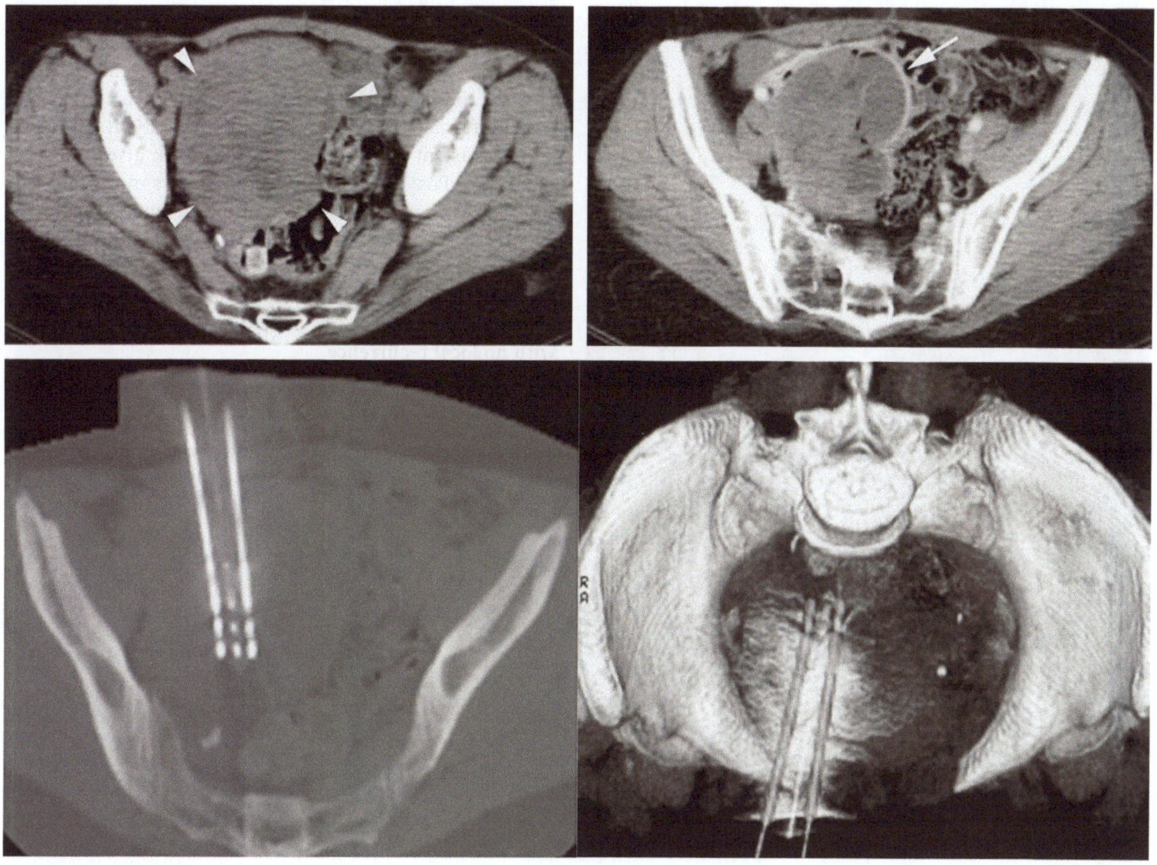

Fig. 2.2.1a–c. CT scan of a 42-year-old female patient presenting post chemotherapy with recalcitrant pain from a large 10.7×8.0×10.0 cm pelvic metastasis (*white arrowheads*) to the right ovary. **b** CT fluoroscopic placement of microwave applicators. Two 7-min ablations performed at 45 W. **c** Immediate post ablation contrast-enhanced CT shows large nonenhancing mass with a thin enhancing rim and internal gas formation; note the large area of coagulation

a pelvic metastatic breast carcinoma in a 42-year-old female patient. In Figure 2.2.2, the MW ablation of a metastatic lesion in the right acetabulum of a 70-year-old male patient is described. The bone metastasis originated from a metastatic bladder carcinoma. As yet, MR-compatible devices are not available for MW ablation.

In the interventional treatment, patients should be admitted to the ward at least 24 h before the intervention in order to check for potential coagulopathy, and to give written informed consent. Percutaneous ablation is typically performed on conscious sedated patients, using for example 100–150 mg pethidine, and 2.5–5 mg midazolam, although a general anesthetic may be required in selected patients. After diagnostic imaging for localization of the tumor, the puncture is planned and the site of applicator insertion is chosen. After disinfection and sterile covering, skin and adjacent subcutaneous regions are anesthetized with 10–20 ml of 1% xylocaine solution. Under constant visualization by US or CT fluoroscopy, the applicator is inserted into the tumor. Additionally, a thermocouple can be placed close to the probe to measure ablation temperature. With the electrode proven in the correct position within the tumor, the MW ablation procedure may be started, which typically lasts up to 5–10 min of ablation time.

2.2.7 Experimental Studies

In several studies, the cellular damage as caused by MW ablation was investigated by ablate-resect experiments with pathological or histological corre-

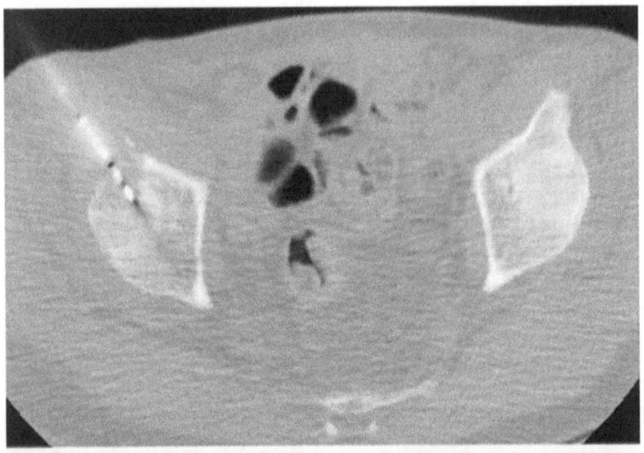
a

Fig. 2.2.2a–c. Microwave ablation of 3-cm metastatic lesion in right acetabulum in a 70-year-old male patient suffering from a metastatic bladder carcinoma. One 10-min microwave ablation with a 3.5-cm active tip antenna was performed. Prior to ablation, the patient presented with persistent pain and inability to walk after radiation therapy. **b** Post ablation CT scan shows nonenhancing 4.5×4.0×3.5 cm thermo-coagulation encompassing the entire metastasis (*arrowhead*). **c** CT scan at 15-month follow-up shows a stable area of lysis measuring 3.5×1.9 cm in the right iliac bone with surrounding sclerosis consistent with post ablation change. The patient remained asymptomatic with no local recurrence

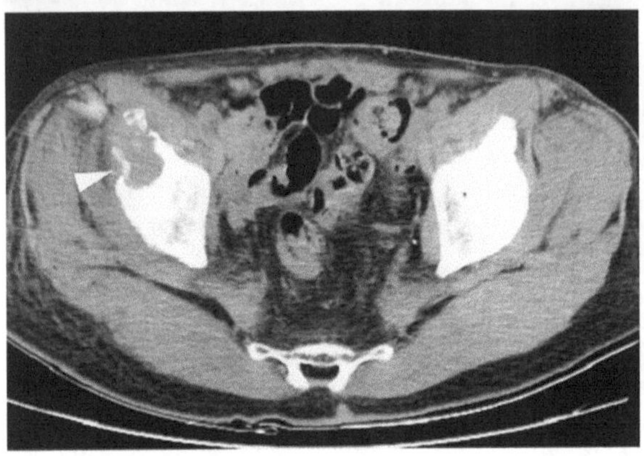
b

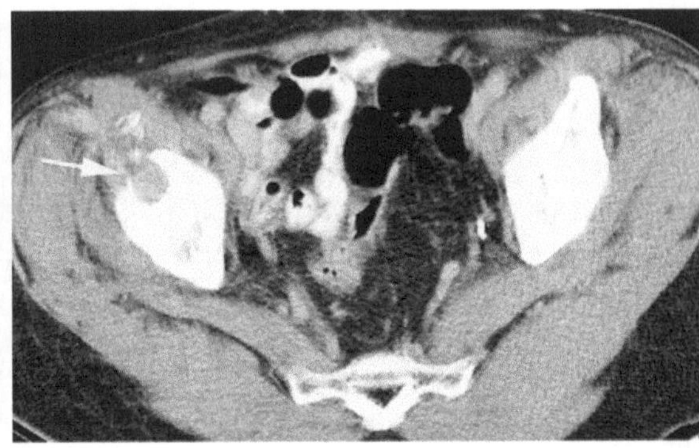
c

lation. Using the aforementioned device of 915 MHz MW frequency, Wright et al. (2005) performed a comparison study to RF ablation in an in vivo hepatic porcine model. Similar pathological appearance and imaging characteristics in CT scans were found for both lesions, caused by MW and by RF thermal energy deposition. A distinctly smaller heat-sink effect close to local blood vessels was detected for MW ablation (3.5%×5.3 deflection), as compared to RF ablation (26.2%×27.9). The laboratory test results were similar between RF-ablation-only animals and MW-ablation-only animals.

Simon et al. (2005) described preliminary results of an ablate-resect study in patients suffering from hepatic or lung malignancies, which was approved by a local institutional review board. In a pilot liver study, patients with hepatic tumors underwent percutaneous MW ablation (915 MHz) before surgical resection. The volumes and diameters of the lesions were measured, and microscopic sections were stained with standard hematoxylin-eosin (H–E) and nicotinamide adenine dinucleotide, reduced (NADH), vital histochemical staining. Three MW antennae were used in a triangular configuration. The mean maximal coagulation necrosis diameter achieved by MW ablation was reported to be 5.5 cm (5.0–6.5 cm), and the ablation volume was 50.4 cm^3 (30.3–58.9 cm^3). Again, no significant heat-sink effect close to large hepatic vessels was found. In the microscopic assessment of the lesions, the H–E staining showed a coagulation necrosis with maximum intensity close to the active tip of the MW antenna. With NADH staining, the uniform absence of viable cells within the ablation zone was demonstrated. Similar results were reported in an ablate-resect study of lung tumors. The mean maximal ablation diameter was reported to be 4.0 cm (3.0–5.0 cm) in the lung, and the coagulation volume was 23.4 cm^3 (9.8–35.4 cm^3).

Recently, a loop antenna for the 915 MHz device was assessed in an in vivo porcine liver model by Shock et al. (2004). Loop antennae were described in combination with an electrocautery device for wire deployment. The loop antenna was reported to create a larger ablation zone (mean ablation diameter 4.3+-0.6 cm) as compared to a single straight MW antenna. However, viable tissue was found in the center of the loop for the single configuration. Complete ablation in the center was described for an orthogonal configuration of two loop antennae.

2.2.8 Clinical Studies

Literature on randomized clinical studies using MW ablation is still sparse. The largest experience in clinical trials with MW ablation as a modality for treatment of malignant diseases is reported from the Asian region using MW devices operating at 2.450 MHz generator frequency.

The first clinical trial on MW ablation therapy was published by Seki et al. (1994). In 18 patients suffering from single unresectable hepatocellular cancer (HCC) smaller than 2 cm, up to 4 MW ablations were performed for treatment. No serious complications were encountered, and no local recurrence was noted in follow-up over 11–22 months. Three patients developed new tumors in sites remote from the treated sites.

Murakami et al. (1995) reported in 1995 their experience in the treatment of nine HCC patients with tumors larger than 3 cm in diameter. Up to 12 MW ablations were performed per tumor, which were reported to be completely ablated on immediate follow-up CT scan. No major complications occurred; however, four of the nine patients developed recurrent tumor at the site of treatment. Lu et al. (2001) described in 2001 a clinical trial with 107 treated HCC nodules in 50 patients using US-guided percutaneous MW ablation. Tumors were divided into two groups, according to whether the tumors were larger or smaller than 2 cm in maximum diameter. Technical success was defined as a lack of enhancing masses at 1-month CT follow-up; 98% of nodules smaller than 2 cm were technically ablated successfully, as were 92% of nodules larger than 2 cm. The 3-year survival rate was 73%.

In 2002, Dong et al. (2003) published a study on MW ablation in a large cohort of 234 patients with 339 HCC lesions treated via MW coagulation therapy with up to 5-year survival rates. Percutaneous interventional treatment was performed with ultrasonographic applicator guidance. A 89.3% rate of technically complete ablations was reported, with a lack of enhancing residual tumor tissue in immediate follow-up CT or MR scan. In 194 nodules, additional post-treatment biopsies were carried out with an absence of viable tumor cells in 180 nodules (92.8%). The 3-year survival rate was 72.9%, the 5-year survival rate 56.7%. No clinical reports have been published so far for the 915-MHz device.

References

Deardorff DL, Diederich CJ, Nau WH (2001) Control of interstitial thermal coagulation: comparative evaluation of microwave and ultrasound applicators. Med Phys 28:104–117

Dewey WC (1994) Arrhenius relationships from the molecule and cell to the clinic. Int J Hyperthermia 10(4):457–483

Dong B, Liang P, Yu X, Su L, Yu D, Cheng Z, Zhang J (2003) Percutaneous sonographically guided microwave coagulation therapy for hepatocellular carcinoma: results in 234 patients. AJR Am J Roentgenol 180:1547–1555

Goldberg SN, Gazelle GS (2001) Radiofrequency tissue ablation: physical principles and techniques for increasing coagulation necrosis. Hepatogastroenterology 48:359–367

Goldberg SN, Gazelle GS, Dawson SL, Rittman WJ, Mueller PR, Rosenthal DI (1995) Tissue ablation with radiofrequency using multiprobe arrays. Acad Radiol 2:670–674

Goldberg SN, Hahn PF, Tanabe KK, Mueller PR, Schima W, Athanasoulis CA, Compton CC, Solbiati L, Gazelle GS (1998) Percutaneous radiofrequency tissue ablation: does perfusion-mediated tissue cooling limit coagulation necrosis? J Vasc Interv Radiol 9:101–111

Haemmerich D, Lee FT Jr (2005) Multiple applicator approaches for radiofrequency and microwave ablation. Int J Hyperthermia 21:93–106

Huber PE, Jenne JW, Rastert R et al (2001) A new noninvasive approach in breast cancer therapy using magnetic resonance imaging-guided focused ultrasound surgery. Cancer Res 61:8441–8447

Ido K, Isoda N, Sugano K (2001) Microwave coagulation therapy for liver cancer: laparoscopic microwave coagulation. J Gastroenterol 36(3):145–152

Lu MD, Chen JW, Xie XY, Liu L, Huang XQ, Liang LJ, Huang JF (2001) Hepatocellular carcinoma: US-guided percutaneous microwave coagulation therapy. Radiology 221:167–172

Matsukawa T, Yamashita Y, Arakawa A, Nishiharu T, Urata J, Murakami R, Takahashi M, Yoshimatsu S (1997) Percutaneous microwave coagulation therapy in liver tumors. A 3-year experience. Acta Radiol 38(3):410–415

Midorikawa T, Kumada K, Kikuchi H, Ishibashi K, Yagi H, Nagasaki H, Nemoto H, Saitoh M, Nakano H, Yamaguchi M, Koh Y, Sakai H, Yoshizawa Y, Sanada Y, Yoshiba M (2000) Microwave coagulation therapy for hepatocellular carcinoma. J Hepatobiliary Pancreat Surg 7:252–259

Murakami R, Yoshimatsu S, Yamashita Y, Matsukawa T, Takahashi M, Sagara K (1995) Treatment of hepatocellular carcinoma: value of percutaneous microwave coagulation. Am J Roentgenol 164:1159–1164

Ohmoto K, Miyake I, Tsuduki M, Shibata N, Takesue M, Kunieda T, Ohno S, Kuboki M, Yamamoto S (1999) Percutaneous microwave coagulation therapy for unresectable hepatocellular carcinoma. Hepatogastroenterology 46:2894–2900

Pennes HH (1948) Analysis of tissue and arterial blood temperatures in the resting human forearm. J Appl Physiol 1:93–122

Pereira PL, Trubenbach J, Schenk M, Subke J, Kroeber S, Schaefer I, Remy CT, Schmidt D, Brieger J, Claussen CD (2004) Radiofrequency ablation: in vivo comparison of four commercially available devices in pig livers. Radiology 232:482–490

Sapareto SA, Dewey WC (1984) Thermal dose determination in cancer therapy. Int J Radiat Oncol Biol Phys 10:787–800
Sato M, Watanabe Y, Ueda S, Iseki S, Abe Y, Sato N, Kimura S, Okubo K, Onji M (1996) Microwave coagulation therapy for hepatocellular carcinoma. Gastroenterology 110:1507–1514
Seki T, Wakabayashi M, Nakagawa T, Itho T, Shiro T, Kunieda K, Sato M, Uchiyama S, Inoue K (1994) Ultrasonically guided percutaneous microwave coagulation therapy for small hepatocellular carcinoma. Cancer 74:817–825
Shibata T, Iimuro Y, Yamamoto Y et al (2002) Small hepatocellular carcinoma: comparison of radio-frequency ablation and percutaneous microwave coagulation therapy. Radiology 223:331–337
Shimada S, Hirota M, Beppu T, Matsuda T, Hayashi N, Tashima S, Takai E, Yamaguchi K, Inoue K, Ogawa M (1998) Complications and management of microwave coagulation therapy for primary and metastatic liver tumors. Surg Today 28:1130–1137
Shock SA, Meredith K, Warner TF, Sampson LA, Wright AS, Winter TC 3rd, Mahvi DM, Fine JP, Lee FT Jr (2004) Microwave ablation with loop antenna: in vivo porcine liver model. Radiology 231:143–149
Simon CJ, Dupuy DE, Mayo-Smith WW (2005) Microwave ablation: principles and applications. Radiographics 25 [Suppl 1]:S69–S83
Vogl TJ, Straub R, Eichler K, Woitaschek D, Mack MG (2002) Malignant liver tumors treated with MR imaging-guided laser-induced thermotherapy: experience with complications in 899 patients (2,520 lesions). Radiology 225:367–377
Wright AS, Lee FT Jr, Mahvi DM (2003) Hepatic microwave ablation with multiple antennae results in synergistically larger zones of coagulation necrosis. Ann Surg Oncol 10:275–283
Wright AS, Sampson LA, Warner TF, Mahvi DM, Lee FT Jr (2005) Radiofrequency versus microwave ablation in a hepatic porcine model. Radiology 236:132–139

Ablative Techniques (Percutaneous)

2

Thermal Ablative Techniques

2.3 Laser Ablation

Martin G. Mack and Thomas J. Vogl

CONTENTS

2.3.1 Introduction

Interstitial laser-induced thermotherapy (LITT) is a minimally invasive technique suitable for local tumor destruction within solid organs, using optical fibers to deliver high-energy laser radiation to the target lesion. Due to light absorption, temperatures of up to 120°C are reached within the tumor, leading to substantial thermocoagulation. MR imaging is used both for placement of the laser applicator in the tumor and for monitoring progress of thermocoagulation. The thermosensitivity of certain MR sequences is the key to real-time monitoring, allowing accurate estimation of the actual extent of thermal damage.

Thus, laser can destroy tumor by direct heating, while greatly limiting damage to surrounding structures. Experimental work has shown that a well-defined area of coagulative necrosis is obtained around the fiber tip, with minimal damage to surrounding structures. Pilot clinical studies have demonstrated that this technique is practical for the palliation of hepatic tumors. The success of LITT is dependent on delivering the optical fibers to the target area, real-time monitoring of the effects of the treatment and subsequent evaluation of the extent of thermal damage. The key to achieving these objectives is the imaging method used.

MR-guided laser-induced thermotherapy offers a number of potential treatment benefits. First, MR imaging provides unparalleled topographic accuracy due to its excellent soft-tissue contrast and high spatial resolution. Secondly, the temperature sensitivity of specially designed MR sequences can be used to monitor the temperature elevation in the tumor and surrounding normal tissues. This enables the exact visualization of the growing coagulative necrosis. On-line MR imaging during LITT is essential for avoiding local complications due to laser treatment. Thirdly, recovery times, lengths of hospital stay, and the risk of infection and other complications can be reduced when compared with conventional palliative surgery. Finally, successful implementation of such minimally invasive procedures would significantly reduce costs in comparison to surgical procedures. A further, indirect advantage is the psychological effect due to avoidance of cosmetic deformities that can result from major reconstructive surgery.

A big advantage of laser ablation over radiofrequency (RF) ablation is that it can be combined with MR because (laser) light is used instead of RF. To generate an MR image an RF pulse is used. If there is any RF source in the MR room there is always interference between the radiofrequencies from the RF generator and the radiofrequencies from the MR scanner. The result is that the MR image is completely destroyed. Even with an MR-compatible RF probe it is necessary to disconnect the probes for every MR scan and this is quite uncomfortable.

Another advantage of the laser is that multiple laser applicators can be used in completely different parts of the liver simultaneously, because the different laser applicators do not interact. Multiple RF probes would interact. Therefore, two or three

M. G. Mack, MD, PD; T. J. Vogl, MD, Professor
Institute for Diagnostic and Interventional Radiology, University Hospital, Johann Wolfgang Goethe University, Theodor-Stern-Kai 7, 60590 Frankfurt am Main, Germany

metastases can be ablated simultaneously with the laser (under local anesthesia on an outpatient basis). With RF it is only possible to ablate one metastasis after another. Therefore, treatment time is significantly shorter with laser.

2.3.2 Technique of LITT

2.3.2.1 Laser System and Application Set

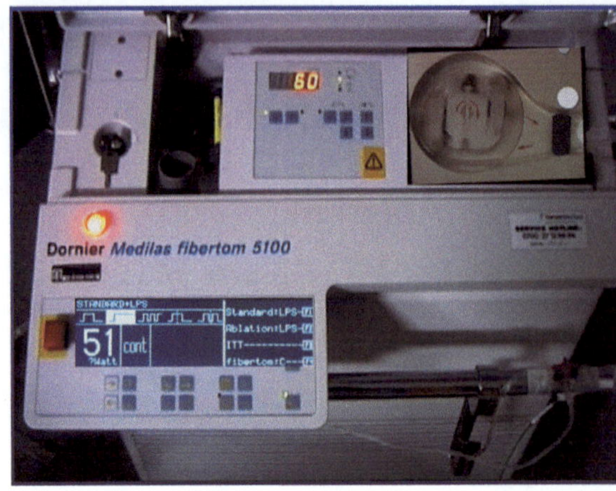

Fig. 2.3.1. The Nd:YAG laser Dornier MediLas 5100

Laser coagulation is performed using a Neodymium-YAG laser (Fig. 2.3.1) (Dornier MediLas 5060 or Dornier MediLas 5100) with a specially developed flexible laser applicator. Furthermore an application kit for percutaneous treatment was developed and optimized for our purposes.

Laser light with a wavelength of 1046 nm is transmitted to tissue with a diffusing applicator. Laser light of this wavelength penetrates deeply into biological tissue, where photon absorption and heat conduction lead to hyperthermic and coagulative effects. The tissue destruction may be immediate or delayed.

The cooled power laser system (SOMATEX, Germany) for MR-guided minimally invasive percutaneous laser-induced thermotherapy of soft-tissue tumors consists of an MR-compatible cannulation needle (length 20 cm, diameter 1.3 mm) with a tetragonally beveled tip and stylet; guide-wire (length 100 cm); 9-French sheath with stylet; and a 7-French double-tube thermostable (up to 400°C) protective catheter (length 40 cm) also with a stylet, which enables internal cooling with saline solution. Cooling of the surface of the laser applicator modifies the radial temperature distribution so that the maximum temperature shifts into deeper tissue layers. The protective catheter prevents direct contact of the laser applicator with the patient and enables complete removal of the applicator even in the unlikely event of damage during treatment. This increases patient safety and simplifies the procedure. The catheter is transparent for laser radiation and resistant to heat (up to 400°C). Marks on the sheath and the protective catheter allow exact positioning of both in the lesion (Fig. 2.3.2).

The system is fully compatible with MR imaging systems. Magnetite markers on the laser applicator allow an easier visualizing and positioning procedure.

The laser itself is installed outside of the examination unit. The laser light is transmitted via a 10-m-long optical fiber. The complete set-up used for LITT is shown in Figure 2.3.3.

Prior to LITT treatment all patients undergo CT and a contrast-enhanced MRI study at least 2 days prior to the intervention. After localization of the tumor with CT, local anesthesia is achieved with 20–30 ml of 1% mepivacaine (Scandicain, AstraZeneca, Wedel, Germany). Distance to the lesion and the puncture angle are calculated electronically.

After CT-guided puncture of the lesion and positioning of the laser application system, the patient is transferred to a conventional MR system.

First of all a magnetite marker is placed for verification of the positioning of the laser application systems. After verifying the correct positioning of the laser application systems in relation to the lesion, the magnetite markers are removed and the laser applicator inserted in the laser application system.

In most cases a 3-cm active length of the laser applicator is used (2 and 4 cm active lengths are also available). For larger lesions the multi-applicator technique (Fig. 2.3.4) and the pull-back technique are used.

All laser applicators per metastases are used simultaneously in order to get synergistic effects. Therefore, in all patients the ablation procedure is performed by using T_1-weighted thermal imaging to monitor the LITT procedures, and in all patients the procedure is modified concerning the duration of ablation. Moreover, the pull-back procedure is calculated on the basis of the thermal imaging. The

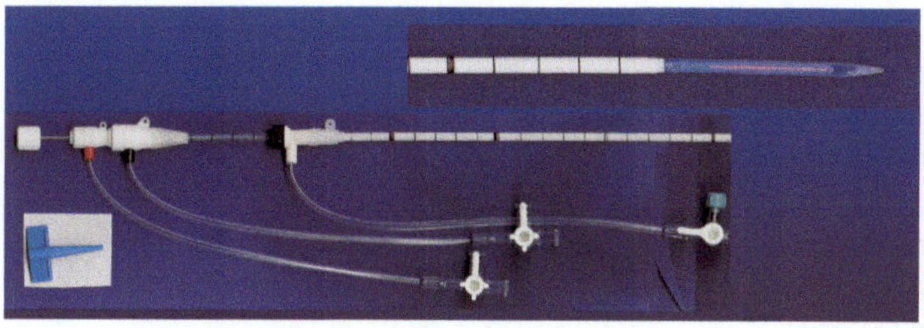

a

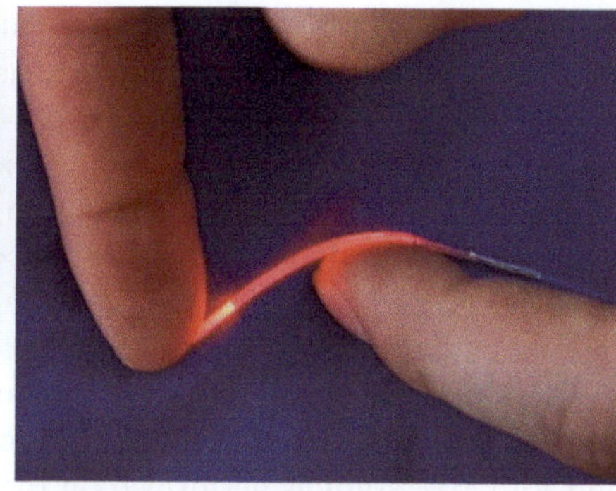

b

Fig. 2.3.2. a Internally cooled power laser application system with laser applicator. **b** The flexible laser applicator

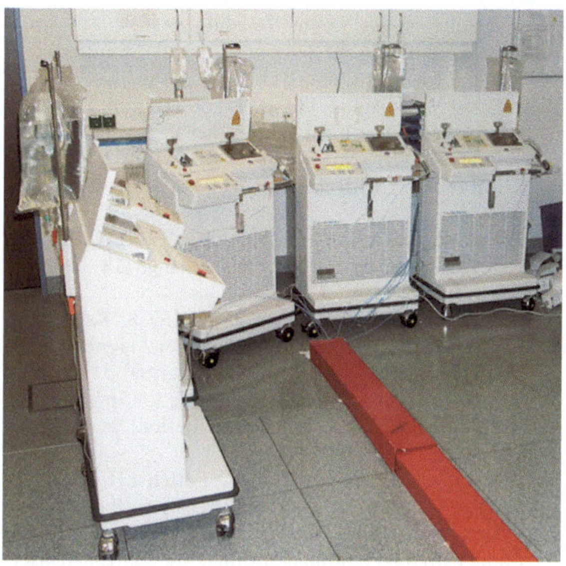

Fig. 2.3.3. The complete interstitial laser-induced thermotherapy (LITT) set-up with the laser systems outside in the control room

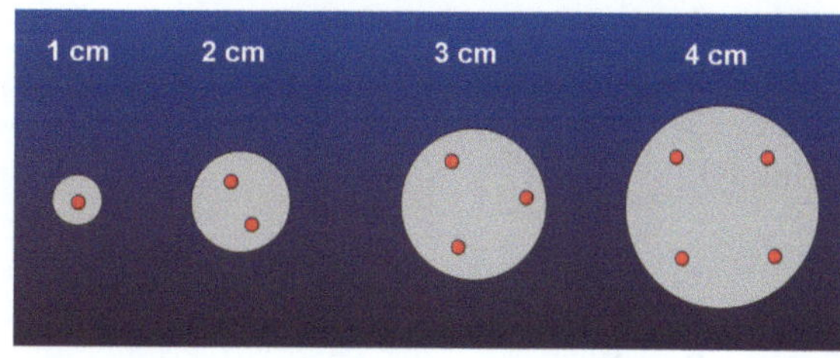

Fig. 2.3.4. The multi-applicator technique for larger lesions

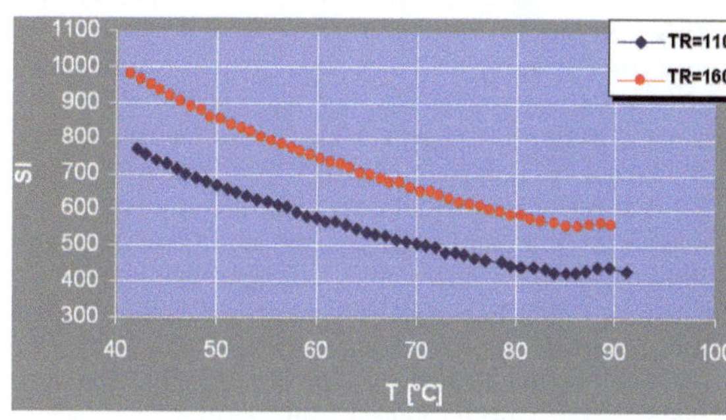

Fig. 2.3.5. The relationship between tissue temperature and signal intensity

pull-back procedure is used to enlarge the coagulation necrosis in the longitudinal axis by pulling back the laser fiber between 1 and 3 cm (depending on the size of the lesion, the relationship to surrounding structures, and the thermal imaging) within the protective catheter. In no case is the ablation procedure performed on a time or energy basis.

The LITT treatment is performed under MR guidance using a 0.5 Tesla scanner (Privilig, Escint, Israel) by T_1-weighted GE sequences (TR/TE=140/12, flip angle=80°, matrix 128 × 256, 5 slices, slice thickness 8 mm, interslice gap 30%, acquisition time 15 s) in axial slice orientation and parallel to the laser applicators. These two sequences are repeated every minute. Increasing tissue temperature results in an increase in the T_1 relaxation time. Finally this results in a decrease of signal intensity (Fig. 2.3.5).

The entire LITT treatment is performed using local anesthesia and intravenously injected analgesics [Pethidin 10–80 mg (Dolantin, Aventis Pharma, Frankfurt, Germany) and/or Piritramid 5–15 mg (Dipidolor, Janssen-CILAG, Neuss, Germany)] and sedation (2–10 mg midazolam, Hoffmann-La Roche, Grenzach-Wyhlen, Germany).

After the procedure the needle track is closed with fibrin glue (Tissucol Duo S, Baxter, Wien, Austria).

2.3.2.2 Follow-Up MR Imaging

Unenhanced and contrast-enhanced (0.1 mmol/kg body weight Gd-DTPA, Magnevist, Schering,

Berlin, Germany) MRI is performed in all cases in order to verify the necrosis obtained. The imaging protocol includes a T_2-weighted breath-hold TSE sequence (TR/TE=3000/92, matrix 154 × 256, flip angle=150°) in transverse slice orientation, a HASTE sequence (TR/TE=1000/60, matrix 178 × 256, flip angle=147°), and a T_1-weighted unenhanced and contrast-enhanced gradient (GE) sequence (FLASH 2D, TR/TE=110/5, matrix 178 × 256, flip angle=90°) in transverse and sagittal slice orientation. The first follow-up MRI study is performed on the day after the LITT treatment. Further follow-up studies are performed every 3 months after the intervention. All follow-up studies are performed at a 1.5 Tesla scanner (Symphony Quantum, Siemens, Erlangen, Germany).

Further Reading

Anzai Y, Lufkin RB, Saxton RE, Fetterman H, Farahani K, Layfield LJ, Jolesz FC, Hanafee WH, Castro DJ (1991) Nd: YAG interstitial laser phototherapy guided by magnetic resonance imaging in an ex vivo model: dosimetry of laser-MR-tissue interaction. Laryngoscope 101:755

Castro DJ, Saxton RE, Layfield LJ, Fetterman HR, Castro DJ, Tartell PB, Robinson JD, To SY, Nishimura E, Lufkin RB et al (1990) Interstitial laser phototherapy assisted by magnetic resonance imaging: a new technique for monitoring laser-tissue interaction. Laryngoscope 100:541

Chapman R (1998) Successful pregnancies following laser-induced interstitial thermotherapy (LITT) for treatment of large uterine leiomyomas by a minimally invasive method. Acta Obstet Gynecol Scand 77:1024

De Poorter J (1995) Noninvasive MRI thermometry with the proton resonance frequency method: study of susceptibility effects. Magn Reson Med 34:359

De Poorter J, De Wagter C, De Deene Y, Thomsen C, Stahlberg F, Achten E (1995) Noninvasive MRI thermometry with the proton resonance frequency (PRF) method: in vivo results in human muscle. Magn Reson Med 33:74

Eyrich GK, Bruder E, Hilfiker P, Dubno B, Quick HH, Patak MA, Gratz KW, Sailer HF (2000) Temperature mapping of magnetic resonance-guided laser interstitial thermal therapy (LITT) in lymphangiomas of the head and neck. Lasers Surg Med 26:467

Fiedler VU, Schwarzmaier HJ, Eickmeyer F, Muller FP, Schoepp C, Verreet PR (2001) Laser-induced interstitial thermotherapy of liver metastases in an interventional 0.5 Tesla MRI system: technique and first clinical experiences. J Magn Reson Imaging 13:729

Gewiese B, Beuthan J, Fobbe F, Stiller D, Muller G, Bose Landgraf J, Wolf KJ, Deimling M (1994) Magnetic resonance imaging-controlled laser-induced interstitial thermotherapy. Invest Radiol 29:345

Harth T, Kahn T, Rassek M, Schwabe B, Schwarzmaier HJ, Lewin JS, Modder U (1997) Determination of laser-induced temperature distributions using echo-shifted TurboFLASH. Magn Reson Med 38:238

Hynynen K, Darkazanli A, Damianou CA, Unger E, Schenck JF (1993) Tissue thermometry during ultrasound exposure. Eur Urol 1:12

Kahn T, Bettag M, Ulrich F, Schwarzmaier HJ, Schober R, Furst G, Modder U (1994) MRI-guided laser-induced interstitial thermotherapy of cerebral neoplasms. J Comput Assist Tomogr 18:519

Le Bihan D, Delannoy J, Levin RL (1989) Temperature mapping with MR imaging of molecular diffusion: application to hyperthermia. Radiology 171:853

Mack MG, Straub R, Eichler K, Engelmann K, Roggan A, Woitaschek D, Böttger M, Vogl TJ (2001) Percutaneous MR imaging-guided laser-induced thermotherapy of hepatic metastases. Abdom Imaging 26:369

Matsumoto R, Oshio K, Jolesz FA (1992) Monitoring of laser and freezing-induced ablation in the liver with T1-weighted MR imaging. J Magn Reson Imaging 2:555

Orth K, Russ D, Duerr J, Hibst R, Steiner R, Beger HG (1997) Thermo-controlled device for inducing deep coagulation in the liver with the Nd:YAG laser. Lasers Surg Med 20:149

Panych LP, Hrovat MI, Bleier AR, Jolesz FA (1992) Effects related to temperature changes during MR imaging. J Magn Reson Imaging 2:69

Peters RD, Chan E, Trachtenberg J, Jothy S, Kapusta L, Kucharczyk W, Henkelman RM (2000) Magnetic resonance thermometry for predicting thermal damage: an application of interstitial laser coagulation in an in vivo canine prostate model [In Process Citation]. Magn Reson Med 44:873

Vogl TJ, Mack MG, Muller P, Phillip C, Bottcher H, Roggan A, Juergens M, Deimling M, Knobber D, Wust P et al (1995) Recurrent nasopharyngeal tumors: preliminary clinical results with interventional MR imaging-controlled laser-induced thermotherapy. Radiology 196:725

Vogl TJ, Mack MG, Hirsch HH, Müller P, Weinhold N, Wust P, Philipp C, Roggan R, Felix R (1997) In-vitro evaluation of MR-thermometry for laser-induced thermotherapy. Fortschr Röntgenstr 167:638

Vogl TJ, Mack MG, Straub R, Roggan A, Felix R (1997) Magnetic Resonance Imaging – guided abdominal interventional radiology: laser-induced thermotherapy of liver metastases. Endoscopy 29:577

Vogl TJ, Mack MG, Roggan A, Straub R, Eichler KC, Muller PK, Knappe V, Felix R (1998) Internally cooled power laser for MR-guided interstitial laser-induced thermotherapy of liver lesions: initial clinical results. Radiology 209:381

Vogl TJ, Muller PK, Mack MG, Straub R, Engelmann K, Neuhaus P (1999) Liver metastases: interventional therapeutic techniques and results, state of the art. Eur Radiol 9:675

Vogl TJ, Eichler K, Straub R, Engelmann K, Zangos S, Woitaschek D, Bottger M, Mack MG (2001) Laser-induced thermotherapy of malignant liver tumors: general principals, equipment(s), procedure(s) – side effects, complications and results. Eur J Ultrasound 13:117

Zhang Y, Samulski TV, Joines WT, Mattiello J, Levin RL, LeBihan D (1992) On the accuracy of noninvasive thermometry using molecular diffusion magnetic resonance imaging. Int J Hyperthermia 8:263

Ablative Techniques (Percutaneous)

2

Vascular Ablative Techniques

2.4 Locoregional Chemotherapy Including Perfusion

Herwart Müller

CONTENTS

Regional chemotherapy is a form of anticancer therapy which has recently made striking advances. The rationale for regional application of cytotoxic agents is to increase local efficacy on one hand and to reduce systemic side-effects on the other hand. Regional administration of anticancer drugs may be recommended, if is known and if it is relatively localized and not disseminated. Many attempts have been made to increase the response by administering high concentrations of anticancer drugs selectively to the tumor tissue. It is advantageous for anticancer treatment if the toxic effects of the cytostatics on normal tissue are minimized by administering the drugs only to the cancer tissue in such a way that the drugs do not reach the normal tissue.

Throughout the last 30 years different application forms and techniques have been established in the field of locoregional chemotherapy. Basis for the development of such complex treatment modalities is a clear knowledge of the pharmacokinetic properties of existing antineoplastic agents allied to recent advances in the understanding of molecular and cell biology transformation. Today, different application forms are available; for example, intra-arterial infusion sometimes in the form of chemoembolization, intracavitary application techniques such as intrapleural infusion or intraperitoneal perfusion as well as isolated perfusion techniques such as extremity perfusion or pelvic stop-flow perfusions. Up to now, only a few of these techniques have reached a level of standardization combined with an efficacy superior to that of conventional systemic chemotherapy to be accepted as a standard treatment by the oncology community.

2.4.1 Pharmacokinetic Principles

Pharmacokinetics can be determined as the knowledge of the various processes connected to the application of a drug such as absorption, distribution, metabolism and excretion. The exact knowledge of these processes is the basis of reaching the maximal effect of each drug used for anticancer treatment.

H. Müller, MD
Oncological Surgery, Hammelburg Hospitals, Ofenthaler Weg 20, 97762 Hammelburg, Germany

2.4.1.1
Dose-Response Relationship

Since the fundamental work of COLLINS, it has been widely assumed that cytotoxic drugs have steep dose-response curves, i.e., there can be a large increase in cytotoxicity with a relatively small increase in drug exposure (COLLINS and DEDRICK 1982). This has two different implications; namely, that the attainment of very high drug concentrations in the target organ being regionally perfused will increase the degree of tumor cells killed, and if less drug is delivered into the systemic vascular compartments there will be reduced exposure of rapidly dividing normal cell populations, such as bone marrow progenitors. This will lead to less toxicity.

Based on this dose-response relationship for cytotoxic drugs the aim of regional chemotherapy will be:

- To increase efficacy in the treated area by raising local drug concentrations.
- To avoid systemic toxicity by decreasing systemic drug exposure.
- If there is no need to prevent systemic toxicity, it will be possible to use combined systemic and regional chemotherapy in order to reach a high local efficacy and systemic drugs level high enough to be effective against micrometastatic cancer.

2.4.1.2
Intraperitoneal Application

The concentration differential between the peritoneal cavity and the systemic circulation arises because the rate of movement of the drug from the peritoneal cavity into the plasma (peritoneal clearance) is generally slow relative to the total body clearance. The pharmacokinetics of intraperitoneal treatment is best understood as a three-compartment model. The drug is administered directly into the tumor-containing cavity (1st compartment). It will then be absorbed into the bloodstream (2nd compartment) and distributed to all other tissues in contact with the blood circulation (3rd compartment). After injection of a drug into the peritoneal cavity, its concentration will gradually fall as the drug leaks into the systemic circulation and is distributed to other tissues as well as being metabolized or excreted from the body. The rate at which the concentration falls is a function of the volume of the peritoneal cavity (V), the surface of the peritoneal membrane through which the drug will diffuse (A), the permeability of the membrane (P) and the difference in free drug concentration between the cavity (C_{pc}) and the plasma (C_{pl}). This is defined quantitatively by the following equation (LOS 2000).

$$\frac{dCpl.}{dt} = \frac{PA(Cp.c. - Cpl.)}{V}$$

This means that the greater the clearance from the systemic circulation and the smaller the clearance from the peritoneal cavity, the greater the concentration difference and the greater the advantage of an intraperitoneal as compared to an intravenous application will be. This advantage directly depends on the drug used for cytostatic therapy.

2.4.1.3
Intra-arterial Application

The greatest advantage of intra-arterial infusion is that the drug is distributed at high concentrations in the regional artery supplying the tumor during the initial circulation after administration. When the drug is transported to the heart, it will be detoxified or excreted before recirculation by being passed through the liver and the kidneys. As a result, its blood concentrations during the next circulation cycle do not differ from the levels achieved after intravenous infusion. The advantage of intra-arterial infusion should be maximized to gain a better response than that obtained after intravenous therapy. To achieve this objective, the following criteria should be met:

- The drug should flow at high concentrations during the initial circulation.
- The drug should adhere to the tumor tissue.
- It should permeate the tissue and be taken up by the tumor cells.
- It should be inactivated or excreted almost completely in a short period of time to reduce systemic toxicity.

The pharmacokinetics of intra-arterially applied cytostatics has been studied in detail by Stephens (STEPHENS 1983). Based on cardiovascular physiology, he described an excellent model to account for the advantage of intra-arterial over intravenous applications. In this model, the intravenously applied dose of a drug should be 100%. If it is assumed that 10% of the dose is distributed in the tumor and the regional artery supplying the blood to the tumor, X% of the dose may show its biological activity when it passes through the tumor. In contrast, if 100% of the dose is given to the regional artery supplying the tumor then 10 times *X*% of the dose should show biological activity against the tumor during the initial circulation. After the first circulation, the drug is distributed almost equally irrespective of whether it is given intra-arterially or intravenously. High concentrations that are achieved during the initial circulation after intra-arterial infusion are decreased depending on the rate of excretion and detoxification. Comparing different modes of application such as bolus intravenous, continuous intravenous or intra-arterial, the advantage of the latter becomes evident (Taguchi 1979). He has demonstrated in an animal study that bolus application of cytostatics into an artery lead to nearly identical drug concentrations as an intravenous bolus administration. Only a continuous arterial infusion can increase local drug exposure 4–5 times higher than both other infusion forms.

2.4.1.4 Isolated Perfusion Techniques

To exemplify the benefit of isolated perfusion techniques our group compared pharmacokinetic data achieved by high-dose intravenous chemotherapy versus isolated abdominal perfusion using a stop-flow perfusion technique. Details of the techniques of this form of application are given later in this chapter. This special technique has shown promising efficacy in patients with heavily pre-treated, recurrent peritoneal metastatic ovarian cancer.

Treosulfan was used in a dosage of 2.600 mg/m^2 for isolated abdominal perfusion; perfusion time was 30 min. In contrast, the maximum tolerated dose of conventional intravenous therapy was defined to 8000 mg/m^2 (Harstrick et al. 1996). High-dose chemotherapy of 10.000–56.000 mg/m^2 treosulfan needs the support of autologous peripheral blood stem cell transplantation (PBSC). Pharmacokinetic data demonstrated a twofold higher peak plasma concentration (C_{max}) after the intraabdominal application of 2.600 mg/m^2 treosulfan, compared to the intravenous infusion of 10.000 mg/m^2 treosulfan. Additionally, the area under the concentration versus time curve (AUC) reached exactly the same values, by using only a quarter of the intravenous route without the need of PBSC support (Hilger et al. 1998) (Fig. 2.4.1).

2.4.2 Application Techniques

2.4.2.1 Intracavitary Application

In the early 1950s, Weissberger for the first time treated ovarian cancer patients with nitrogen mustard intraperitoneally and demonstrated an impressive control of malignant ascites (Weissberger et al. 1955). Unfortunately, this study and other early clinical investigations were unable to demonstrate any therapeutic impact of the intraperitoneal approach on peritoneal tumor masses. In spite of the convincing pharmacokinetic and experimental data indicating that intraperitoneal chemotherapy is more

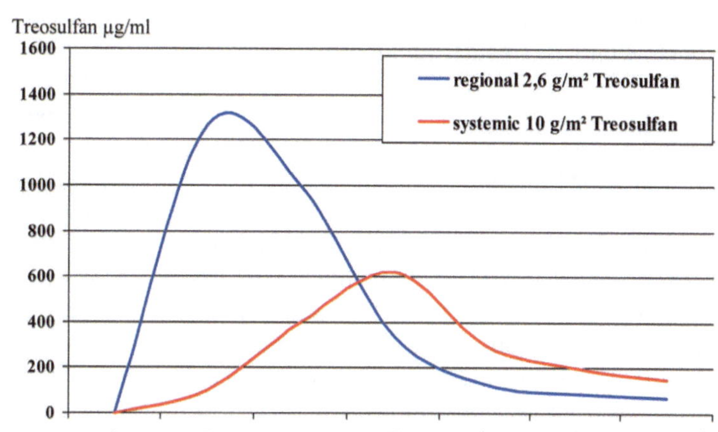

Fig. 2.4.1. Pharmacokinetic data of isolated abdominal perfusion using 2600 mg/m^2 treosulfan versus high-dose systemic chemotherapy using 10.000 mg/m^2

effective than systemic administration of cytostatics in patients with cancer restricted to the peritoneal cavity, it was still unclear up to 1995 whether intraperitoneal treatment would be superior to intravenous treatment in terms of survival. Alberts et al. (1995) presented a carefully controlled prospective trial showing that median survival of patients with minimal disease ovarian cancer (tumors <2 cm) was 8 months longer after intraperitoneal cisplatin plus iv cyclophosphamide than after iv cisplatin plus iv cyclophosphamide. Results of this study were confirmed by a large Intergroup Study in 2001 showing a survival advantage for the group of patients treated by intraperitoneal chemotherapy (iv paclitaxel/intraperitoneal carboplatin) of 28 as compared to 22 months (Markman et al. 2001).

Intraperitoneal application of cytostatics is always combined with an increase in local drug exposure, but this high drug concentration can lead to local side-effects and complications such as pain or cramps induced by a chemical peritonitis or formation of adhesions. These adhesions can prohibit a uniform diffusion of applied drug into all areas of the peritoneal cavity. Keeping in mind that drugs infused in the peritoneum invade only the first cell layers up to a depth of 1.0–1.5 mm of the tissue repetitive use of intraperitoneal chemotherapy is definitely restricted. There are two completely different situations when intraperitoneal application of cytostatic drugs is worthwhile doing. In the palliative setting this treatment form should be used to reduce mutilating ascites in patients with widespread peritoneal carcinosis. With a more curative intent the intraperitoneal chemotherapy can be used to eliminate microscopic disease after cytoreductive surgery including peritonectomy procedures. At the end of such an operation when all or almost all visible tumor formations have been resected it is a unique and unparalleled situation that cytostatics have to eliminate singular tumor cells.

2.4.2.2 Intra-arterial Infusion

In 1950, Klopp et al. began to infuse anticancer drugs directly into arteries supplying the tumors to minimize systemic adverse reactions and to achieve higher concentrations of the drug in tumor tissue. Since then, a large variety of different application forms has been established for intra-arterial infusion in different application areas. The easiest access to arteries supplying the tumor is the transient insertion of catheters via percutaneous angiography with Seldinger technique. Using this technique, catheterization of many different arteries of the body is readily possible in different areas.

A problem of such angiographic catheterization of different arteries supplying the tumor is that it will be necessary to repeat the treatment and procedure. This will lead to restrictions in the patient's daily life, which was the reason for implanting catheter devices that can be used repeatedly.

Despite the advantages of such implantable devices with regard to secure placement and application whilst avoiding restrictions to the patient's life, such catheters have several drawbacks. Moreover, an operation is necessary. There is also the risk of arterial thrombosis and infections. Last but not least, the catheter tip may be displaced. Several different catheter devices have been produced and several different implantation techniques have been published in recent years. This has led to an improvement in success rate and lower morbidity.

2.4.2.3 Regional Perfusion Techniques

In 1958, Creech et al. used extracorporeal circulation to perfuse anticancer drugs locally in organs which could be separated from the systemic circulation. They attempted active intervention to eradicate all tumor cells and to decrease systemic adverse reactions more completely than can be achieved by arterial infusion therapy. This technique has been established primarily for primary or recurrent tumors located in the pelvic area. Up to now the technique of isolated perfusion has been established for different areas of the body such as the limbs, the liver, the thoracic region, the abdomen or the pelvis.

2.4.2.3.1 Stop-Flow Perfusions

Depending on the anticancer agent used and its dosage, a varying degree of leakage can occur, leading to a more or less pronounced systemic toxicity. Accepting this leakage, it will be possible to use special balloon catheter techniques to establish such isolated perfusions. Such balloon-assisted, minimally invasive perfusions are called "stop-flow" perfusions. This technique leads to a considerable reduction in side-effects and morbidity (Figs. 2.4.2–2.4.4).

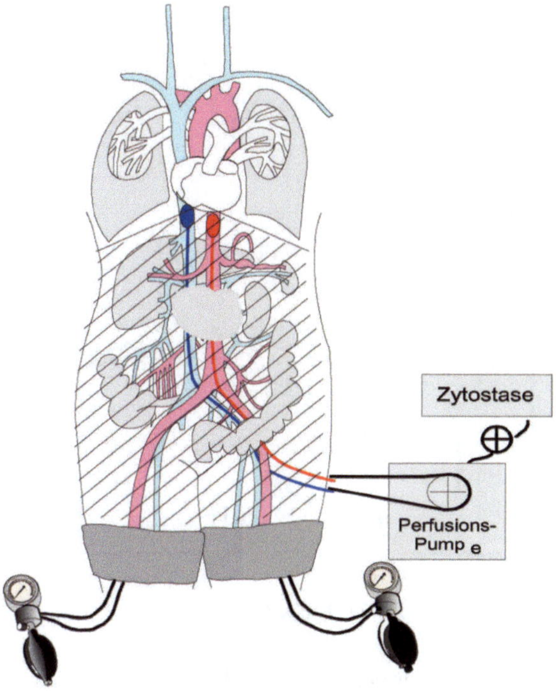

Fig. 2.4.2. Scheme of isolated abdominal perfusion

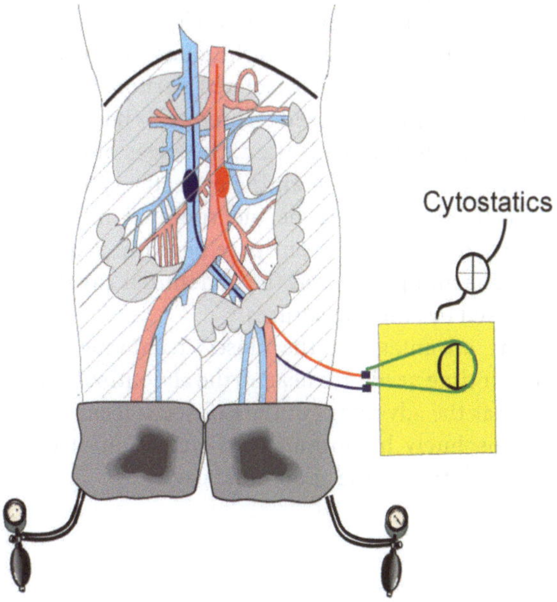

Fig. 2.4.3. Scheme of isolated pelvic perfusion

An abdominal perfusion can be established with two special balloon catheters, which are placed in the aorta and vena cava via an inguinal approach under general anesthesia (Fig. 2.4.2). The balloons are placed under X-ray control in such a way that when leveling the diaphragm they ensure complete occlusion of both vessels. Additionally, two Esmarch

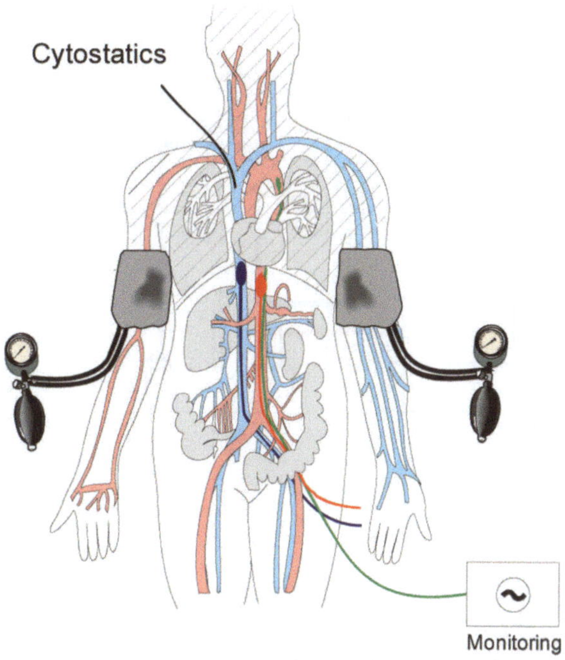

Fig. 2.4.4. Scheme of isolated thoracic perfusion

bandages are insufflated at both roots of the legs. Via these inserted catheters, an isolated circuit of the abdominal region can be established for 30 min using a specific pump system.

Using the same technique and equipment an isolated perfusion circuit can be established if the catheter tips are placed just above the aortic bifurcation and iliac confluence (Fig. 2.4.3).

By placing the bandages on both roots of the upper limbs and the catheters at the level of the diaphragm a dramatic reduction of systemic circulation can be achieved, which is called isolated thoracic perfusion (Fig. 2.4.4). Pharmacokinetic evaluations in different mouse models have shown that using thoracic as well as lung perfusion techniques cytostatic drug concentrations of melphalan, doxorubicin, cisplatin, 5-fluorouracil and mitomycin are 6–10 times higher compared with systemic administration (Hendriks et al. 1999; Ng et al. 1996).

2.4.2.3.2 Isolated Extremity Perfusion (ILP)

The technique of isolated extremity perfusion (ILP) was established by Creech and Krementz in 1958 (Creech et al. 1958). Isolation of extremity is achieved by cross-clamping major vessels, cannulation of artery and vein and connection to an extracorporeal circuit (Fig. 2.4.5). To minimize

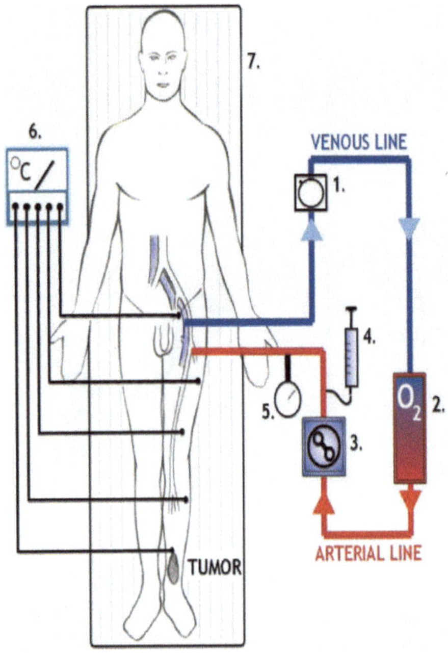

Fig. 2.4.5. Scheme of isolated extremity perfusion

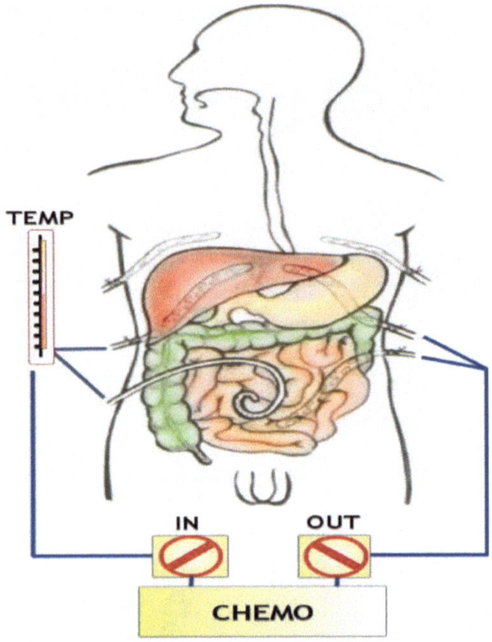

Fig. 2.4.6. Scheme of peritoneal perfusion

leakage collateral vessels are ligated and a tourniquet is placed around the groin. Using this technique regional drug concentrations of 15–25 times higher than following systemic application can be achieved (Benckhuijsen et al. 1988). Many different drugs, cytostatics such as adriamycin or DTIC as well as immunotherapeutic agents such as interferon gamma, have been used for ILP as monotherapy or in combination. Due to its efficacy and low local toxicity profile melphalan is now used as the cytostatic agent of choice for ILP. In 1969 Stehlin modified the technique integrating regional hyperthermia into the concept. Performing isolated extremity perfusions under hyperthermic conditions efficacy of this technique could be increased, but this was combined with an increase in side-effects and complications as well. So Wieberdinck established (Wieberdinck et al. 1982) a classification system for acute tissue reactions which has widely been accepted.

2.4.2.3.3 Hyperthermic Peritoneal Perfusion (HIPEC)

After cytoreductive surgery is complete closed suction drains will be placed in each quadrant of the abdomen as well as an inflow drain to apply the drug solution. These drains are connected to a specific device that allows establishment of an isolated circuit under heated conditions. Flow rates are a 1500 ml/min and higher, and temperature in the abdominal cavity between 41.5 and 43.0°C (Fig. 2.4.6).

Two different surgical techniques are currently in use to establish such isolated peritoneal perfusion: an open and a closed technique. When an open (Coliseum) technique is used, the edges of the skin are secured to a self-retaining retractor system and a plastic sheet has to be incorporated into these sutures to create an open space beneath. When the closed technique is used the abdominal cavity will be closed by running sutures.

The advantage of the closed technique is the shorter time needed to heat up the abdominal cavity, whereas the advantage of the Coliseum technique is the absolutely homogeneous distribution of cytostatic solution in the abdominal cavity.

2.4.3 Clinical Indications

2.4.3.1 Pancreas Carcinoma

Pancreatic cancer is the fifth leading cause of cancer-related mortality in the Western World. In fact, the annual mortality rate almost approximates the annual incidence rate, which reflects the generally short survival time associated with pancreatic cancer, most often less than 1 year. Surgical resection is the only hope of cure for this tumor disease, but in only about 15% of all patients complete surgical resection is possible. Most of these patients are at an advanced stage with locally inoperable tumors or metastases, in many cases defined to the lymph nodes or the liver. Median survival rates are dropping down from 17 months in the case of complete resection to about 4–6 months in cases of existing metastases. These data illustrate not only the aggressiveness of pancreatic carcinoma, but also the insufficiency of systemic chemotherapy. This opens the way to other modalities and application forms.

In 1999 Beger et al. published the results of a phase II trial of intra-arterial chemotherapy applied via an angiographically placed celiac axis catheter in 26 patients with locally advanced and inoperable pancreatic cancer. As cytostatics they used a combination of mitoxantrone, CDDP and 5-fluorouracil. Compared to historical controls patients treated with intra-arterial chemotherapy survived longer, with a median of 23 months compared to 10.5 months.

A survival advantage of an intra-arterial approach for inoperable pancreatic cancer patients was documented by Aigner et al. (1998) in a small randomized trial. In this study mitomycin, mitoxantrone and CDDP were used as standard intravenous treatment as well as in the experimental arm using an intra-arterial infusion. Here the cytostatics were mixed with amilomer which is a micro-embolizing substance. The survival advantage was 33 vs 11 weeks with significant improvement of performance status in the experimental arm. A problem of this study was the small number of treated patients.

Similar results have been documented by Lygidakis et al. (1998) in a comparative study with a large number of patients ($n=238$). In this study, a very sophisticated therapy was used for intra-arterial treatment consisting of a combination of immunotherapeutic agents (interleukin-2, interferon γ) plus cytostatic agents (gemcitabine, carboplatin and mitoxantrone mixed with lipiodol). This therapy has been compared with best supportive care, leading to a statistically significant survival benefit of 16.0 vs 6.8 months.

Other groups confirmed the positive effect of an intra-arterial treatment on performance status and sometimes on overall survival. Treatment modalities are inhomogeneous, sometimes using a continuous infusion, sometimes a micro-embolization and sometimes cytostatics in combination with immune activating drugs. These different intra-arterial treatment strategies published in the literature are far from being standardized, so up to now acceptance by the oncology community is considerably low for this regional approach in the treatment of pancreatic cancer.

Most studies published in the literature confirm the efficacy of intra-arterial therapy especially for patients with locally advanced disease. Due to the increase in local drug exposure regional chemotherapy should be used as part of inductive treatment in locally unresectable situations. Our own results favor this approach reaching a resectability rate of 19.5% after regional induction therapy in 251 patients (unpublished data).

2.4.3.2 Bronchial Carcinoma

Non small cell lung cancer (NSCLC) remains the leading cause of cancer deaths in both men and women in the Western World. NSCLC accounts for approximately 75% of all lung carcinomas and 35% of patients with NSCLC will present with stage IIIA or IIIB disease. The majority of these patients with mediastinal involvement are not amenable to surgical resection, and primary radiation therapy alone results in 5-year actuarial survival of only 3%–7% and a median survival time of 6–11 months (Jeremic et al. 1996). Combined modality therapy is now considered the standard of care for those patients with unresectable tumors and a good performance status.

The majority of these patients ultimately die of distant metastases. Recent efforts to improve their intermediate and long-term survival have therefore focused on neoadjuvant chemotherapy with or without radiotherapy as an induction regimen followed by surgical resection. The theoretical advantages of the neoadjuvant approach include systemic as well as local effects such as:

- Early control of distant micrometastatic disease
- Prevention of visible tumor seeding at surgery
- An increase in resectability of malignant lesions technically unresectable at diagnosis
- A reduction of tumor mass before definitive radiotherapy
- Decreased incidence of positive margins at surgery
- Increased chance of using less radical surgery with organ preservation

Moreover, early chemotherapy has been associated with greater efficacy and improved drug delivery to tumor cells via the intact vascular system. Disadvantages of the neoadjuvant approach include morbidity and mortality related to the side-effects of induction chemotherapy and an increase in surgical morbidity and mortality as well as a delay in time to definitive surgery. Since local control remains a substantial problem in patients with unresectable stage III NSCLC, strategies designed to enhance local control are likely to enable further improvements in the long-term outcome of patients with this disease.

Okada et al. (2000) demonstrated in his series of 51 patients an advantage in survival for all NSCLC patients with bulky nodal involvement after induction therapy and resection. These results could be confirmed by Stathopulos et al. (1999) in a larger trial with 359 patients, but their resectability rate was very low, at 6.2%. This stands in contrast to other studies reaching resectability rates of up to 88% after induction chemotherapy in patients with NSCLC stage III-A bulky disease.

In a pilot study published in 2002 by our group (Müller 2002), high efficacy of regional chemotherapy using isolated thoracic perfusion as the form of regional application inductive therapy of advanced NSCLC could be demonstrated. In this study a combination of regional and systemic chemotherapy has been used leading to an acceptable toxicity profile. The resectability rate in this trial of bulky stage N2 disease was 73%. Very interesting in this study was the improvement in lung function parameters after thoracic perfusion, which opens the way to curative resections also in patients with reduced condition and impaired lung function (Fig. 2.4.7).

2.4.3.3 Extremity Sarcoma

There are two different tumor entities which can be treated by use of the isolated perfusion technique: malignant melanoma and sarcoma of the extremities. Both entities are difficult to treat by conventional systemic chemotherapy, especially in advanced disease. Response rates observed with ILP in patients with advanced and regional metastatic melanoma were higher than those associated with any other treatment modality. This combined with the fact that about a quarter of patients with histologicly prooven complete remission after ILP had a disease-free interval of more than 10 years, promoted the use of ILP. Nevertheless this technique did not become widely used and several major cancer centers did not include it in their therapeutic armamentarium. Reasons for that are the use of a heart-lung machine, the specific knowledge of the surgeon in the field of oncology as well as vascular surgery, the long operation time and the need for very close multidisciplinary cooperation.

Recently standardization of this technique was reached in respect to surgical technique, administered drugs, indications, and degree of hyperthermia. This standardization opened the way for multi-institutional studies to be conducted for more precise evaluation of efficacy and complications.

In 1992 Lienard and co-workers added a new agent to the list of drugs used for ILP – tumor necrosis factor alpha (TNF-α). This drug is able to produce very fast and effective tumor necrosis. This effect is caused by the suppression of specific adhesion molecules on the surface of endothelial cells within the

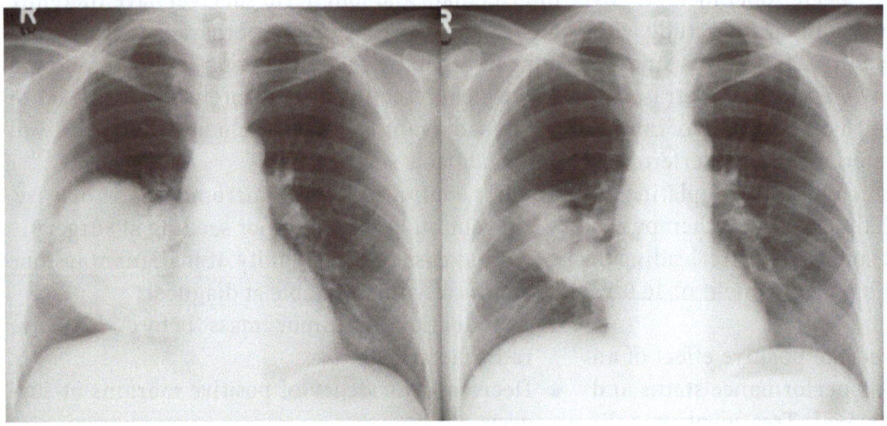

Fig. 2.4.7. Chest X-ray examination of a patient with locally inoperable bronchial carcinoma (adenocarcinoma) before and after two ITP as an inductive treatment

tumor and on macrophages and leucocytes. This suppression of adhesion molecules such as integrin $\alpha V\beta 3$ will lead to apoptosis of endothelial cells within the tumor. This mechanism is defined to the tumor vasculature only and the normal vascular system is spared. The dosage of TNF-α needed to induce an anti-tumor effect is 10–20 times higher than the maximal tolerated dose, which will be about 200 mg/m^2. Administration of a dosage higher than that will lead to severe side-effects such as hypotension, tachycardia, coagulopathy, and thrombocytopenia - conditions typically associated with septic shock and multi-organ failure. To increase local drug exposure and to overcome this problem of severe side-effects the application of the drug into an isolated circuit is needed.

As it became evident that amputation is not mandatory in patients with soft-tissue sarcoma, and that comparable survival rates can be achieved with adequate tumor resection, limb preservation became a major goal. However, when the tumor is large, expanding into more than one compartment, when it is invading major blood vessels or nerves, or when there is a multifocal appearance, amputation or mutilating surgery are still considered almost inevitable.

Several treatment modalities have been developed to facilitate limb-sparing in patients with advanced tumors. Neoadjuvant therapies, mainly radiation or combined chemo- and radiotherapy, have led to a significant reduction in amputation rates, although 8%–15% of patients with extremity sarcoma still undergo amputation.

Prior to the era of TNF-based perfusion, ILP was not a viable option for tumor reduction in soft-tissue sarcoma due to poor response rates. However, promising results following the introduction of high-dose TNF in ILP led to a phase II multicenter study to determine the effect of ILP with TNF and melphalan in patients with nonresectable sarcoma confined to the limb. Here the response rate was 82% with 18% complete responses. These excellent results have been confirmed by other centers.

These results were obtained in a selected group of patients with very extensive disease. All were candidates for amputation with large tumor size and high-grade differentiation. In this group of patients, who have a grave prognosis anyway, the value of limb preservation is even more enhanced. Limb salvage can be achieved in about 85% of these patients. This high rate is the most valuable and proven benefit of ILP with TNF in advanced sarcoma patients.

2.4.3.4 Peritoneum

Most cancers that occur within the abdomen or pelvis will disseminate by three different routes: these are hematogenous metastases, lymphatic metastases and through peritoneal spaces to surfaces of the abdominal cavity. In a substantial number of patients with abdominal or pelvic malignancy surgical treatment failure is isolated to the resection site or to peritoneal surfaces.

In the past cancer spread to the lining of the abdomen and pelvis has been regarded as a terminal condition. Peritoneal carcinomatosis is the most common terminal feature of abdominal cancers. For gastrointestinal surgeons and medical oncologists it is a vexing condition because, although the disease is limited to the abdominal cavity, complete surgical removal seems to be impossible and systemic chemotherapy is of limited effect in this setting only. The only options available for these patients are limited to palliative surgery such as limited resection, by-pass procedures and diverting enterostomies plus systemic chemotherapy. These treatments have been recommended to help alleviate suffering, but no positive effect on survival could be documented. Recently Sadeghi and co-workers (2000) confirmed in a prospective, multi-institutional study a 6-month survival for these patients

Due to rapid tumor progression peritoneal carcinosis is combined with a fast deterioration in general condition. This makes clinicians abandon further aggressive treatments. Recently, a curative approach appropriate for selected patients has been reported in the peer-reviewed literature. This treatment calls for the complete removal of all visible cancer from the abdomen and pelvis followed by intraoperatively given intraperitoneal chemotherapy. The aim of this therapeutic endeavor is to eliminate macroscopic tumor formation by cytoreductive surgery and microscopic tumor remnants by intraoperative chemotherapy.

2.4.3.4.1 Surgical Technique

Cytoreductive surgery means complete removal of all visible tumors in the peritoneal cavity by use of multivisceral resection of bulky tumor formation plus resection of infiltrated peritoneum, called peritonectomy. These peritonectomy procedures are used in the areas of visible cancer progression in an attempt to leave the patient with only microscopic residual disease. Here small tumor nodes are removed by use of electro-evaporation techniques; larger tumors or confluent infiltrations are removed by segmental resection of peritoneum.

There are different peritonectomy procedures that are used to eliminate cancer on visceral intra-abdominal surfaces or to strip cancer from parietal peritoneal surfaces. One or all of these procedures may be required, depending on the distribution and volume of peritoneal disease.

- Central peritonectomy with resection of midline scars of previous operations and ventral hepatic ligaments
- Greater omentectomy, including resection of the gastrocolic ligament and splenectomy
- Peritoneal stripping of right and left hemi-diaphragm
- Dissection of Glisson's capsule
- Lesser omentectomy, including cholecystectomy and dissection of the hepato-duodenal ligament
- Stripping of the omental bursa
- Peritoneal stripping at the lateral abdominal wall
- Peritoneal stripping of mesentery
- Stripping of the pelvic walls

Bulky involvement of visceral peritoneum frequently requires resection of a portion of the stomach, small intestine or colorectum. In order to adequately perform cytoreductive surgery a specific preparation technique should be used, called lasermode electrosurgery. This technique allows the minimizing of blood loss, and due to a rim of heated necrosis cancer cells are less likely to adhere at resected areas.

2.4.3.4.2 Rationale

In the past the use of intraperitoneal chemotherapy had shown limited success. Two major impediments to greater benefits of this application form exist. First of all an intracavitary instillation allows a limited penetration of drug into tumor nodules. High drug concentrations can be documented in the first 1.0–1.5 mm only.

The second problem associated with intraperitoneal chemotherapy is the nonuniform drug distribution. Due to the fact that the majority of patients treated by drug instillation into the peritoneal cavity have had prior surgery, adhesions create multiple barriers to the free access of fluid. This inhomogeneous distribution will lead to the problem of insufficient exposure for some areas and the problem of high or even extensive exposure of other areas of the peritoneal cavity. This "over treatment" is combined with side-effects and complications.

Nevertheless intraperitoneal chemotherapy is an effective tool in the treatment of peritoneal carcinosis and combined with high response rates for microscopic residual disease. For cytotoxic drugs with high molecular weight elimination out of the abdominal cavity is prolonged, leading to an increase in local drug exposure. This means that application of specific cytotoxic drugs – with high molecular weight – into the peritoneal cavity will lead to an extensive pharmacological advantage (Table 2.4.1). The use of this application form under specific conditions, here in the perioperative period, will overcome the problems of inhomogeneous exposure.

The present knowledge of cell-kill kinetics with cytotoxic drugs indicates that, due to a larger proportion of the cell growth fraction, micrometastases are more susceptible to chemotherapy than macroscopic ones. This means that cancer cells free in the peritoneal cavity as a result of cytoreductive surgery represent an ideal target for a locally intensified chemotherapeutic intervention. To intensify the efficacy of cytotoxic agents a locoregional application form can be used under hyperthermic conditions. Hyperthermia is used in order to maximize the cytotoxic effect of drugs and to increase the amount of drug penetrating the tumor formations.

Table 2.4.1. Advantage of intraperitoneal versus intravenous application of cytostatics depending on the measured area under the curve (AUC)

Cytostatic	Molecular weight	Advantage of AUC intravenous vs. intraperitoneal
Irinotecan	677	1 : 18
Oxaliplatin	397	1 : 25
Cisplatin	300	1 : 20
Mitomycin	334	1 : 75
5-Fluorouracil	130	1 : 250
Doxorubicin	544	1 : 500
Mitoxantrone	445	1 : 640
Paclitaxel	854	1 : 1000

2.4.3.4.3
Clinical Results

A wide variety of solid tumors are able to disseminate to peritoneal surfaces. Some of these grow in just the abdominal cavity and lack the capacity to produce distant metastases. These malignancies, such as mucinous adenocarcinoma of the colon or appendix, grow at the surface of the peritoneum not infiltrating deeper tissue. Due to these reasons this tumor type is an excellent candidates for a cytoreductive approach.

2.4.3.4.3.1
Pseudomyxoma Peritonei Syndrome

Numerous phase II studies showing a high cure rate with epithelial malignancy of the appendix with peritoneal dissemination (pseudomyxoma peritonei syndrome) and a lack of other successful treatment alternatives have led to a consensus regarding the management of this condition. For this very rare tumor disease long-lasting positive effects have been documented with 5-year survival rates of 86% (Sugarbaker 2001) and 96% (Deraco et al. 2002).

2.4.3.4.3.2
Recurrent Ovarian Cancer

Over the past 30 years it has become largely established that optimal debulking surgery of metastatic epithelial ovarian cancer has a favorable impact on the survival of patients with advanced staged disease. Optimal surgery followed by platinum-based systemic chemotherapy is the cornerstone in the management of ovarian cancer. However, the majority of patients have advanced disease at time of presentation, hampering an optimal effect of primary cytoreduction. Furthermore, a considerable number of patients present with residual disease after front-line chemotherapy or relapse after complete clinical response.

For second-line treatment no definite therapy has yet been defined. The combination of secondary cytoreduction plus hyperthermic peritoneal perfusion constitutes a feasible and effective option for this subset of patients. Several phase II trials have been published showing a positive effect of second cytoreductive surgery on survival of patients with recurrent or persistent epithelial ovarian cancer. At this moment the role intraoperative hyperthermic peritoneal perfusion is not clear and has to be determined in a prospective randomized trial.

2.4.3.4.3.3
Gastric Cancer

In patients with gastric cancer with peritoneal seeding, gastrectomy plus perioperative intraperitoneal chemotherapy represents a palliative treatment option associated with a small likelihood of long-term survival. Eight different phase III studies reported a survival advantage when perioperative intraperitoneal chemotherapy is added to surgery in patients with primary gastric cancer. Stage III patients projected the greatest survival advantage·

2.4.3.4.3.4
Mesothelioma

Although long-term survival has been less conclusively demonstrated with peritoneal mesothelioma, the prolonged benefit recently reported with this disease suggests that the routine application of an aggressive locoregional approach is the preferred strategy. The lack of any other successful strategy that competes with comprehensive treatment is an important factor in the recommendation of this approach as a standard of care.

2.4.3.4.3.5
Colorectal Cancer

Currently, recommendations for routine application of comprehensive treatment in colorectal cancer with peritoneal seeding are less secure. Certainly, systemic chemotherapy does not provide any patient with a hope for cure. The combined approach when used in peritoneal carcinomatosis from colorectal cancer is supported by results from numerous phase II studies at different institutions. The 5-year survival rate of approximately 30% is consistent in all reports.

Verwaal and co-workers demonstrated in a prospective randomized trial at National Cancer Institute of Amsterdam the superiority of an aggressive approach using a combination of cytoreductive surgery plus hyperthermic peritoneal perfusion plus consolidation chemotherapy over a more paaliative approach of by-pass surgery plus chemotherapy (Verwaal et al. 2003). The median survival with combined treatment was 22.3 months and for the control it was 12.6 months ($p = 0.032$). The morbidity and mortality associated with this treatment compares favorably with that reported for the surgical management of large surgical procedures for gastrointestinal cancer. It may be suggested that sufficient data have accumulated to move this strategy from clinical research to standard of practice.

The survival reported by numerous groups is comparable with that observed with other abdominopelvic malignancy such as retroperitoneal and visceral sarcoma and liver metastases from colorectal cancer. The survival is far superior to that for some cancers that are routinely resected, such as pancreatic cancer, gallbladder cancer, and cholangiocarcinoma. By analogy with other standard of practice management plans, the efficacy of these peritoneal carcinosis treatments and the morbidity and mortality are acceptable.

References

Aigner KR, Gailhofer S, Kopp S (1998) Regional versus systemic chemotherapy for advanced pancreatic cancer: a randomized study. Hepatogastroenterology 45:1125–1129

Alberts DS, Liu PY, Hannigan EV et al (1995) Phase III study of intraperitoneal (IP) cisplatin (CDDP) / intravenous (IV) cyclophosphamide (CPA) vs. IV CDDP/IV CPA in patients with optimal disease stage III ovarian cancer: a SWOG - GOG - ECOG Intergroup study (INT 0051). Proc Am Soc Clin Oncol 14:273

Beger HG, Gansauge F, Buchler MW, Link KH (1999) Intra-arterial adjuvant chemotherapy after pancreaticoduodenectomy for pancreatic cancer: significant reduction in occurrence of liver metastasis. World J Surg 23:946–949

Benckhuijsen C, Kroon BB, van Geel AN et al (1988) Regional perfusion treatment with melphalan for melanoma in a limb: an evaluation of drug kinetics. Eur J Surg Oncol 14:157–163

Collins JM, Dedrick RL (1982) In: Chabner W (ed) Pharmacokinetics of anticancer drugs – pharmacologic principles of cancer treatment. Saunder, Philadelphia, pp 77–79

Creech O, Krementz ET, Ryan RF et al (1958) Chemotherapy of cancer: regional perfusion utilizing an extracorporeal circuit. Ann Surg 148:616–632

Deraco M, Gronchi A, Mazzaferro V et al (2002) Feasibility of peritonectomy associated with intraperitoneal hyperthermic perfusion in patients with pseudomyxoma peritonei. Tumori 88(5):370–375

Harstrick A, Wilke H, Eberhardt W et al (1996) A phase I dose escalation trial of intravenous treosulfan in refractory cancer. Onkologie 19:153–156

Hilger RA, Harstrick A, Eberhardt W et al (1998) Clinical pharmacokinetics of intravenous treosulfan in patients with advanced solid tumours. Cancer Chemother Pharmacol 42:99–104

Jeremic B, Shibamoto Y, Acimovic L, Milisavljevic S (1996) Hyperfractionated radiation therapy with or without concurrent low-dose daily carboplatin/ etoposide for Stage III non-small-cell lung cancer -a randomized study. J Clin Oncol 14:1065–1070

Klopp CT, Alford T, Bateman JB et al (1950) Fractionated intra-arterial cancer chemotherapy with methyl bis amine hydrochloride; a preliminary report. Ann Surg 132:811–832

Lienard D, Ewaienko P, Delmotti JJ et al (1992) High-dose recombinant tumor necrosis factor alpha in combination with interferon gamma and melphalan in isolation perfusion of the limbs for melanoma and sarcoma. J Clin Oncol 10:52–60

Los G (2000) Intraperitoneal chemotherapy. In: Kerr DJ, Mc Ardle CS (eds) Regional chemotherapy – theory and practice. Harwood, Chur, pp 9–27

Lygidakis NJ, Spentzouris N, Theodoracopoulos M et al (1998) Pancreatic resection for pancreatic carcinoma combined with neo- and adjuvant locoregional targeting immunochemotherapy – a prospective randomized study. Hepatogastroenterology 45(20):396–403

Markman M, Bundy BN, Alberts DS et al (2001) Phase III trial of standard-dose intravenous cisplatin plus paclitaxel versus moderately high-dose carboplatin followed by intravenous paclitaxel and intraperitoneal cisplatin in small-volume stage III ovarian carcinoma: an intergroup study of Gynaecologic Oncology Group, Southwestern Oncology Group, and Eastern Cooperative Oncology Group. J Clin Oncol 19(4):1001–1007

Müller H (2002) Combined regional and systemic chemotherapy for advanced and inoperable non-small cell lung cancer. Eur J Surg Oncol 28(2):165–171

Ng B, Hochwald SN, Burt ME (1996) Isolated lung perfusion with doxorubicin reduces cardiac and host toxicities associated with systemic administration. Ann Thorac Surg 61:969–972

Okada M, Tsubota N, Yoshimura M, Miyamoto Y, Matsuoka H (2000) Induction therapy for non-small cell lung cancer with involved mediastinal nodes in multiple stations. Chest 118(1):123–128

Sadeghi B, Arvieux C, Glehen O et al (2000) Peritoneal carcinomatosis from non-gynecologic malignancies: results of the EVOCAPE 1 multicentric prospective study. Cancer 88(2):358–363

Stathopoulos GP, Dafni UG, Malamos NA, Rigatos S, Kouvatseas G, Moschopoulos N (1999) Induction chemotherapy in non small cell lung cancer stage IIIa-b and IV and second-line treatment. Anticancer Res 19(4C):3543–3548

Stehlin JS (1969) Hyperthermic perfusion with chemotherapy for cancers of the extremities. Surg Gynecol Obstet 129:305–308

Stephens FO (1983) Pharmacokinetics of intra-arterial chemotherapy. Vascular perfusion in cancer therapy. In: Schwemmle K, Aigner K (eds) Recent results in cancer research, vol. 86. Springer, Berlin Heidelberg New York

Sugarbaker PH (2001) Cytoreductive surgery and peri-operative intraperitoneal chemotherapy as a curative approach to pseudomyxoma peritonei syndrome. Eur J Surg Oncol 27(3):239–243

Taguchi T (1979) Attainability of anticancer drugs into the tumour. Jpn J Cancer Clin 25:782–788

Verwaal VJ, van Ruth S, de Bree E et al (2003) Randomized trial of cytoreduction and hyperthermic intraperitoneal chemotherapy versus systemic chemotherapy and palliative surgery in patients with peritoneal carcinomatosis of colorectal cancer. J Clin Oncol 21:3737–3743

Weissberger AS, Levine B, Stoorasli JP (1955) Use of nitrogen mustard in treatment of serious effusions of neoblastic origin. J Am Med Assoc 159:1704–1707

Further Reading

Alexakis N, Halloran C, Raraty M, Ghaneh P, Sutton R, Neoptolemos JP (2004) Current standards of surgery for pancreatic cancer [review]. Br J Surg 91(11):1410–1427

Alexander HR, Fraker DL, Bartlett DL (1996) Isolated limb perfusion for malignant melanoma. Semin Surg Oncol 12:416–426

Carmignani CP, Sugarbaker PH (2004) Comprehensive approach to advanced primary and recurrent ovarian cancer: a personal experience [review]. Expert Rev Anticancer Ther 4(3):477–487

Cavanagh D, Hovadhanakul P, Comas MR (1975) Regional chemotherapy – a comparison of pelvic perfusion and intra- arterial infusion in patients with advanced gynecologic cancer. Am J Obstet Gynecol 123(4):435–441

Collins JM (1984) Pharmacological rational for regional drug delivery. J Clin Oncol 2(5):498–504

De Leyn P, Vansteenkiste J, Deneffe G et al (1999) Result of induction chemotherapy followed by surgery in patients with stage IIIA N2 NSCLC: importance of pre-treatment mediastinoscopy. Eur J Cardiothorac Surg 15(5):608–614

Dillman RO, Hemdon J, Seagren SL et al (1996) Improved survival in stage III nonsmall cell lung cancer. seven-year follow-up of Cancer and Leukemia Group B (CALGB) 8433 trial. J Natl Cancer Inst 88:1210–1215

Eggermont AMM, Schraffordt-Koops H, Klausner JM et al (1996) Isolated limb perfusion with tumor necrosis factor and melphalan for limb salvage in 186 patients with locally advanced soft-tissue extremity sarcomas: the cumulative multicenter European experience. Ann Surg 224:756–765

Feldman AL, Libutti SK, Pingpank JF et al (2003) Analysis of factors associated with outcome in patients with malignant peritoneal mesothelioma undergoing surgical debulking and intraperitoneal chemotherapy. J Clin Oncol 21:4560–4567

Glehen O, Gilly FN, Sugarbaker PH (2003a) New perspectives in the management of colorectal cancer: what about peritoneal carcinomatosis? Scand J Surg 92:178–179

Glehen O, Mithieux F, Osinsky D et al (2003b) Surgery combined with peritonectomy procedures and intraperitoneal chemohyperthermia in abdominal cancers with peritoneal carcinomatosis: a phase II study. J Clin Oncol 21:799–806

Guadagni S, Aigner KR, Palumbo G et al (1998) Pharmacokinetics of mitomycin C in pelvic stopflow infusion and hypoxic pelvic perfusion with and without hemofiltration: a pilot study of patients with recurrent unresectable rectal cancer. J Clin Pharmacol 38(10):936–944

Guadagni S, Fiorentini G, Palumbo G et al (2001) Hypoxic pelvic perfusion with mitomycin C using a simplified balloon- occlusion technique in the treatment of patients with unresectable locally recurrent rectal cancer. Arch Surg 136(1):105–112

Gutman M, Inbar M, Shlush-Lev D et al (1997) High dose tumor necrosis factor alpha and melphalan administered via isolated limb perfusion for advanced soft tissue sarcoma results in a >90% response rate and limb preservation. Cancer 79:1129–1137

Hendriks JM, Van Schil PE, Van Oosterom AA, Kuppen PJ, Van Marck E, Eyskens E (1999) Isolated lung perfusion with melphalan prolongs survival in a rat model of metastatic pulmonary adenocarcinoma. Eur Surg Res 31:267–271

Kecmanovic DM, Pavlov MJ, Kovacevic PA et al (2003) Cytoreductive surgery for ovarian cancer. Eur J Surg Oncol 29(4):315–320

Klein ES, Davidson B, Apter S, Azizi E, Ben-Ari GY (1994) Total abdominal perfusion (TAP) in the treatment of abdominal metastatic melanoma. J Surg Oncol 57(2):134–137

Link KH, Leder G, Formentini A et al (1999) Surgery and multimodal treatments in pancreatic cancer – a review on the basis of future multimodal treatment concepts. Gan To Kagaku Ryoho 26(1):10–40

Lygidakis NJ, Sgourakis G, Aphinives P (1999) Upper abdominal stop-flow perfusion as a neo and adjuvant hypoxic regional chemotherapy for resectable gastric carcinoma. A prospective randomized clinical trial. Hepatogastroenterology 46(27):2035–2038

Lygidakis NJ, Jain S, Sacchi M, Vrachnos P (2005) Adenocarcinoma of the pancreas – past, present and future [review]. Hepatogastroenterology 52(64):1281–1292

Müller H, Guadagni S (2001) Regional plus systemic chemotherapy: an effective treatment in recurrent non-small cell lung cancer. Eur J Surg Oncol 27(2):190–195

Smeenk RM, Verwaal VJ, Zoetmulder FA (2006) Toxicity and mortality of cytoreduction and intraoperative hyperthermic intraperitoneal chemotherapy in pseudomyxoma peritonei-a report of 103 procedures. Eur J Surg Oncol 32(2):186–190

Sperti C, Pasquali C, Pastorelli D et al (2003) Adenocarcinoma of the pancreas: the rationale for neoadjuvant therapy [review]. Acta Biomed Ateneo Parmense 74 [Suppl 2]:91–95

Sugarbaker PH (1991) Early postoperative intraperitoneal adriamycin as an adjuvant treatment for advanced gastric cancer with lymph node or serosal invasion. In: Sugarbaker PH (ed) Management of gastric cancer. Kluwer, Boston, pp 277–284

Sugarbaker PH (1999) Successful management of microscopic residual disease in large bowel cancer. Cancer Chemother Pharmacol 43:S15–S25

Sugarbaker PH (2003) Carcinomatosis – is cure an option? J Clin Oncol 21:762–764

Sugarbaker PH, Welch LS, Mohamed F et al (2003a) A review of peritoneal mesothelioma at the Washington Cancer Institute. Surg Oncol Clin N Am 12:605–621

Sugarbaker PH, Yu W, Yonemura Y (2003b) Gastrectomy, peritonectomy, and perioperative intraperitoneal chemotherapy: the evolution of treatment strategies for advanced gastric cancer. Semin Surg Oncol 21:233–248

Vaglini M, Cascinelli F, Chiti A et al (1996) Isolated pelvic perfusion for the treatment of unresectable primary or recurrent rectal cancer. Tumori 82(5):459–462

Vrouenraets BC, Klaase JM, Kroon BB et al (1995) Long-term morbidity after regional isolated perfusion with melphalan for melanoma of the limbs. The influence of acute regional toxic reactions. Arch Surg 130:43–47

Wanebo HJ, Belliveau JF (1999) A pharmacokinetic model and the clinical pharmacology of cis-platinum, 5-fluorouracil and mitomycin-C in isolated pelvic perfusion. Cancer Chemother Pharmacol 43(5):427–434

Wanebo HJ, Chung MA, Levy AI, Turk PS, Vezeridis MP, Belliveau JF (1996) Preoperative therapy for advanced pelvic malignancy by isolated pelvic perfusion with the balloon-occlusion technique. Ann Surg Oncol 3(3):295–303
Wieberdinck K, Benckhuijsen C, Braat RP et al (1982) Dosimetry in isolation perfusion of the limbs by assessment of perfused tissue volume and grading of toxic tissue reactions. Eur J Cancer Clin Oncol 18:905–910
Yonemura Y, Bandou E, Kinoshita K, Kawamura T, Takahashi S, Endou Y, Sasaki T. (2003) Effective therapy for peritoneal dissemination in gastric cancer. Surg Oncol Clin N Am 12:635–648
Zanon C, Clara R, Chiappino I et al (2004) Cytoreductive surgery and intraperitoneal chemohyperthermia for recurrent peritoneal carcinomatosis from ovarian cancer. World J Surg 28(10):1040–1045

Ablative Techniques (Percutaneous)

2

Vascular Ablative Techniques

2.5 Transarterial Chemoembolization (TACE) in Primary and Secondary Liver Tumors

Stephan Zangos, Katrin Eichler, and Thomas J. Vogl

CONTENTS

2.5.1 Introduction

Primary and secondary malignant hepatic tumors are a major health problem worldwide. While metastases are common in western countries, primary liver cancers are frequently diagnosed in Asia and Africa. However, recent data suggest that the incidence and mortality of hepatocellular carcinoma (HCC) in Western nations are on the rise (Taylor-Robinson et al. 1997; Llovet et al. 2003). Likewise, the liver is the most common site for metastases. In 25%–50% of patients with malignancies liver metastases were observed at autopsy (Bernardino et al. 1982). The most frequent primary sites are colon, breast, pancreas, and lung. In the case of colorectal metastatic disease, the liver is the only metastatic site in 20%–30% of patients (Sasson and Sigurdson 2002).

S. Zangos, MD; K. Eichler, MD; T. J. Vogl, MD, Professor
Institute for Diagnostic and Interventional Radiology, University Hospital, Johann Wolfgang Goethe University, Theodor-Stern-Kai 7, 60590 Frankfurt, Germany

Malignant liver tumors have only a very poor prognosis. Surgical resection is considered the only potentially curative option. But local ablative treatments, such as MR-guided or laser interstitial thermotherapy (LITT) (Vogl et al. 2002), microwave coagulation (Midorikawa et al. 2000) or radiofrequency ablation (Allgaier et al. 1999; Livraghi 2003), are also more frequently used techniques and may replace surgical resection in the near future. However, only a few patients are candidates for these treatments. The degree of hepatic tumor manifestation is a life-threatening prognostic indicator in these patients (Fiorentini et al. 2000).

Transarterial chemoembolization (TACE) of the liver for unresectable liver tumors, although controversially discussed, is being used with increasing frequency. Below, anatomical factors, technical realization of the chemoembolization, as well as the results and complications of chemoembolization are discussed.

2.5.2 Mechanism

While normal liver tissue receives 75% of its blood supply from the portal vein and 25% from the hepatic artery, liver tumors are almost exclusively supplied by the hepatic artery (Breedis and Young 1954; Wang et al. 1994). This different blood supply is used for the chemoembolization of liver tumors. The liver parenchyma is rarely damaged by TACE because it obtains the majority of its blood supply from the portal vein, while blood supply to hepatic tumors originates predominantly from the hepatic artery (Breedis and Young 1954). Therefore, embolization of the hepatic artery can lead to selective necrosis of the liver tumor leaving normal liver parenchyma virtually unaffected (Jaeger et al. 1996). TACE is based on the synergistic effect of arterial occlusion and local chemotherapy, which makes the tissue hypoxic and enhances the effectiveness of the chemotherapeutics (Kennedy et al. 1980; Pan et al. 1984). The dwell time for the drug is markedly prolonged, with measurable drug levels present in the tumor for as long as a month after chemoembolization. The selective delivery of the chemotherapeutic agents into the liver arteries increases the drug concentration in the liver tissue 10- to 100-fold compared to systemic application. TACE produces a high concentration of the chemotherapeutic agent in the tumor rim but lower levels in the tumor center and the normal liver (Daniels et al. 1988). Likewise, increased vascular permeability has been shown, with anoxic damage promoting chemotherapy penetration into the tumor (Wallace et al. 1990). Up to 85% of the administered drug is trapped in the liver, minimizing systemic toxicity (Soulen 1994). In conclusion, TACE reduces the maximum plasma concentration, lengthens the half-life and increases the average concentration of cytostatic agents in the tumor compared with intravenous administration of cytostatics. For these reasons TACE can be considered a safe therapeutic tool for liver tumors without significant long-term worsening of liver function (Bianco et al. 1996; Caturelli et al. 2000).

2.5.2.1 Patient Selection

Chemoembolization can be used in patients with ether primary or metastatic malignant hepatic tumors who are not surgical candidates (Table 2.5.1). Surgery is not feasible in advanced malignant disease involving both lobes of the liver, or complicating factors such as cirrhosis or failure of systemic chemotherapy. Likewise, TACE should be reserved for those patients who have liver-dominant disease, because the predominant effect is local.

A response to chemoembolization can be expected in liver tumors, such as HCC, metastases from colorectal tumors, metastases from neuroendocrine tumors, metastases from ocular melanoma, and gastrointestinal sarcomas (Gates et al. 1999; Vogl et al. 2000, 2003; Zangos et al. 2001; Kress et al. 2003; Roche et al. 2003). Other tumor types showed only a little response after chemoembolization. In every patient the advantages of treatment should be balanced against possible risks.

To ensure adequate treatment compliance the patients had to be in a good physical and mental state and must be able to undergo angiography. Before each treatment laboratory values such as white blood cell count, elementary bodies, hemoglobin, bilirubin, creatinine, transaminases, choline esterase, and coagulation should be monitored. There should be no medical condition that is likely to be life threatening within 3 months.

Contraindications for the TACE are poor performance status (Karnofsky status ≤50%), nutritional impairment, neoplastic ascites, high serum bilirubin level (> 3 mg%), poor hepatic synthesis (serum albumin < 2.0 mg/dl) and renal failure (serum creatinine > 2 mg%). There should be an adequate amount of residual uninvolved liver tissue. A tumor burden of more than 50%–75% resulting in an inadequate liver function is regarded as a contraindication for performing TACE (Therasse et al. 1993; Gates et al. 1999). Likewise florid infections or myelosuppression (white blood cell count < 2000/ml, elementary bodies < 100,000/μl) are classified as contraindications for TACE.

Partial or complete thrombosis of the main portal vein is often classified as an exclusion criterion for the procedure. Nevertheless, portal vein thrombosis should not be considered an absolute contraindication to hepatic chemoembolization. Hepatic chemoembolization can be performed in these patients safely in the presence of adequate collateral circulation (Pentecost et al. 1993).

Table 2.5.1. Indications for liver chemoembolization

Indications
• Unresectable liver tumor
• Failure of systemic chemotherapy
• No available effective systemic chemotherapy
• Liver-dominant disease
• Symptomatic liver lesions
• Adequate medical status
Contraindications
• Poor performance status (Karnofsky status ≤75%)
• Extensive liver involvement >75%
• Poor hepatic synthesis (albumin <2 mg/dl)
• Bilirubin > 3 mg %
• Florid infections

2.5.2.2 Imaging Technique Before and After TACE

For the documentation of tumor size, tumor location and tumor vascularization unenhanced and contrast-enhanced MR or CT images should be obtained before planning the TACE treatment. Thereby exposure of the liver vessels should be performed for pre-interventional evaluation of the anatomy and patency of the vessels.

Lipiodol retention in the tumor and liver parenchyma can be verified with nonenhanced CT examinations using spiral technique 24–72 h after TACE. An extrahepatic uptake of chemoembolization materials can be eliminated on these images; however, evaluation of the tumor size is often difficult. While some investigators recommend continuing follow-up with nonenhanced CT scans (Gates et al. 1999), we have found that nonenhanced MR scans allows optimal control of the treatment response during the treatment cycles. Follow-up examinations should be performed with contrast-enhanced CT or MR imaging (Vogl et al. 2000; Zangos et al. 2001) to document remaining tumor viability and newly developed liver lesions. Some authors use dynamic CT for a quantification of the hemodynamic changes after TACE (Tsushima et al. 1998).

Doppler sonographic monitoring can also give information concerning changes in the perfusion of a tumor following chemoembolization and, in conjunction with CT and clinical findings, provide indications for further tumor embolization (Steger et al. 1998; Hosoki et al. 1999; Cioni et al. 2000).

2.5.2.3 TACE Technique

TACE treatments should be performed after exclusion of contraindications, and detailed information about the patient has been obtained, along with written consent. All patients have to stop eating 6 h before the treatments. Fluids and necessary medications can be consumed until 2 h before the intervention.

A premedication regime consisting of an opioid, an antiemetic as well as a glucocorticoid should be administered intravenously before the TACE treatment to reduce the acute side-effects of TACE.

All angiographies should be performed using the digital subtraction angiography (DSA) technique. The resultant angiogram can be reviewed with high-contrast resolution and without delay. During catheter and guidewire manipulation pulsed fluoroscopy at 7 frames/s (FMS) should be used if available for radiation dose reduction. Most diagnostic and therapeutic interventions are performed using nonionic contrast media (300 mg/ml iodine).

An angiographic survey of the abdominal vessels should be performed after the introduction of a 4- to 5-French Pigtail catheter using a femoral approach during the first TACE course. Catheters most often used in hepatic arterial studies from the femoral approach are those with downward or reverse curves such as Cobra, sidewinder, or MK-2 shapes (Fig. 2.5.1). To document the vascular supply of the liver, conventionally diagnostic hepatic and mesenteric angiography are performed. Selective superior mesenteric arteriography (Fig. 2.5.2) should be per-

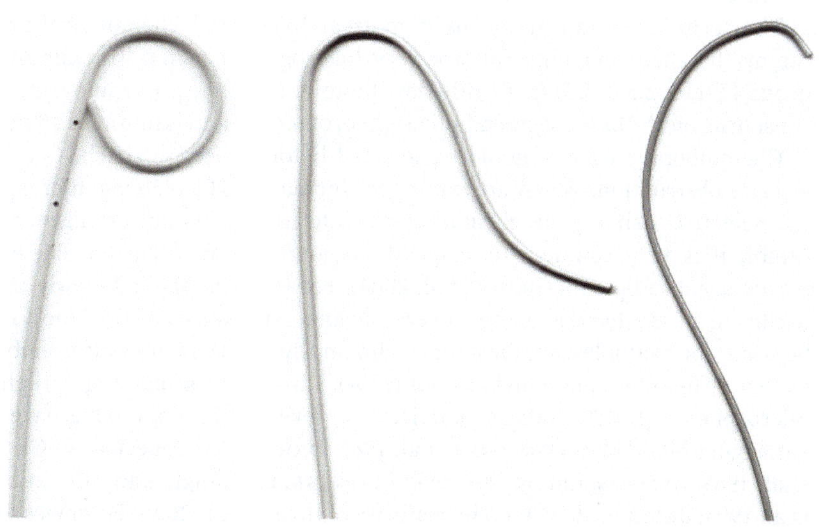

Fig. 2.5.1. Photograph shows catheters frequently used for chemoembolization, including pigtail, sidewinder, and cobra catheter

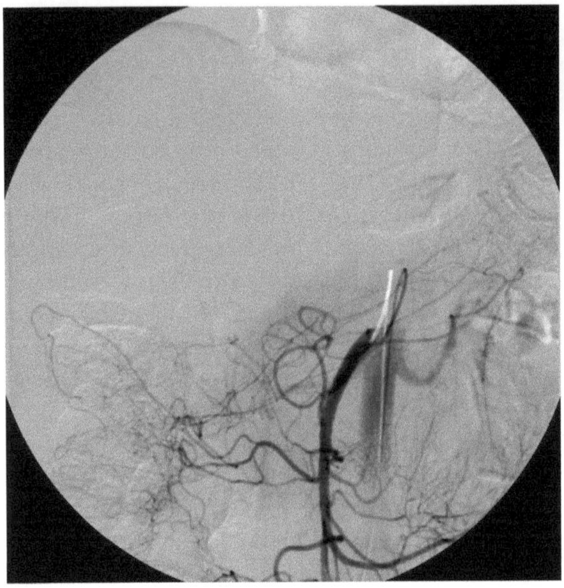

Fig. 2.5.2. Selective superior mesenteric arteriogram shows normal anatomical blood supply

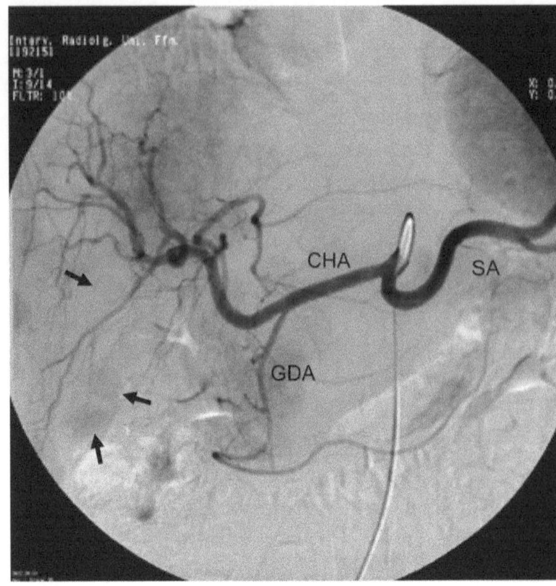

Fig. 2.5.3. Celiac angiogram obtained before chemoembolization shows normal anatomy, including common hepatic artery (*CHA*), splenic artery (*SA*) and gastroduodenal artery (*GDA*). Additional multiple small hypervascular tumors (*arrows*) can be documented

formed with late-phase imaging of the portal venous anatomy with an injection flow of between 3 and 8 ml/s to document the patency of the portal vein. If a catheter is placed in the celiac trunk, the angiography should be performed with an injection rate of between 3 and 8 ml/s (Fig. 2.5.3). Afterwards the catheter is placed selectively in the hepatic artery and advanced beyond the gastroduodenal artery. If possible, the tip of the catheter is advanced further into segmental arteries near to the tumor. Some authors prefer the use of 3-Fr microcatheters for superselective embolization of liver tumors. However, the use of microcatheters aggravates the procedure and increases the cost of treatment.

The techniques and agents used to treat liver tumors by chemoembolization are very heterogeneous (Tables 2.5.2, 2.5.3). To this day, there is no consensus on the best chemoembolization protocol.

Chemotherapy agents should be injected before arterial obstruction. When attempting to increase the selective delivery of chemotherapy into the tumor, it is very common to suspend the angioplastic agent in lipiodol (Bruix et al. 2004). For the occlusion of the hepatic artery several agents can be used, for example metallic coils, Gelfoam, lipid particles (lipiodol), polyvinyl alcohol (PVA), starch microspheres (DMS), collagen particles, or event autologous blood clots (Wollner et al. 1986; Inoue et al. 1989; Allison and Booth 1990; Martinelli et al. 1994; Bruix et al. 2004). The majority of investigators have explored the role of chemoembolization with lipiodol in combination with different chemotherapy therapies (Tellez et al. 1998). Lipiodol results in the obstruction of the peripheral vascular bed, and it is cleared more rapidly from the normal liver parenchyma due to the increased blood flow rate and the phagocytic action of the Kupffer cells (Choi et al. 1992; Tellez et al. 1998). Commonly used chemotherapeutic agents include 5-fluorouracil, mitomycin c, doxorubicin, and cisplatin (Tellez et al. 1998; Bruix et al. 2004).

In our department we perform selective arterial chemoembolization with a mixture of mitomycin C (maximum of 10 mg/m^2, Medac, Hamburg, Germany) as a chemotherapeutic agent and a maximum of 15 ml lipiodol, an iodized oil (Guerbet, Sulzbach, Germany), followed by injection of 200–450 mg microspheres (Spherex, Pharmacia and Upjohn, Erlangen, Germany) for additional vascular occlusion. The embolization suspension should be applied slowly under fluoroscopic control until stasis of the blood flow can be observed. Devascularization after embolization can be confirmed by terminal angiographic study of the hepatic artery. Several reports have described better response rates for repeated TACE procedures in comparison to single administration (Tellez et al. 1998; Vogl et al. 2000; Huppert et al. 2004). For that reason we

Table 2.5.2. Results of chemoembolization in hepatocellular cancer (literature review). (*A, Adria* Adriamycin, *ADMOS* doxorubicin+mitomycin+lipiodol, *CDDP* cisplatin, *Collag* bovine collagen, *CTLS* CDDP+pirarubicin, *DSM* degradable starch microspheres, *Epi* epirubicin, *F 5-FU* 5-fluorouracil, *FUDR* 5-fluorodeoxyuridine, *Gel* gelfoam, *Lipi* lipiodol, *M, Mito* mitomycin, *Mo* months, *N/A* not available, *Neuroend TM* neuroendocrine tumors, *PVA* polyvinyl alcohol, *STZ* streptozotocin)

References (Year)	Patients	Agents	Survival rates
Bismuth et al. (1992)	291	Doxo/Lipiodol/	2 years: 49% Child-Pugh A
		Gel	29% Child-Pugh B
			9% Child-Pugh C
Raoul et al. (1992)	4	Doxo	N/A
	7	Doxo/Lipiodol	
	7	Doxo/Lipiodol/Gel	
Stuart et al. (1993)	52	Doxo/Lipi/Gel/Ethanol	1 year: 60%
Park et al. (1993)	87	Doxo/Lipiodol/Gel	1 year: 75%/2 years: 55%
Mondazzi et al. (1994)	84	Doxo/Lipiodol/Gel	1 year: 60% / 2-years: 31%
Colella et al. (1998)	171	K.A.	3 years: 32%
Pelletier et al. (1998)	37	CDDP/Lipi/Lecithin/Gel	
		Tamoxifen	1 year: 51% / 3-years: 21%
Allgaier et al. (1998)	33	Mito/Lipiodol	MÜ: 8 months
Savastano et al. (1999)	182	Epi/Lipiodol/Gel	1 year: 83%/ 3-years: 40%
Ueno et al. (2000)	26	ADMOS	1 year: 59%/3 years: %
	70	CDDP-ADMOS	1 year: 70%/3 years: 16%
	56	CTLS	1 year: 72%/3 years:30%
Lladò et al. (2000)	143	Doxo/Lipiodol	1 year: 61%/2 years: 32%
			3 years: 16%
Vogl et al. (2000)	37	Adria/CDDP/Lipi/DSM	Median 387 days
Gattoni et al. (2000)	62	Doxo/Lipiodol/spongostan	1 year: 78%/3 years: 40%
Lo et al. (2002)	40	CDDP/Lipi/gelatin sponge particles	1 year, 57%; 2 years, 31%; 3 years, 26%
Chen et al. (2002)	473	Epi/Lipiodol	1 year: 79.2%, 2 years: 51.8%, 3 years: 34.9%
Sumie et al.(2003)	21	Epi/Lipiodol	1 year: 76.2%, 2 years: 33.3%, 3 years: 28.6%
Huppert et al. (2004)	91	Epi/Lipiodol	1 year: 72.7% Okuda I
			22.8% Okuda II and III

perform three separate courses of chemoembolization at 4-week intervals.

2.5.2.4 Anatomical Variants and Hemodynamic Features of the Hepatic Artery

The classic common hepatic artery (CHA) lies in the hepatoduodenal ligament to the left of the common bile duct and anterior to the portal vein (Lee et al. 2002). In general, the CHA divides into a right and left hepatic artery (Fig. 2.5.4). However, the anatomy of the arterial supply of the liver often shows congenital variations. Common variants of the hepatic artery are having the origin of the left hepatic artery from the left gastric artery (LGA; Fig. 2.5.4b) and having the right hepatic artery (RHA) (Figs. 2.5.4c, 2.5.5) branching off the superior mesenteric artery (SMA) (Lee et al. 2002). A full understanding of the potential variations and the ability to achieve selective cannulation is required to allow complete treatment with chemoembolization.

2.5.3 Complications

Knowledge of the complications of TACE treatment is important for correct diagnosis and appropriate

Table 2.5.3. Results of chemoembolization in liver metastasis (literature review). (*A, Adria* Adriamycin, *CDDP* cisplatin, *Collag* bovine collagen, *DSM* degradable starch microspheres, *Epi* epirubicin, *F, 5-FU* 5-fluorouracil, *FUDR* 5-fluorodeoxyuridine, *Gel* gelfoam, *M, Mito* mitomycin, *N/A* not available, *Neuroend TM* neuroendocrine tumors, *PVA* polyvinyl alcohol, *STZ* streptozotocin)

References	Agents	Primary tumor	Patients	Survival rates
Wollner et al. (1986)	Mito/DSM	Colorectal CA	15	Median 7 months
Kobayashi et al. (1987)	Adria/Mito/Lipiodol	Colorectal CA	7	N/A
Starkhammar et al. (1987)	Mito/DSM	Colorectal CA	11	N/A
Inoue et al. (1989)	Adria/Mito	Colorectal CA	33	Median 337 days
Taniguchi et al. (1989)	A/AM/FAM Lipiodol	Colorectal CA	20	Median 12.5 months
Yamashita et al. (1989)	FUDR-C8/Lipiodol	Colorectal CA	13	Median 13.7 months
Meakem et al. (1992)	CDDP/Adria/Mito/Collag	Colorectal CA	11	N/A
Kameyama et al. (1992)	CDDP/Lipiodol	Colorectal CA	11	N/A
Lang and Brown (1993)	Adria/Lipiodol	Colorectal CA	46	Median 23 months
Feun et al. (1994)	CDDP/Lipiodol	Colorectal CA	6	N/A
Soulen (1994)	CDDP/Adria Mito/Lipiodol	Colorectal CA	30	1 year: 70%
Tellez et al. (1998)	CDDP/Mito Gel/Kollag	Colorectal CA	30	Median 8.6 months
Salman et al. (2002)	PVA/FU/interferon	Colorectal CA	24	Median 11 months/8 months with extrahepatic disease
Wasser et al. (2005)	Mito/DSM	Colorectal CA	21	Median 13.8 months
Mavligit et al. (1988)	CDDP/PVA	Melanoma	30	Median 11 months
Agarwala et al. (2004)	CDDP /PVA	Melanoma		N/A
Therasse et al. (1993)	Adria/Lipiodol	Neuroend. TM	23	Median 24 months
Diamandidou et al. (1998)	microencapsulated CDDP	Neuroend. TM	20	N/A
Falconi et al. (1999)	Lipiodol FU/DCB/DSM	Neuroend. TM	28	Median 35.4 months
Dominguez et al. (2000)	STZ /Lipiodol/ Gelatine	Neuroend. TM	15	N/A
Fiorentini et al. (2004)	Mito/ CDDP/ Epi Lipiodol Gel	Neuroend. TM		Median 22 months
Li et al. (2005)		Breast cancer		1 year: 63 %

management. Sakamato et al. described a complication rate of 4.4%, for a total of 2300 procedures, which were related to the use of chemoembolic agents or the manipulation of a catheter or guidewire (Sakamoto et al. 1998). These complications included acute hepatic failure, liver infarction or abscess, intrahepatic bilioma, multiple intrahepatic aneurysms, cholecystitis, splenic infarction, gastrointestinal mucosal lesions, pulmonary embolism or infarction, tumor rupture, variceal bleeding, and iatrogenic dissection or perforation of the celiac artery and its branches.

A common symptom after TACE is the so-called postembolization syndrome, consisting of transient abdominal pain, fever, abnormal fatigue, nausea, and emesis. These symptoms continue for some days and can be treated orally with antiemetics and analgesics (Zangos et al. 2001; Vogl et al. 2003). Prophylactic antibiotics must not be routinely used because the fever is caused by tissue necrosis and is a predictor of treatment response (Castells et al. 1995). In the liver a degree of tumor infarction after TACE is probably unavoidable and small amounts of gas are commonly seen. However, long-lasting fever can be a sign of an abscess and consistent therapeutic treatment may be required in these cases (Fig. 2.5.6). A very rare complication after TACE is the rupture of the treated hepatocellular carcinoma (HCC) (Sakamoto et al. 1999).

Extrahepatic uptake of chemoembolization material can be documented on noncontrast CT images (Fig. 2.5.7). Asymptomatic deposition of chemoembolization material may be seen in the lung, stomach, pancreas, duodenum, gallbladder, diaphragm, and the spleen (Gates et al. 1999).

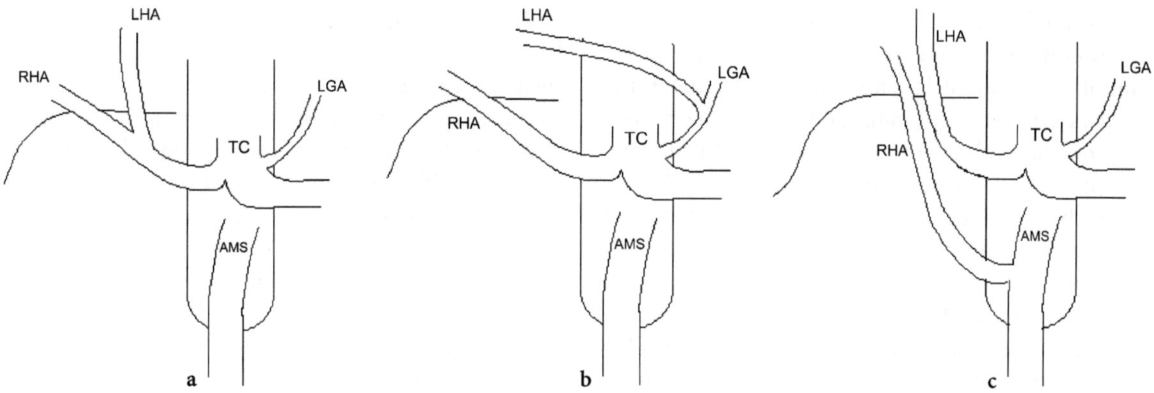

Fig. 2.5.4a–c. Common variations in hepatic arterial supply. **a** Conventional celiac (*TC*) and hepatic arterial anatomy (55%). **b** Replaced left hepatic artery (*LHA*) arising from the left gastric artery (*LGA*) (20%). **c** Replaced right hepatic artery (*RHA*) arises from the superior mesenteric artery (*SMA*) (6%)

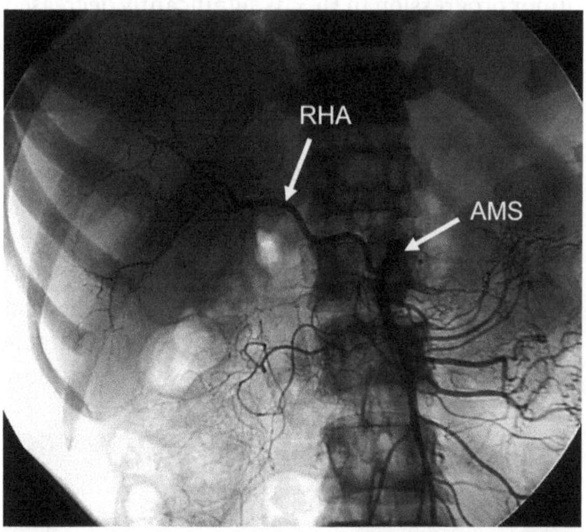

Fig. 2.5.5. Replaced right hepatic artery (*RHA*) from the superior mesenteric artery (*AMS*)

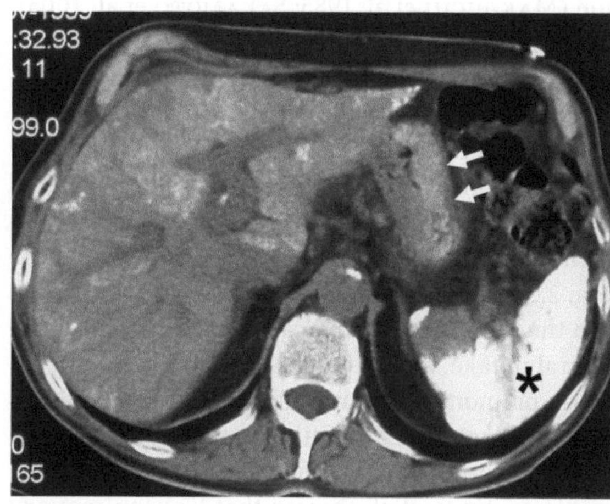

Fig. 2.5.7. Nonenhanced CT scan obtained 1 day after chemoembolization shows ethiodized oil in stomach (*arrows*) and spleen (*star*)

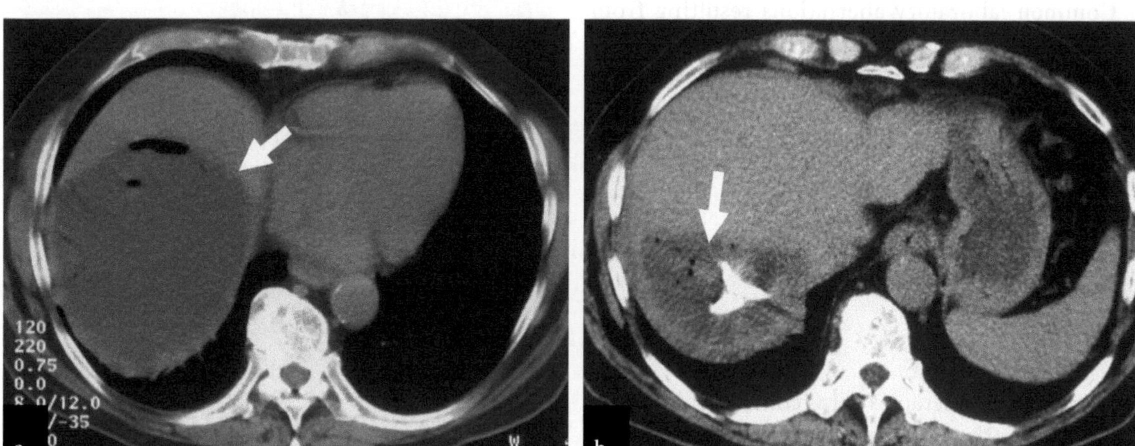

Fig. 2.5.6a,b. Nonenhanced CT scan obtained 4 weeks after chemoembolization shows extensive gas in a treated tumor due to abscess formation (**a**). This abscess was treated with drainage and intravenous antibiotics (**b**)

Although gastric uptake is uncommon and asymptomatic, the gastric deposition of chemoembolization material can cause peptic ulceration (Hirakawa et al. 1988). For that reason these patients should receive prophylactic histamine$_2$-receptor blockers for 1 month after TACE. Even when the gallbladder does receive some chemoembolization material, there is usually no clinically significant complication of this procedure. Patients with post-TACE infarction of the gallbladder can be treated conservatively if they are kept under close observation (Kuroda et al. 1983). Unusually an emphysematous cholecystitis can arise from the chemoembolization (Takayasu et al. 1985; Gates et al. 1999). Some authors have reported abscess formation or bilioma as a result of biliary infarction (Makuuchi et al. 1985; Sakamoto et al. 2003). TACE can also induce bilious pleuritis as a rare complication, which should be considered as an adverse effect of TACE in patients with a dilated hepatic duct (Ichikawa et al. 1997). Splenic artery reflux of the chemoembolization agent can cause focal splenic infarction.

In some tumors small arteriovenous shunts (Fig. 2.5.8) allow chemoembolization agent to pass into the hepatic veins and can thence cause lung or pleural uptake. Even though some authors reported acute pulmonary complications following TACE (Samejima et al. 1990; Chung et al. 1993; Tajima et al. 2002), it is unlikely that this uptake can cause problems. Vogl et al. showed that transpulmonary chemoembolization (TPCE) can be performed as a treatment for unresectable lung metastases without major side-effects or complications (Vogl et al. 2005).

Common laboratory aberrations resulting from TACE include transient elevation of lactate dehydrogenase (LDH), bilirubin, and alkaline phosphatase with an accompanying drop in the hemoglobin and platelet counts (Tellez et al. 1998).

2.5.4 Discussion

Regional liver therapies are considerably more common now than they were a decade ago. Kato et al. described in 1981 the first arterial chemoembolization with a microencapsulated anticancer drug in different organs (Kato et al. 1981).

Nevertheless, assessing the efficacy of TACE can be difficult because multiple factors can be used to measure the success. These factors include patient survival, tumor size reduction, generation of tumor necrosis, lipiodol retention, biological response, quality of life, and improvement of the symptoms. This is the challenging problem when interpreting the published data.

Various studies have demonstrated an improvement in long-term patient survival after TACE. Unfortunately, most studies did not compare patients with TACE with untreated control subjects. As such, these data are inherently confounded, leaving these randomized trials unable to accurately assess the effect of TACE on survival (Ramsey et al. 2002).

Prospective studies (Table 2.5.2) have shown that tumor progression in HCC is significantly decreased in patients treated by TACE than in untreated controls (Bruix et al. 2004). Camma et al. (2002) described, in patients with unresectable HCC, that chemoembolization can improve significantly the overall 2-year survival compared with nonactive treatment, but the magnitude of the benefit is relatively small.

Llovet and Bruix (2003) reviewed 61 randomized trials to assess the evidence of the impact of medical treatments on survival of patients with unresectable HCC. Arterial embolization improved 2-year sur-

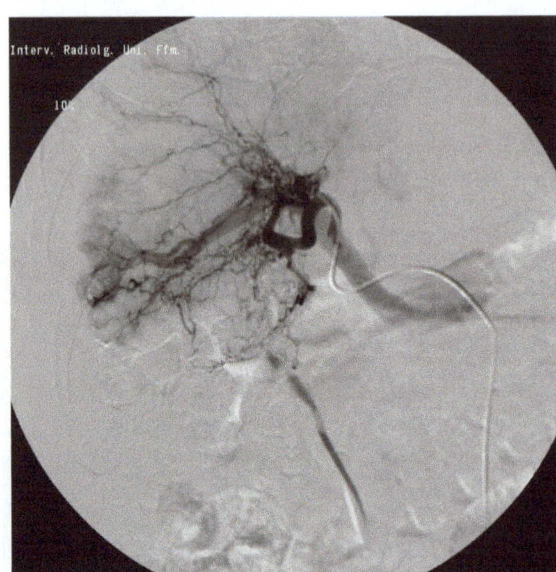

Fig. 2.5.8. Selective hepatic arteriogram shows a hypervascular hepatocellular carcinoma (*HCC*) in the right lobe with transtumoral arterioportal shunting. Before starting the chemoembolization, embolization of these shunts is necessary to prevent serious side-effects

vival compared to control group in patients with HCC. Sensitivity analysis showed a significant benefit of chemoembolization with cisplatin or doxorubicin but none with embolization alone. Overall, treatment induced objective responses in 35% of patients (range, 16%–61%). Tamoxifen showed no antitumoral effect and no survival benefits, and only low-quality scale trials suggested 1-year improvement in survival. So the authors conclude that chemoembolization improves survival of patients with unresectable HCC and may become the standard treatment. Treatment with tamoxifen does not modify the survival of patients with advanced disease (Llovet and Bruix 2003).

Likewise, different authors (Table 2.5.3) described TACE as a feasible treatment modality for patients with liver metastases who have experienced failure with other systemic treatments (Tellez et al. 1998). Patt et al. (1981) published one of the first studies suggesting a palliative role for hepatic arterial infusion and arterial occlusion in patients with colorectal carcinoma and metastases to the liver. The overall tumor response rate was 43.4% and median overall survival was 11 months. They observed an increased median survival to 15 months in those patients who underwent arterial occlusion hepatic arterial occlusion.

While TACE of liver metastases has been investigated in numerous studies for two decades, the results from clinical trials do not allow definitive conclusions to be made about the role of chemoembolization in the treatment of colorectal cancer (CRC) liver metastases. The clinical value of TACE in liver metastases remains controversial. Nevertheless different authors describe promising results for the treatment of liver metastases.

Tellez and colleges showed that chemoembolization is a feasible treatment modality in patients with liver metastasis from CRC who have experienced failure with other systemic treatments. It results in high response rates with transient mild-to-moderate toxicity. Patients who are able to undergo repetitive chemoembolization procedures may receive the most clinical benefit (Tellez et al. 1998). Salman et al. (2002) resumed that embolization of the liver as second-line therapy in patients with liver-predominant metastases is safe and effective. Median survivals are comparable to those following other second-line therapies.

In contrast to this, Popov et al. described that TACE for liver metastases from CRC performed with an injection of iodinated oil (lipiodol) with mitomycin C (3 mg/ml) did not appear to bring any benefit; furthermore, significant liver toxicity compromises the safety of such procedures (Popov et al. 2002). Our results with out patient treatment of 245 patients do not agree with this result and prove that TACE results in an extremely low rate of side-effects (Zangos et al. 2001). A combination of TACE with local ablative treatment may present a potentially curative treatment option for huge unresectable tumors (Vogl et al. 2003). Repetitive high-concentration regional chemotherapy by use of chemoembolization combined with continuously administered 5-fluorouracil (5-FU) and supplemented with granulocyte-macrophage colony-stimulating factor (GM-CSF) cytokine is an effective tool in the therapy of disseminated colorectal liver metastases as front-line as well as a second-line treatment (Muller et al. 2003).

You and colleagues (2005) evaluated the combination of systemic chemotherapy and chemoembolization. Chemoembolization was performed using a mixture of 10 ml lipiodol, 1500 mg 5-FU and 15 mg leucovorin. Two weeks following chemoembolization, patients underwent systemic chemotherapy with 2600 mg/m^2 5-FU continuous infusion for 24 h and received 150 mg leucovorin (intravenous bolus). The course of chemotherapy was repeated weekly for 24 weeks. The median disease-free interval was 12 months and the median survival time was 16 months. In conclusion the authors suggested that the results of this study are of sufficient interest to justify future randomized trials (You et al. 2005).

The cost-effectiveness of TACE for the treatment of CRC liver metastases varies considerably according to the anticipated survival benefit. A survival benefit of nearly 5 months for TACE treatment should be gained to meet the moderate cost-effectiveness standard of $50,000 per life year (Abramson et al. 2000).

Promising results have been published for liver metastases of other different original tumors. Neuroendocrine tumors, particularly those of gastrointestinal tract origin, have a predisposition for metastasizing to the liver, causing parenchymal substitution and paraneoplastic syndrome (Fiorentini et al. 2004). TACE is thought to be an effective symptomatic and antiproliferative treatment in patients with liver metastases of neuroendocrine tumors.

Roche et al. reported the outcome in 14 patients with liver metastases from endocrine tumors who underwent TACE performed with doxorubicin emulsified in lipiodol and gelatin sponge particles as the first-line nonsurgical treatment. An objective

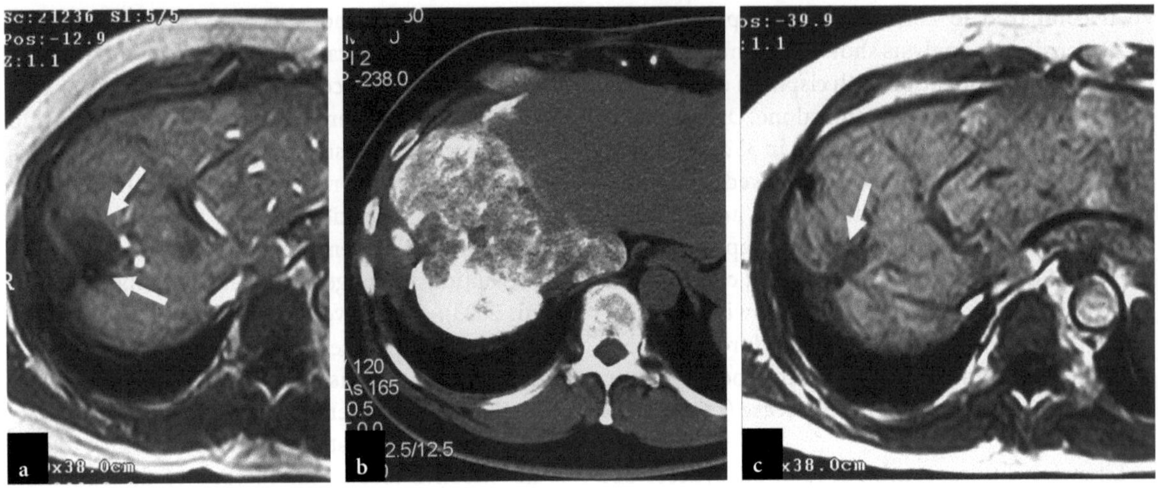

Fig. 2.5.9a–c. Patient with a new colorectal liver metastasis after hemihepatectomy. Unenhanced transverse GRE T_1-weighted MR images demonstrate a 20×35 mm target lesion (*arrows*) at the resection border before treatment (**a**). Unenhanced transverse CT scan obtained after the first TACE course demonstrates low intratumoral lipiodol uptake (**b**). A massive shrinking of the treated lesion (*arrow*) could be observed on unenhanced transverse T_1-weighted GRE MR scan after the third course of TACE (**c**)

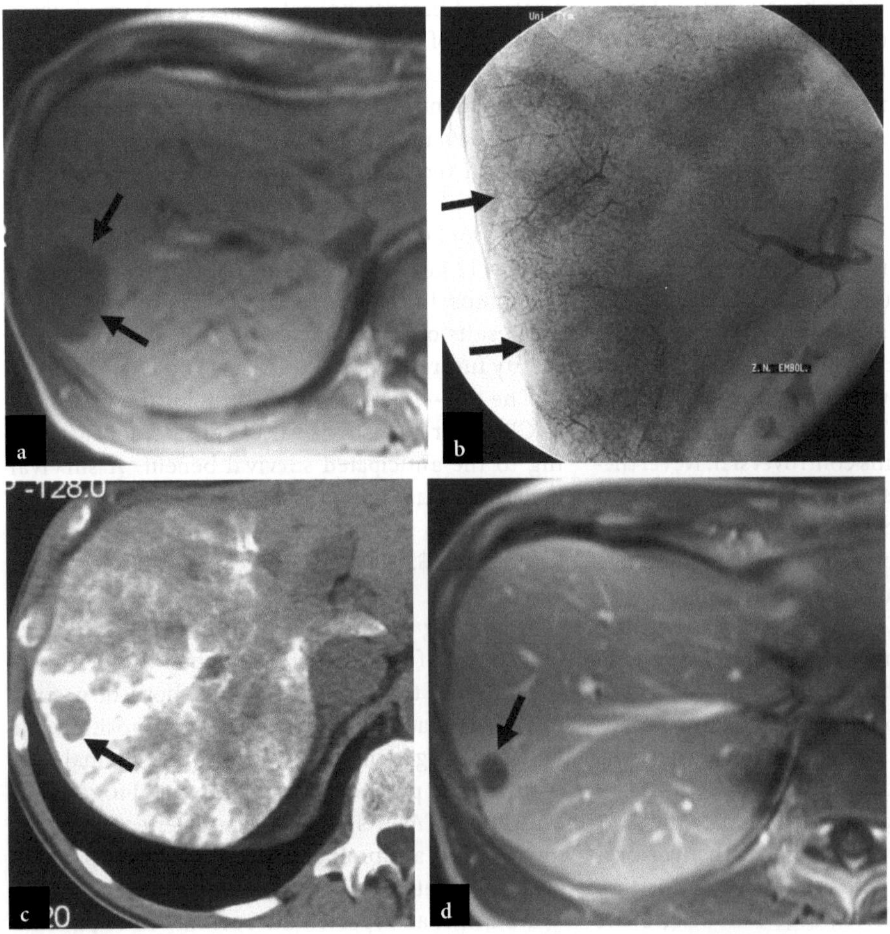

Fig. 2.5.10a–d. Unenhanced MR images shows a colorectal metastasis in the right liver lobe (**a**). Angiographic imaging after chemoembolization showed a second lesion (*arrow*) and high lipiodol uptake in the treated lesions (**b**). After the third course of TACE, shrinking of the lesion could be archived (**c**). Contrast-enhanced MR imaging after 8 weeks shows necrosis (*arrow*) of the lesion (**d**). Nevertheless, residual tumor in the periphery cannot be excluded definitely

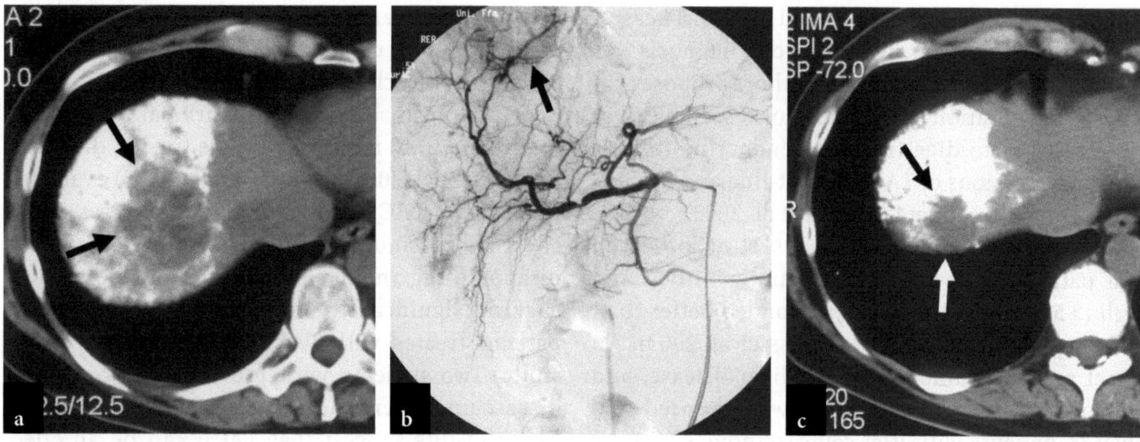

Fig. 2.5.11a–c. Nonenhanced CT scan in a patient with liver metastases (*arrows*) from breast cancer shows after the first TACE course only moderate intra-tumoral lipiodol uptake (**a**) The hepatic angiogram shows hypervascular tumor staining in the liver dome (**b**). Nevertheless conspicuous shrinking of the tumor (*arrows*) can be observed after the third course of TACE (**c**)

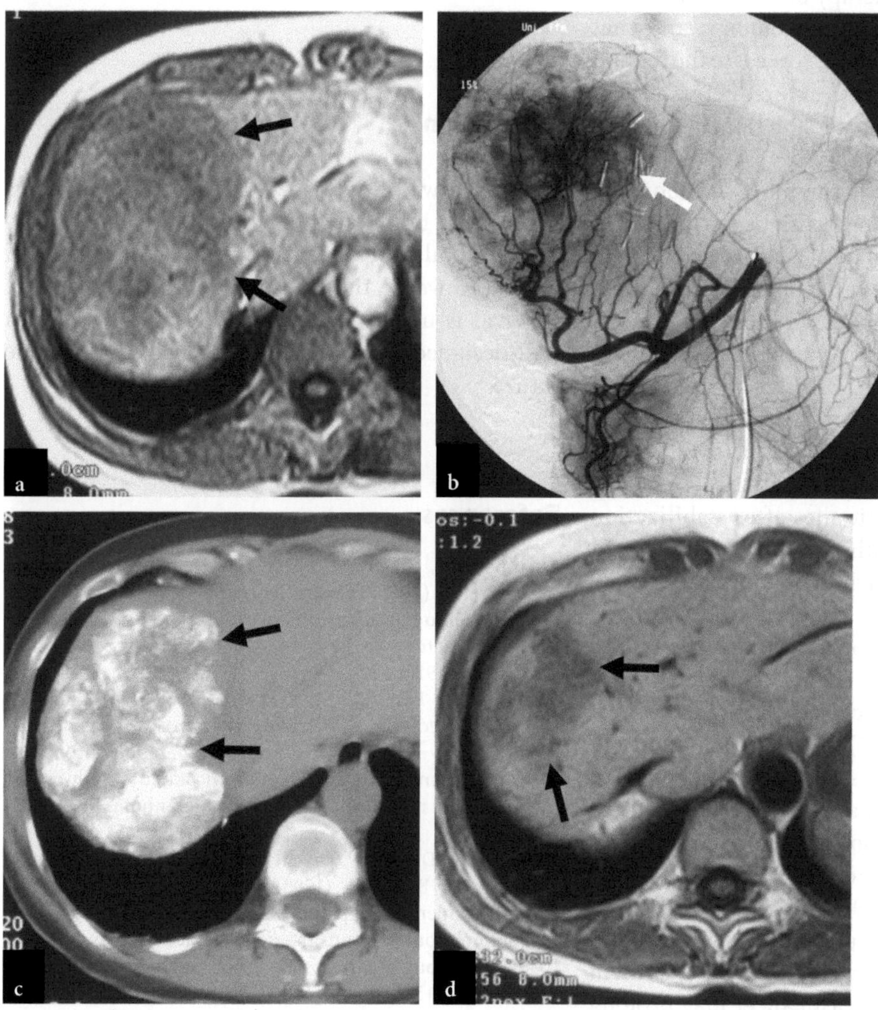

Fig. 2.5.12a–d. Nonenhanced MR imaging shows large HCC in the right liver lobe (**a**). Hepatic angiogram documents the hypervascularization of the tumor (**b**). Nonenhanced CT obtained after the first TACE course documents high lipiodol retention (*arrows*) within the tumor (**c**). The tumor decreases in size after the third course of TACE treatment (*arrows*) (**d**)

morphological response was noted in 12 of 14 cases. The 5- and 10-year survival rate from diagnosis was 83% and 56%, respectively. The authors propose that long-term palliation is possible in unresectable liver metastases from digestive neuroendocrine tumors with a few sessions of TACE as first-line and eventually exclusive treatment (Roche et al. 2003).

In a retrospective study Kress et al. observed that patients with low (< 50%) tumor burden and high (> 50%) lipiodol uptake responded better than end-stage patients to TACE (Kress et al. 2003). An intact primary tumor, extensive liver disease, and bone metastases were associated with reduced survival in patients with islet cell carcinomas (Gupta et al. 2005). Fiorentini et al. (2004) conclude that chemoembolization will improve the clinical condition of a significant percentage of patients with liver metastases, that future therapy of carcinoid tumors will be based on specific tumor biology, and that treatment will be customized for each individual patient combining the use of cytoreductive procedures including radiofrequency ablation, laser treatment, and chemoembolization.

In melanoma the liver is the most common site for systemic metastases. TACE can be performed in patients with liver metastases to improve the survival. Agarwala et al. observed that TACE produces a modest response rate in patients with ocular melanoma and liver metastases (Agarwala et al. 2004). Chemoembolization using 1,3-bis(2-chloroethyl)-1-nitrosourea (BCNU) dissolved in ethiodized oil is a useful palliative treatment for the control of hepatic metastases in uveal melanoma patients. However, progression in extrahepatic sites after stabilization of hepatic metastases requires further improvement in the therapeutic approach to this disease (Patel et al. 2005).

Liver metastases from breast cancer are associated with poor prognosis. Intravenous chemotherapy is commonly used and can result in regression of tumor lesions (Li et al. 2005). Li et al. (2005) reported the results of TACE and systemic chemotherapy for patients with liver metastases from breast cancer and evaluated the prognostic factors. The 1-, 2- and 3-year survival rates for the TACE group were 63.04%, 30.35%, and 13.01%, and those for the systemic chemotherapy group were 33.88%, 11.29%, and 0%. These data showed that TACE treatment of liver metastases from breast cancer may prolong survival in certain patients. This approach offers new promise for the curative treatment of patients with metastatic breast cancer (Li et al. 2005).

A new indication of TACE is the treatment of unresectable cholangiocarcinoma. Normally, patients with cholangiocarcinoma carry only a poor prognosis, with median survival times ranging from 6 to 12 months from the time of diagnosis (Burger et al. 2005). Burger et al. (2005) evaluated the value of TACE in the treatment of unresectable cholangiocarcinoma. Palliative therapies have been disappointing and have not been shown to prolong survival significantly. The median survival for 17 patients treated with TACE was 23 months in this study. Two patients with previously unresectable disease underwent successful resection after TACE. These results suggest that TACE can be an effective palliative therapy in patients with unresectable cholangiocarcinoma.

2.5.5 Conclusion

TACE is a well established procedure for patients with HCC, but in patients with liver metastases TACE can also be an effective palliative treatment option. However, the true effect of TACE on patient survival is unclear and needs to be assessed with well-designed randomized controlled trials in the future.

References

Abramson R, Rosen M, Perry L, Brophy D, Raeburn S, Stuart K (2000) Cost-effectiveness of hepatic arterial chemoembolization for colorectal liver metastases refractory to systemic chemotherapy. Radiology 216:485–491

Agarwala SS, Panikkar R, Kirkwood JM (2004) Phase I/II randomized trial of intrahepatic arterial infusion chemotherapy with cisplatin and chemoembolization with cisplatin and polyvinyl sponge in patients with ocular melanoma metastatic to the liver. Melanoma Res 14:217–222

Allgaier HP, Deibert P, Olschewski M, Spamer C, Blum U, Gerok W, Blum HE (1998) Survival benefit of patients with inoperable hepatocellular carcinoma treated by a combination of transarterial chemoembolization and percutaneous ethanol injection-a single-center analysis including 132 patients. Int J Cancer 79:601–605

Allgaier HP, Deibert P, Zuber I, Olschewski M, Blum HE (1999) Percutaneous radiofrequency interstitial thermal ablation of small hepatocellular carcinoma. Lancet 353:1676–1677

Allison DJ, Booth A (1990) Arterial embolization in the management of liver metastases. Cardiovasc Intervent Radiol 13:161–168

Bernardino ME, Thomas JL, Barnes PA, Lewis E (1982) Diagnostic approaches to liver and spleen metastases. Radiol Clin North Am 20:469–485

Bianco S, Merkel C, Savastano S et al (1996) Short-term effects of transcatheter arterial chemoembolisation on metabolic activity of the liver of cirrhotic patients with hepatocellular carcinoma. Gut 39:325–329

Bismuth H, Morino M, Sherlock D, Castaing D, Miglietta C, Cauquil P, Roche A (1992) Primary treatment of hepatocellular carcinoma by arterial chemoembolization. Am J Surg 163:387–394

Breedis C, Young G (1954) The blood supply of neoplasms in the liver. Am J Pathol 30:969–985

Bruix J, Sala M, Llovet J (2004) Chemoembolization for hepatocellular carcinoma. Gastroenterology 127:S179–188

Burger I, Hong K, Schulick R, Georgiades C, Thuluvath P, Choti M, Kamel I, Geschwind JF (2005) Transcatheter arterial chemoembolization in unresectable cholangiocarcinoma: initial experience in a single institution. J Vasc Interv Radiol 16:353–361

Camma C, Schepis F, Orlando A, Albanese M, Shahied L, Trevisani F, Andreone P, Craxi A, Cottone M (2002) Transarterial chemoembolization for unresectable hepatocellular carcinoma: meta-analysis of randomized controlled trials. Radiology 224:47–54

Castells A, Bruix J, Ayuso C, Bru C, Montanya X, Boix L, Rodes J (1995) Transarterial embolization for hepatocellular carcinoma. Antibiotic prophylaxis and clinical meaning of postembolization fever. J Hepatol 22:410–415

Caturelli E, Siena DA, Fusilli S, Villani MR, Schiavone G, Nardella M, Balzano S, Florio F (2000) Transcatheter arterial chemoembolization for hepatocellular carcinoma in patients with cirrhosis: evaluation of damage to nontumorous liver tissue-long-term prospective study. Radiology 215:123–128

Chen MS, Li JQ, Zhang YQ, Lu LX, Zhang WZ, Yuan YF, Guo YP, Lin XJ, Li GH (2002) High-dose iodized oil transcatheter arterial chemoembolization for patients with large hepatocellular carcinoma. World J Gastroenterol 8:74–78

Choi BI, Kim HC, Han JK, Park JH, Kim YI, Kim ST, Lee HS, Kim CY, Han MC (1992) Therapeutic effect of transcatheter oily chemoembolization therapy for encapsulated nodular hepatocellular carcinoma: CT and pathologic findings. Radiology 182:709–713

Chung JW, Park JH, Im JG, Han JK, Han MC (1993) Pulmonary oil embolism after transcatheter oily chemoembolization of hepatocellular carcinoma. Radiology 187:689–693

Cioni D, Lencioni R, Bartolozzi C (2000) Therapeutic effect of transcatheter arterial chemoembolization on hepatocellular carcinoma: evaluation with contrast-enhanced harmonic power Doppler ultrasound. Eur Radiol 10:1570–1575

Colella G, Bottelli R, De Carlis L et al (1998) Hepatocellular carcinoma: comparison between liver transplantation, resective surgery, ethanol injection, and chemoembolization. Transpl Int 11:S193–196

Daniels JR, Sternlicht M, Daniels AM (1988) Collagen chemoembolization: pharmacokinetics and tissue tolerance of cis-diamminedichloroplatinum(II) in porcine liver and rabbit kidney. Cancer Res 48:2446–2450

Diamandidou E, Ajani JA, Yang DJ, Chuang VP, Brown CA, Carrasco HC, Lawrence DD, Wallace S (1998) Two-phase study of hepatic artery vascular occlusion with microencapsulated cisplatin in patients with liver metastases from neuroendocrine tumors. AJR Am J Roentgenol 170:339–344

Dominguez S, Denys A, Madeira I, Hammel P, Vilgrain V, Menu Y, Bernades P, Ruszniewski P (2000) Hepatic arterial chemoembolization with streptozotocin in patients with metastatic digestive endocrine tumours. Eur J Gastroenterol Hepatol 12:151–157

Falconi M, Bassi C, Bonora A, Sartori N, Procacci C, Talamini G, Mansueto GC, Pederzoli P (1999) Role of chemoembolization in synchronous liver metastases from pancreatic endocrine tumours. Dig Surg 16:32–38

Feun LG, Reddy KR, Yrizarry JM et al (1994) A phase I study of chemoembolization with cisplatin and lipiodol for primary and metastatic liver cancer. Am J Clin Oncol 17:405–410

Fiorentini G, Poddie DB, Giorgi UD et al (2000) Global approach to hepatic metastases from colorectal cancer: indication and outcome of intra-arterial chemotherapy and other hepatic-directed treatments. Med Oncol 17:163–173

Fiorentini G, Rossi S, Bonechi F, Vaira M, De Simone M, Dentico P, Bernardeschi P, Cantore M, Guadagni S (2004) Intra-arterial hepatic chemoembolization in liver metastases from neuroendocrine tumors: a phase II study. J Chemother 16:293–297

Gates J, Hartnell GG, Stuart KE, Clouse ME (1999) Chemoembolization of hepatic neoplasms: safety, complications, and when to worry. Radiographics 19:399–414

Gattoni F, Dova S, Uslenghi CM (2000) Three-year follow-up of 62 cirrhotic patients with hepatocellular carcinoma treated with chemoembolization. Minerva Chir 55:31–37

Gupta S, Johnson MM, Murthy R et al (2005) Hepatic arterial embolization and chemoembolization for the treatment of patients with metastatic neuroendocrine tumors. Cancer 104:1590–1602

Hirakawa M, Iida M, Aoyagi K, Matsui T, Akagi K, Fujishima M (1988) Gastroduodenal lesions after transcatheter arterial chemo-embolization in patients with hepatocellular carcinoma. Am J Gastroenterol 83:837–840

Hosoki T, Yosioka Y, Matsubara T, Minamitani K, Higashi M, Ohtani M, Choi S, Mitomo M, Tono T (1999) Power Doppler sonography of hepatocellular carcinoma treated by transcatheter arterial chemoembolization. Assessment of the therapeutic effect. Acta Radiol 40:639–643

Huppert PE, Lauchart W, Duda SH, Torkler C, Kloska SP, Weinlich M, Benda N, Pereira P, Claussen CD (2004) Chemoembolization of hepatocellular carcinomas: which factors determine therapeutic response and survival?. Rofo 176:375–385

Ichikawa T, Yamada T, Takagi H, Abe T, Ito H, Sakurai S, Nagamine T, Mori M (1997) Transcatheter arterial embolization-induced bilious pleuritis in a patient with hepatocellular carcinoma. J Gastroenterol 32:405–409

Inoue H, Kobayashi H, Itoh Y, Shinohara S (1989) Treatment of liver metastases by arterial injection of adriamycin/mitomycin C lipiodol suspension. Acta Radiol 30:603–608

Jaeger HJ, Mehring UM, Castaneda F, Hasse F, Blumhardt G, Loehlein D, Mathias KD (1996) Sequential transarterial chemoembolization for unresectable advanced hepatocellular carcinoma. Cardiovasc Intervent Radiol 19:388–396

Kameyama M, Imaoka S, Fukuda I, Nakamori S, Sasaki Y, Fujita M, Hasegawa Y, Iwanaga T (1992) Delayed washout of intratumor blood flow is associated with good response to intraarterial chemoembolization for liver metastasis of colorectal cancer. Surgery 114:97–101

Kato T, Nemoto R, Mori H, Takahashi M, Tamakawa Y, Harada M (1981) Arterial chemoembolization with microencapsulated anticancer drug. An approach to selective cancer chemotherapy with sustained effects. J Am Med Assocama 245:1123–1127

Kennedy KA, Rockwell S, Sartorelli AC (1980) Preferential activation of mitomycin C to cytotoxic metabolites by hypoxic tumor cells. Cancer Res 40:2356–2360

Kobayashi H, Inoue H, Shimada J, Yano T, Maeda T, Oyama T, Shinohara S (1987) Intra-arterial injection of adriamycin/mitomycin C lipiodol suspension in liver metastases. Acta Radiol 28:275–280

Kress O, Wagner HJ, Wied M et al (2003) Transarterial chemoembolization of advanced liver metastases of neuroendocrine tumors – a retrospective single-center analysis. Digestion 68:94–101

Kuroda C, Iwasaki M, Tanaka T, Tokunaga K, Hori S, Yoshioka H, Nakamura H, Sakurai M, Okamura J (1983) Gallbladder infarction following hepatic transcatheter arterial embolization. Angiographic study. Radiology 149:85–89

Lang EK, Brown CL Jr (1993) Colorectal metastases to the liver: selective chemoembolization. Radiology 189:417–422

Lee K, Sung K, Lee D, Park S, Kim K, Yu J (2002) Transcatheter arterial chemoembolization for hepatocellular carcinoma: anatomic and hemodynamic considerations in the hepatic artery and portal vein. Radiographics 22:1077–1091

Li XP, Meng ZQ, Guo WJ, Li J (2005) Treatment for liver metastases from breast cancer: results and prognostic factors. World J Gastroenterol 11:3782–3787

Livraghi T (2003) Radiofrequency ablation, PEIT, and TACE for hepatocellular carcinoma. J Hepatobiliary Pancreat Surg 10:67–76

Lladò L, Virgili J, Figueras J et al (2000) A prognostic index of the survival of patients with unresectable hepatocellular carcinoma after transcatheter arterial chemoembolization. Cancer 88:50–57

Llovet J, Bruix J (2003) Systematic review of randomized trials for unresectable hepatocellular carcinoma: chemoembolization improves survival. Hepatology 37:429–442

Llovet J, Burroughs A, Bruix J (2003) Hepatocellular carcinoma. Lancet 362:1907–1917

Lo CM, Ngan H, Tso WK, Liu CL, Lam CM, Poon RT, Fan ST, Wong J (2002) Randomized controlled trial of transarterial lipiodol chemoembolization for unresectable hepatocellular carcinoma. Hepatology 35:1164–1171

Makuuchi M, Sukigara M, Mori T, Kobayashi J, Yamazaki S, Hasegawa H, Moriyama N, Takayasu K, Hirohashi S (1985) Bile duct necrosis: complication of transcatheter hepatic arterial embolization. Radiology 156:331–334

Martinelli DJ, Wadler S, Bakal CW, Cynamon J, Rozenblit A, Haynes H, Kaleya R, Wiernik PH (1994) Utility of embolization or chemoembolization as second-line treatment in patients with advanced or recurrent colorectal carcinoma [see comments]. Cancer 74:1706–1712

Mavligit GM, Charnsangavej C, Carrasco CH, Patt YZ, Benjamin RS, Wallace S (1988) Regression of ocular melanoma metastatic to the liver after hepatic arterial chemoembolization with cisplatin and polyvinyl sponge. J Am Med Assoca 260:974–976

Meakem TJd, Unger EC, Pond GD, Modiano MR, Alberts DR (1992) CT findings after hepatic chemoembolization. J Comput Assist Tomogr 16:916–920

Midorikawa T, Kumada K, Kikuchi H et al (2000) Microwave coagulation therapy for hepatocellular carcinoma. J Hepatobiliary Pancreat Surg 7:252–259

Mondazzi L, Bottelli R, Brambilla G, Rampoldi A, Rezakovic I, Zavaglia C, Alberti A, Ideo G (1994) Transarterial oily chemoembolization for the treatment of hepatocellular carcinoma: a multivariate analysis of prognostic factors. Hepatology 19:1115–1123

Müller H, Nakchbandi V, Chatzisavvidis I, von Voigt C (2003) Repetitive chemoembolization with melphalan plus intra-arterial immuno-chemotherapy within 5-fluorouracil and granulocyte-macrophage colony-stimulating factor (GM-CSF) as effective first- and second-line treatment of disseminated colorectal liver metastases. Hepatogastroenterology 50:1919–1926

Pan SS, Andrews PA, Glover CJ, Bachur NR (1984) Reductive activation of mitomycin C and mitomycin C metabolites catalyzed by NADPH-cytochrome P-450 reductase and xanthine oxidase. J Biol Chem 259:959–966

Park JH, Han JK, Chung JW, Han MC, Kim ST (1993) Postoperative recurrence of hepatocellular carcinoma: results of transcatheter arterial chemoembolization. Cardiovasc Intervent Radiol 16:21–24

Patel K, Sullivan K, Berd D, Mastrangelo MJ, Shields CL, Shields JA, Sato T (2005) Chemoembolization of the hepatic artery with BCNU for metastatic uveal melanoma: results of a phase II study. Melanoma Res 15:297–304

Patt YZ, Chuang VP, Wallace S, Hersh EM, Freireich EJ, Mavligit GM (1981) The palliative role of hepatic arterial infusion and arterial occlusion in colorectal carcinoma metastatic to the liver. Lancet 1:349–350

Pelletier G, Ducreux M, Gay F et al (1998) Treatment of unresectable hepatocellular carcinoma with lipiodol chemoembolization: a multicenter randomized trial. Groupe CHC. J Hepatol 29:129–134

Pentecost MJ, Daniels JR, Teitelbaum GP, Stanley P (1993) Hepatic chemoembolization: safety with portal vein thrombosis. J Vasc Interv Radiol 4:347–351

Popov I, Lavrnic S, Jelic S, Jezdic S, Jasovic A (2002) Chemoembolization for liver metastases from colorectal carcinoma: risk or a benefit. Neoplasma 49:43–48

Ramsey DE, Kernagis LY, Soulen MC, Geschwind JF (2002) Chemoembolization of hepatocellular carcinoma. J Vasc Interv Radiol 13:S211–221

Raoul JL, Heresbach D, Bretagne JF, Ferrer DB, Duvauferrier R, Bourguet P, Messner M, Gosselin M (1992) Chemoembolization of hepatocellular carcinomas. A study of the biodistribution and pharmacokinetics of doxorubicin. Cancer 70:585–590

Roche A, Girish BV, de Baere T, Baudin E, Boige V, Elias D, Lasser P, Schlumberger M, Ducreux M (2003) Transcatheter arterial chemoembolization as first-line treatment for hepatic metastases from endocrine tumors. Eur Radiol 13:136–140

Sakamoto I, Aso N, Nagaoki K et al (1998) Complications associated with transcatheter arterial embolization for hepatic tumors. Radiographics 18:605–619

Sakamoto Y, Kita Y, Takayama T, Kawauchi N, Minagawa M, Makuuchi M (1999) Rupture of hepatocellular carcinoma after transcatheter arterial embolization: an unusual case. Hepatogastroenterology 46:453–456

Sakamoto I, Iwanaga S, Nagaoki K et al (2003) Intrahepatic biloma formation (bile duct necrosis) after transcatheter arterial chemoembolization. AJR Am J Roentgenol 181:79–87

Salman HS, Cynamon J, Jagust M, Bakal C, Rozenblit A, Kaleya R, Negassa A, Wadler S (2002) Randomized phase II trial of embolization therapy versus chemoembolization therapy in previously treated patients with colorectal carcinoma metastatic to the liver. Clin Colorectal Cancer 2:173–179

Samejima M, Tamura S, Kodama T, Yuuki Y, Takasaki J, Sekiva R, Koga Y, Watanabe K (1990) Pulmonary complication following intra-arterial infusion of lipiodol-adriamycin emulsion for hepatocellular carcinoma, report of a case. Nippon Igaku Hoshasen Gakkai Zasshi 50:24–28

Sasson AR, Sigurdson ER (2002) Surgical treatment of liver metastases. Semin Oncol 29:107–118

Savastano S, Miotto D, Casarrubea G, Teso S, Chiesura-Corona M, Feltrin GP (1999) Transcatheter arterial chemoembolization for hepatocellular carcinoma in patients with Child's grade A or B cirrhosis: a multivariate analysis of prognostic factors. J Clin Gastroenterol 28:334–340

Soulen MC (1994) Chemoembolization of hepatic malignancies. Oncology (Huntingt) 8:77–84; discussion 84, 89–90 passim

Starkhammar H, Hakansson L, Morales O, Svedberg J (1987) Intra-arterial mitomycin C treatment of unresectable liver tumours. Preliminary results on the effect of degradable starch microspheres. Acta Oncol 26:295–300

Steger W, Vogl TJ, Hosten N, Steger S, Hidajat N, Felix R (1998) Doppler sonographic monitoring control of perfusion of hepatocellular carcinoma after arterial chemoembolization. Rofo Fortschr Geb Rontgenstr Neuen Bildgeb Verfahr 168:49–56

Stuart K, Stokes K, Jenkins R, Trey C, Clouse M (1993) Treatment of hepatocellular carcinoma using doxorubicin/ethiodized oil/gelatin powder chemoembolization. Cancer 72:3202–3209

Sumie S, Yamashita F, Ando E, Tanaka M, Yano Y, Fukumori K, Sata M (2003) Interventional radiology for advanced hepatocellular carcinoma: comparison of hepatic artery infusion chemotherapy and transcatheter arterial lipiodol chemoembolization. AJR Am J Roentgenol 181:1327–1334

Tajima T, Honda H, Kuroiwa T, Yabuuchi H, Okafuji T, Yosimitsu K, Irie H, Aibe H, Masuda K (2002) Pulmonary complications after hepatic artery chemoembolization or infusion via the inferior phrenic artery for primary liver cancer. J Vasc Interv Radiol 13:893–900

Takayasu K, Moriyama N, Muramatsu Y, Shima Y, Ushio K, Yamada T, Kishi K, Hasegawa H (1985) Gallbladder infarction after hepatic artery embolization. AJR Am J Roentgenol 144:135–138

Taniguchi H, Takahashi T, Yamaguchi T, Sawai K (1989) Intraarterial infusion chemotherapy for metastatic liver tumors using multiple anti-cancer agents suspended in a lipid contrast medium. Cancer 64:2001–2006

Taylor-Robinson SD, Foster GR, Arora S, Hargreaves S, Thomas HC (1997) Increase in primary liver cancer in the UK, 1979–94. Lancet 350:1142–1143

Tellez C, Benson AB 3rd, Lyster MT, Talamonti M, Shaw J, Braun MA, Nemcek AA Jr, Vogelzang RL (1998) Phase II trial of chemoembolization for the treatment of metastatic colorectal carcinoma to the liver and review of the literature. Cancer 82:1250–1259

Therasse E, Breittmayer F, Roche A, De Baere T, Indushekar S, Ducreux M, Lasser P, Elias D, Rougier P (1993) Transcatheter chemoembolization of progressive carcinoid liver metastasis. Radiology 189:541–547

Tsushima Y, Unno Y, Koizumi J, Kusano S (1998) Hepatic perfusion changes after transcatheter arterial embolization (TAE) of hepatocellular carcinoma: measurement by dynamic computed tomography (CT). Dig Dis Sci 43:317–322

Ueno K, Miyazono N, Inoue H, Nishida H, Kanetsuki I, Nakajo M (2000) Transcatheter arterial chemoembolization therapy using iodized oil for patients with unresectable hepatocellular carcinoma: evaluation of three kinds of regimens and analysis of prognostic factors. Cancer 88:1574–1581

Vogl TJ, Trapp M, Schroeder H, Mack M, Schuster A, Schmitt J, Neuhaus P, Felix R (2000) Transarterial chemoembolization for hepatocellular carcinoma: volumetric and morphologic CT criteria for assessment of prognosis and therapeutic success-results from a liver transplantation center. Radiology 214:349–357

Vogl TJ, Straub R, Eichler K, Woitaschek D, Mack MG (2002) Malignant liver tumors treated with MR imaging-guided laser-induced thermotherapy: experience with complications in 899 patients (2,520 lesions). Radiology 225:367–377

Vogl TJ, Mack MG, Balzer JO, Engelmann K, Straub R, Eichler K, Woitaschek D, Zangos S (2003) Liver metastases: neoadjuvant downsizing with transarterial chemoembolization before laser-induced thermotherapy. Radiology 229:457–464

Vogl TJ, Wetter A, Lindemayr S, Zangos S (2005) Treatment of unresectable lung metastases with transpulmonary chemoembolization: preliminary experience. Radiology 234:917–922

Wallace S, Carrasco CH, Charnsangavej C, Richli WR, Wright K, Gianturco C (1990) Hepatic artery infusion and chemoembolization in the management of liver metastases. Cardiovasc Intervent Radiology 13:153–160

Wang LQ, Persson BG, Bergqvist L, Bengmark S (1994) Influence of dearterialization on distribution of absolute tumor blood flow between hepatic artery and portal vein. Cancer 74:2454–2459

Wasser K, Giebel F, Fischbach R, Tesch H, Landwehr P (2005) Transarterial chemoembolization of liver metastases of colorectal carcinoma using absorbable starch microspheres (Spherex). Our own investigations and review of the literature. Radiologe 45:633–643

Wollner IS, Walker-Andrews SC, Smith JE, Ensminger W (1986) Phase II study of hepatic arterial degradable starch microspheres and mitomycin. Cancer Drug Deliv 3:279–284

Yamashita Y, Takahashi M, Bussaka H, Fukushima S, Kawaguchi T, Nakano M (1989) Intraarterial infusion of 5-fluoro-2-deoxyuridine-C8 dissolved in a lymphographic agent in malignant liver tumors. A preliminary report. Cancer 64:2437–2444

You YT, Changchien CR, Huang JS, Ng KK (2005) Combining systemic chemotherapy with chemoembolization in the treatment of unresectable hepatic metastases from colorectal cancer. Int J Colorectal Dis 21(1):33–37

Zangos S, Mack MG, Straub R, Engelmann K, Eichler K, Balzer J, Vogl TJ (2001) Transarterial chemoembolization (TACE) of liver metastases. A palliative therapeutic approach. Radiologe 41:84–90

Ablative Techniques (Percutaneous)

Actinic Ablative Techniques

2.6 CT-Guided HDR Brachytherapy: Challenging the Limits of Thermal Ablation

KONRAD MOHNIKE and JENS RICKE

CONTENTS

K. MOHNIKE, MD
Klinik für Radiologie und Nuklearmedizin, Universitätsklinikum Magdeburg AöR, Leipziger Strasse 44, 39120 Magdeburg, Germany
J. RICKE, MD
Professor, Klinik für Radiologie und Nuklearmedizin, Universitätsklinikum Magdeburg AöR, Leipziger Strasse 44, 39120 Magdeburg, Germany

2.6.1 Background

The impact of surgical resection on prognosis and patient outcome in certain malignancies in the absence of extrahepatic disease is unchallenged. Percutaneous, image-guided tumor ablation has developed and stands today as a genuine, dedicated and widely used procedure for patients with otherwise non-resectable primary or secondary liver malignancies. Procedures based on thermal tissue effects (e.g., thermal ablation and cryoablation) were initially developed with the intention of treating hepatic malignancies. Visual guidance by computed tomography (CT), magnetic resonance imaging (MRI) or ultrasound is necessary for all percutaneous approaches to the liver.

In the majority of cases, local ablation of non-resectable primary or secondary malignancies is accomplished by image-guided thermal ablative techniques [e.g., radiofrequency ablation (RF) and laser-induced thermotherapy (LITT)]. However, in clinical practice, disadvantages of thermal ablation have been found; for example, a size limitation of approximately 5 cm, adjacent large vessels being responsible for adverse cooling effects, and the close proximity to the liver hilum. Furthermore, it is difficult to achieve effective local thermal ablation in tumors that have a high level of perfusion (typically hepatocellular carcinomas), because of cooling effects (RHIM 2003; PECH et al. 2004), even though successful treatment series in combination with transarterial chemoembolization or the instillation of ethanol (QIAN et al. 2003; SAKR et al. 2005; ZANGOS et al. 2007) or in rare cases alone (EICHLER et al. 2001), have been published.

Intraoperative radiotherapy (IORT) in a single high dose has been used to treat non-resectable liver metastases with good levels of safety and efficacy. The typical doses applied range between 15 and 30 Gy with reference to the tumor margin, accepting dose inhomogeneity in the target volume depending on the particular irradiation technique (Nauta et al. 1987; Dritschilo et al. 1988; Holt et al. 1988; Thomas et al. 1993; Antoch et al. 2004).

However, the intraoperative approach has some drawbacks. First, IORT is an open procedure with significant invasiveness and procedure-related co-morbidity. Second, administering the radiation dose in the target volume is hampered by the fact that applicator placement is guided by manual palpation or sonographic monitoring (Dritschilo et al. 1986, 1988). In this situation, neither adequate coverage of the target volume fraction nor exact sparing of adjacent critical tissues, such as hepatic reserve capacity, bile duct or intestine, can be guaranteed.

To overcome these technical limitations of IORT we developed a technique for high-dose-rate (HDR) irradiation of liver metastases using an afterloading method with a ^{192}iridium source sited using CT-guided percutaneous applicator placement with dosimetry using three-dimensional CT data sets.

CT-guided interstitial brachytherapy – like LITT and RF – is based on percutaneous image-guided insertion of dedicated catheters, which enables circumscribed high-dosage brachytherapy in almost all body regions. Single, unfractionated applications of very high radiation dosages are applied to the planned target volume, which encloses the visible tumor boundaries (clinical target volume) as well as the safety margin. Therapeutic cytotoxic effects develop and are potent over weeks and months (Ricke et al. 2005a). The tumor is retained by the applicators, therefore any movements by the patient or alterations in their position have a negligible impact on achieving the exact dosimetry. Indications for local treatment are not limited by size or a location near to the liver hilum, gall bladder or large vessels (Ricke 2004; Ricke et al. 2002, 2003, 2004a, 2004b).

The indications for this treatment include large liver metastases from colorectal or other primary and hepatocellular carcinomas or cholangiocarcinoma in patients who present with absolute or relative contraindications for surgical resection. The treatment is given either as part of multimodal therapeutic management or, increasingly, as the sole therapy as a bridging procedure if, for any reason, systemic chemotherapy is not in favor at the time. It is feasible to use the technique to treat primary or secondary lung malignancies and lymph node metastases, and promising results have been achieved after the failure of second-line and third-line chemotherapy (Bergk et al. 2005; Ricke et al. 2004c, 2004d, 2004e, 2005b; Amthauer et al. 2006; Streitparth et al. 2006; Wieners et al. 2006).

2.6.2 Basics

2.6.2.1 Positioning of Applicators and Treatment Planning

The placement of the applicators is performed at fluoroscopy CT. After placing the patient in the appropriate position, the metastasis is punctured using an 18G needle and then angiography sheaths of 6F diameter are inserted over a stiff angiography guide wire. Finally, 16G brachytherapy catheters are placed in the sheaths. For treatment planning purposes, a spiral CT of the liver enhanced by intravenous application of iodide contrast medium is acquired using the breath-hold technique, and the data are then sent to the treatment planning unit.

The catheter's position and tumor boundaries are determined from the 3D CT dataset using dedicated software integrated into the planning unit of the treatment control device.

The HDR after-loading system employs a ^{192}iridium source (10 Ci or 370 GBq). The source diameter is <1 mm. Dwell positions are located every 5 mm. In most cases, a reference dose of between 15 and 25 Gy is prescribed, which, by definition, is identical to the minimum dose enclosing the lesion, and is applied as a single dose. No maximum dose constraints are given inside the tumor volume. To preserve liver function after irradiation, we prescribe that one-third of the liver parenchyma must receive <5 Gy. The irradiation time is typically 20–40 min (Figs. 2.6.1, 2.6.4).

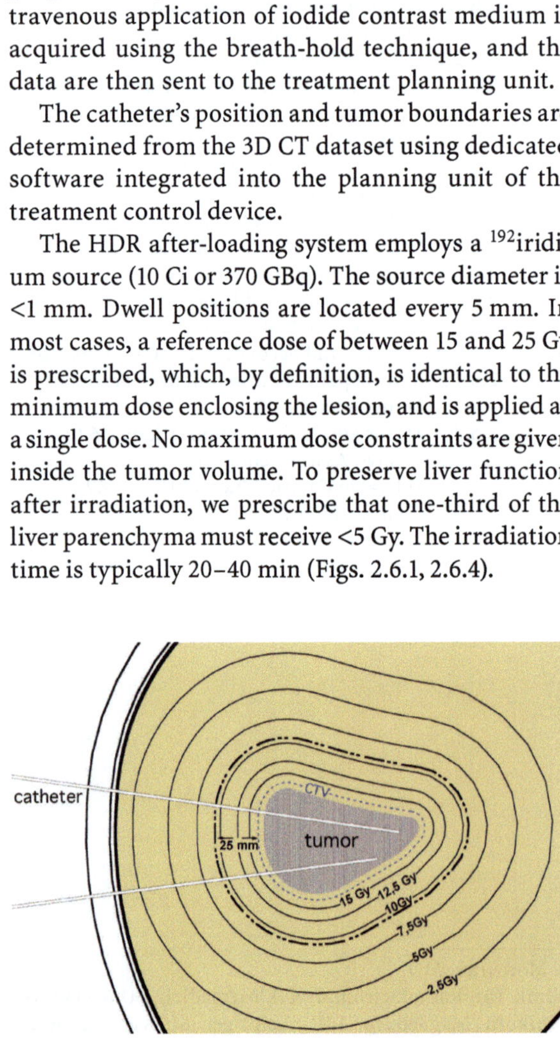

Fig. 2.6.1. Schematic of isodoses in CT-guided HDR brachytherapy of a liver lesion. Visible tumor volume, clinical target volume (tumor volume and safety margin) and 10-Gy isodoses are displayed (courtesy of M. Seidensticker)

2.6.2.2 MRI Guidance

The CT-guided insertion of catheters has some major drawbacks. During the intervention, only non-enhanced fluoroscopy can be used to determine the target, often visually correlated with and corrected using MRI prints. Unfortunately, sometimes it is necessary to reposition the catheters after recording the contrast-enhanced CT dataset. Moreover, tumor volume is systematically underestimated in contrast-enhanced CT compared to MRI (Figs. 2.6.2, 2.6.3) (Pech et al. 2006). For this reason, MRI guidance using open systems will become the state of the art in the future.

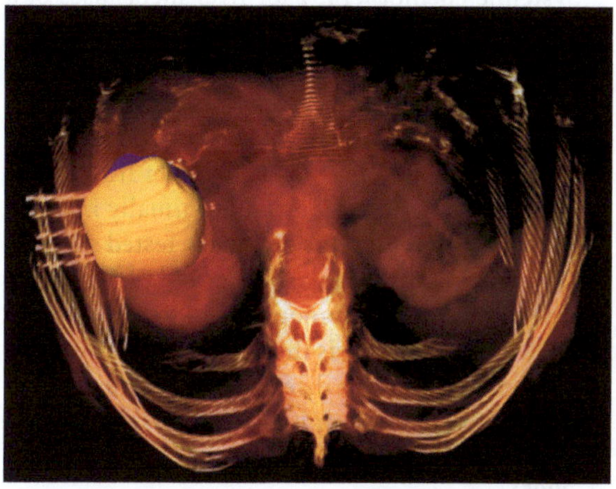

Fig. 2.6.2. Three-dimensional presentation of the same tumor volume: CE-CT (*purple*), T_1-weighted MRT without enhancement (*blue*)

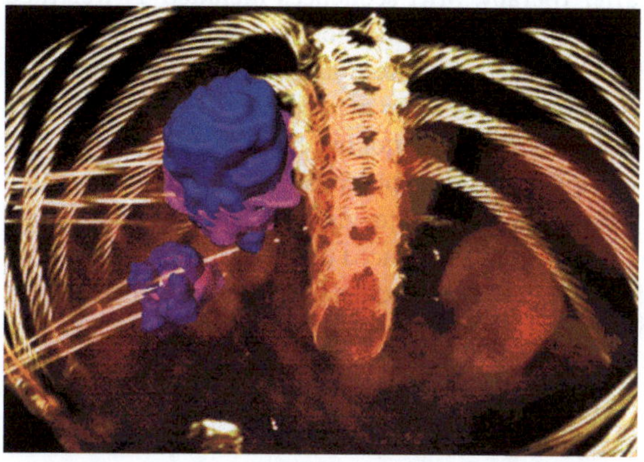

Fig. 2.6.4. Treatment planning with BrachyVision®

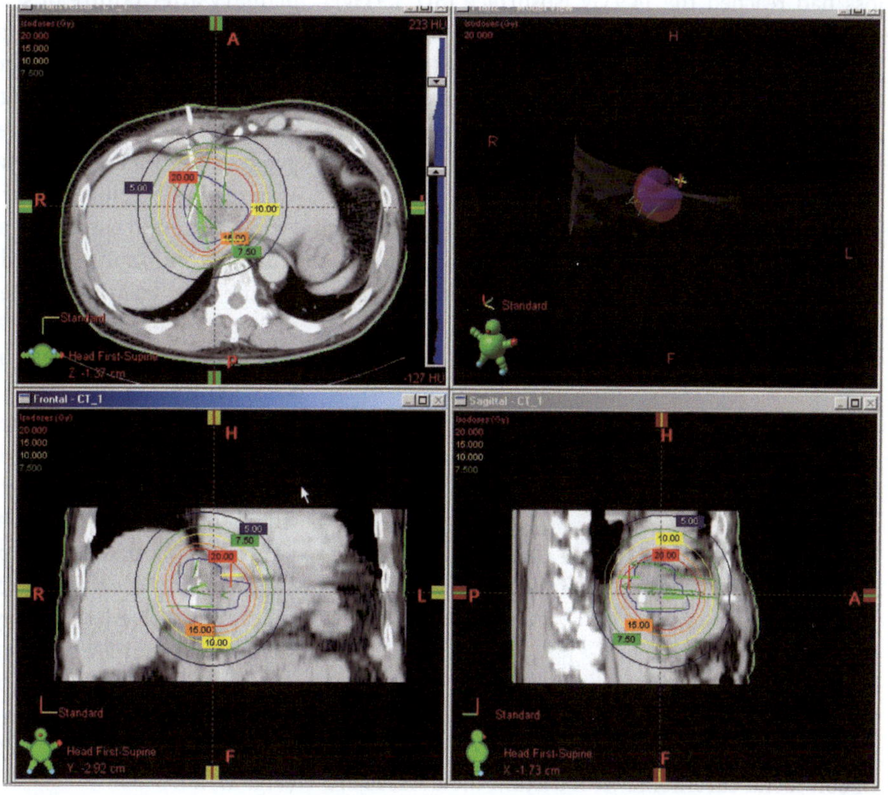

Fig. 2.6.3. Consequence of systematic underestimation: reference dose is not reached at every point of the tumor margin

2.6.2.3 Assessment of Hepatocyte Tolerance to Single-Fraction HDR Irradiation in Vivo

A patient's tolerance of liver irradiation is influenced mainly by the liver's functional reserve capacity. To investigate this, 25 liver metastases were treated using CT-guided interstitial brachytherapy. MRI was performed 1 day before and 3 days, 6, 12, and 24 weeks after therapy. MRI sequences included T_1-weighted GRE enhanced by hepatocyte-targeted Gd-BOPTA. All MRI data sets were merged with 3D-dosimetry data and evaluated by two radiologists. The reviewers indicated the border of hyperintensity on T_2-weighted images (edema) or hypointensity on T_1-weighted images (loss of hepatocyte function). A dose–volume histogram was produced using all of the 3D data. We estimated the threshold dose for either edema or loss of function as the D_{90}, i.e., the dose achieved in at least 90% of the pseudolesion volume.

Between 3 days and 6 weeks, the extent of the edema increased significantly from the 12.9 Gy to the 9.9 Gy isosurface (SD 3.3 and 2.6 Gy, respectively). No significant change was detected between 6 and 12 weeks. After 24 weeks, the edematous tissue had shrunk significantly to the 14.7 Gy isosurface (SD 4.2 Gy). Three days post brachytherapy the D_{90} for hepatocyte function loss had reached the 14.9 Gy isosurface (SD 3.9 Gy). At 6 weeks, the same zone had increased significantly to the 9.9 Gy isosurface (SD 2.3 Gy). After 12 and 24 weeks, the volume of functional loss had decreased significantly to the 11.9 Gy and 15.2 Gy isosurfaces, respectively (SD 3 and 4.1 Gy) Wochen bis zur 15.2 Gy Isodose (SD 4.1) (Fig. 2.6.1). The 95% interval of the minimally tolerated dose for hepatocytes at 6 weeks was 7.6–12.2 Gy; this is accounted for by variations inherent to the technique of CT-guided brachytherapy, including the heterogeneous dose rates delivered by the different catheters arrays employed

2.6.3 First Results in Treatment of Liver Malignancies of Different Etiologies

2.6.3.1 Colorectal Liver Malignancies

Criteria to determine the duration of chemotherapy in colorectal carcinoma with distant metastases are not yet defined. We do not know whether continuous, long-term chemotherapy until the desired result of complete remission extends overall survival compared to a discontinuous scheme. Furthermore, a successful scheme may be made less effective by dose-limiting toxicity or may even have to be stopped. Then again, it may be decided to use a less effective strategy with fewer side-effects for patients who are in poor general condition.

Systemic chemotherapy for liver metastases of a limited extent has uncertain results and is expensive, and its toxicity has a negative impact on the patient's quality of life. These factors support the use of well-tolerated, localized treatment when visible, non-resectable liver metastases of limited extent are first diagnosed. Several minimally invasive approaches to liver lesions have been tested successfully recently, in particular RF and LITT, and have resulted in high local tumor control rates. CT-guided HDR brachytherapy is thought to be of additional value in more extensive disease, or when the tumor's location is unfavorable or if the specific setting at the hospital is appropriate (Vogl et al. 2004; Mulier et al. 2005).

At our institution, we implemented for evaluation purposes a phase III trial in unselected patients with unresectable liver malignancies of a colorectal primary after failure of second-line chemotherapy or where there were absolute or relative contraindications to chemotherapy (comorbidity, age, general condition) with promising results. Some patients were treated twice or more if limited intrahepatic progression was seen following the first treatment. Where possible, local recurrences were also treated twice, although these repeated treatments were excluded from analysis. Median overall survival after the first treatment after the longest follow-up of 3 years was 24 months (95% confidence interval: 20.19–28.77 months), and median progression-free survival was 7.8 months. The data to date indicate that the reference dosages should be 20–25 Gy, especially in the long run (Fig. 2.6.5). The cost of supplies are approximately 100€ per session. Careful examination of the results, looking at the comparability of unselected patients (who have had other tumor-specific therapies following brachytherapy), showed that they are promising, which suggests that HDR brachytherapy and other local ablative therapies have a place in the oncologist's armamentarium (Ricke et al. 2004b, 2004d, 2005a, 2005b; Ruhl and Ricke 2006; Wieners et al. 2006) (Fig. 2.6.6).

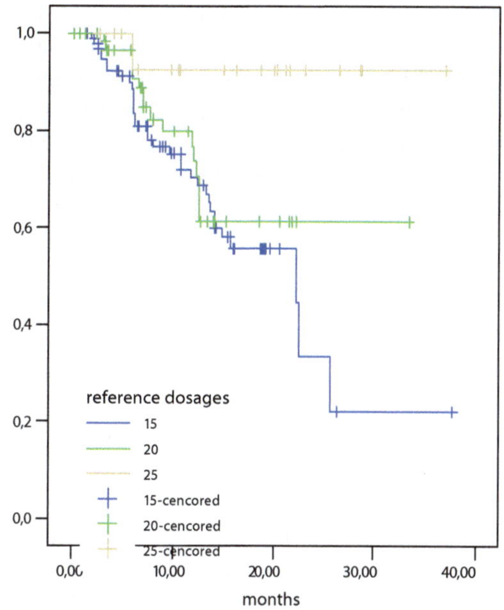

Fig. 2.6.5. Colorectal liver metastases: local control in months depended on reference dose (n=199)

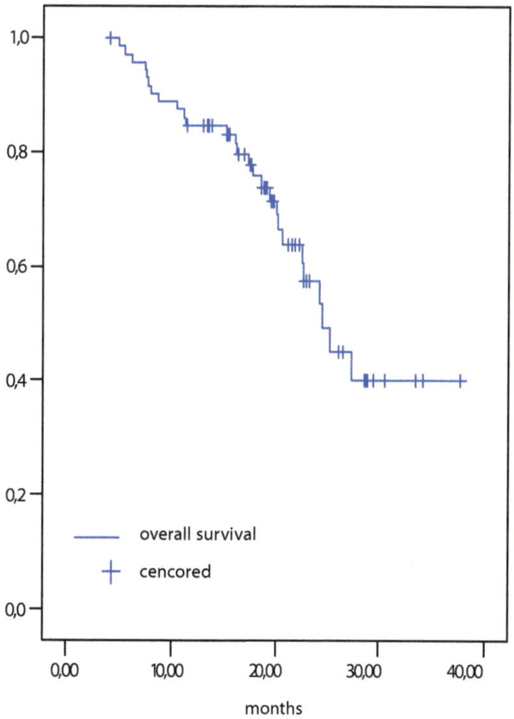

Fig. 2.6.6. Colorectal liver metastases: overall survival after treatment in months

2.6.3.2 Hepatocellular Carcinomas

Since systemic chemotherapies have not been proven to be beneficial in the treatment of hepatocellular carcinomas (HCC) (Nowak et al. 2004), various regional or local tumor ablation techniques have emerged as the most common therapeutic alternatives.

Transarterial chemoembolization (TACE) has widely been proposed as the palliative treatment of choice. However, most data indicate a limited benefit from TACE in patients with advanced liver cirrhosis (Llovet et al. 2003). In the past percutaneous tumor ablation by radiofrequency (RFA) or laser-induced thermo therapy (LITT) has supplemented ethanol injection. Any of these methods has limitations with respect to tumor size, perfusion and localization, as described above.

This prospective phase II trial included 29 consecutive patients with 34 unresectable intrahepatic HCC manifestations. The study population comprised 20 men and 9 women; the medium age was 66 years (43–79 years); 23 patients had liver cirrhosis grade Child A, and six Child B. Pre-interventional ascites was present in 7 patients (24%). The mean tumor diameter was 4.5 cm (1.5–10.5 cm). The median minimal dose inside the tumor volume was 20 Gy (12–25 Gy) applied as a single fraction. We used 1–13 brachytherapy applicators per tumor. During follow-up, MRI was performed 3 days, 6 weeks and every 3 months post treatment, supplemented by clinical examinations and serological liver function tests. Primary endpoints were local tumor control after 12 months as well as safety. Secondary endpoints were progression-free survival and overall survival.

Local tumor control was 93% after 12 months in surviving patients. A progression-free survival was observed in 79% of patients after 6 months and 54% after 12 months. Overall survival was 100% after 6 months and 88% after 12 months (Wieners 2007) (Fig. 2.6.7).

2.6.3.3 Liver Metastases of Breast Carcinomas

We prospectively analyzed 22 patients with breast cancer and 49 hepatic metastases. All patients were pretreated with systemic chemotherapy in several cycles. Reference doses were at minimum 12 Gy, at maximum 25 Gy, and median follow-up 10 months (range: 2–37 months). Three local recurrences (6%)

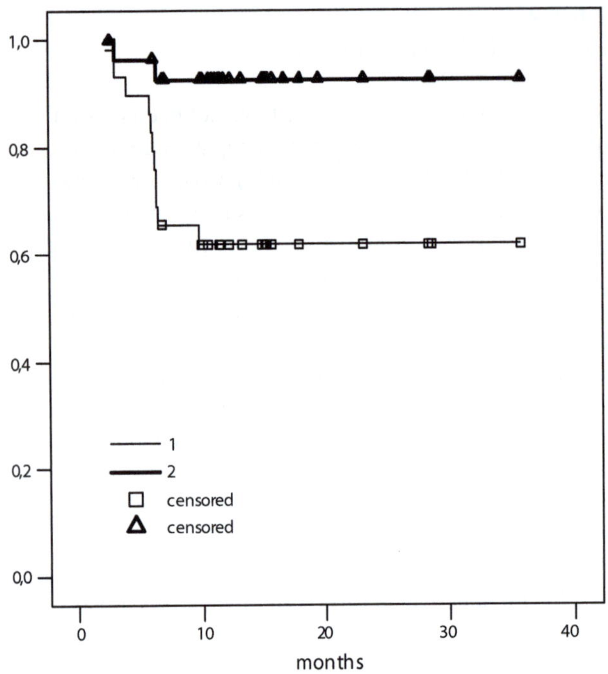

Fig. 2.6.7. Hepatocellular carcinoma (*HCC*): local control (*1*) and progression-free survival (*2*)

were seen during follow-up at 3, 6, and 9 months after the intervention, leading to a local tumor control rate of 94% after 6 months and 89% after 12 months, with no differences between groups.

Progression-free survival was 45% after 6 months and 23% after 12 months; overall survival was 95% after 6 months and 72% after 12 months.

2.6.4 Extrahepatic Malignancies

2.6.4.1 Primary and Secondary Lung Lesions

Thermal ablation of lung malignancies has been evaluated recently (Rose et al. 2002; Hosten et al. 2003; Suh et al. 2003; Ahmed et al. 2004; Akeboshi et al. 2004; Diederich and Hosten 2004; Knappe and Mols 2004; Lencioni et al. 2004; Vogl et al. 2004b, 2004c; de Baere et al. 2006; Hiraki et al. 2006a, 2006b; Kishi et al. 2006). In this setting, only CT guidance seems to be valuable for the insertion of therapeutic tools and therapeutic monitoring.

This prospective phase I trial included 15 patients with 30 lung malignancies (28 metastases and 2 NSCLC), with a median follow-up of 5+ months and a local tumor control rate of 97% (Ricke et al. 2005b). Median lesion diameter was 2 cm (0.6–11 cm), and the reference dose 20 Gy for all lesions (Ricke 2005).

2.6.4.2 Extrahepatic, Extrapulmonary Secondary Malignancies

This prospective study included 19 patients of median age 66 years (49–77 years). Underlying primaries comprised colorectal carcinomas in six patients, renal cell carcinoma in three patients, pancreatic carcinoma in three patients, cervical cancer in two, endometrial cancer in two, and NSCLC, breast cancer and sarcoma each in one patient. All patients had undergone extensive pretreatments.

The median tumor diameter was 6 cm (2–15 cm). Tumor locations included the hepatoduodenal ligament, mesentery, adrenal gland, mesogastrium, and local recurrences after rectal or pancreatic cancer. The minimal median dose in the target volume was 11 Gy (4–18 Gy). Median follow-up was 7 months (1–16). Four patients (21%) died during the follow-up period. Local tumor control was 76.5% after 6 months; progression-free survival, 47% after 6 months (Wieners 2006).

2.6.5 Minor and Major Complications

Typical side-effects comprise moderate gastric and intestinal toxicity, mostly effectively prevented by peri-nterventionally given antiemetic drugs and commonly limited to the day of treatment. For sedation and pain management during the intervention we administrate fentanyl and midazolam i.v.

The general condition is moderately affected and a raised temperature for up to 1 week after the intervention are frequent complications, as are a moderate leukocytosis, and elevated C-reactive protein and liver enzymes.

In comparison with other conditions, HCC has significant major complications strongly linked to the presence of cirrhosis, with a 10% rate of major complications, including bleeding requiring treatment and major pleural effusion and other events correlated with the comorbidity of these patients. Surprisingly, no clinically relevant radiation-induced liver disease was seen, even in cases of advanced cirrhosis. A lack of liver function in the months after treatment was strongly correlated with progressive intrahepatic disease.

2.6.5.1 In Vivo Assessment of the Tolerable Gastric Mucosal Dose

This study included 33 consecutive patients with liver malignancies in segments II and/or III treated by CT-guided HDR brachytherapy. The prescribed minimal doses in the target volume ranged from 15 to 25 Gy applied as a single fraction. All patients received gastric protection post treatment (pantoprazole 40 mg/day for 3 months and Magaldrat if required). For further analysis, the contours of the gastric wall in every CT slice were defined employing Brachyvision® Software (Fig. 2.6.2). Dose–volume histograms were calculated for each individual treatment and correlated with clinical data derived from questionnaires assessing Common Toxicity Criteria (CTC). In addition, all patients presenting symptoms of upper gastrointestinal toxicity were examined endoscopically.

Summarizing all patients, the minimum dose applied to 1 ml of the gastric wall ($D_{1\,\mathrm{ml}}$) ranged from 6.3 Gy to 34.2 Gy; the median dose was 14.3 Gy. Toxicity was present in 18 patients (55%), nausea in 16 (69%), emesis in 9 (27%), cramping in 13 (39%), weight loss in 12 (36%), gastritis in 4 (12%), and ulceration in 5 patients (15%). Ulceration CTC Grades 2 and 1 occurred in 2 (6%) and 3 (9%) patients, respectively. None of the patients showed a toxicity of Grade 3 or higher. A threshold dose $D_{1\,\mathrm{ml}}$ of 11 Gy was found to lead to general gastric toxicity and 15.5 Gy to statistically relevant gastric ulceration (Streitparth 2006).

2.6.6 Coming Soon...

In recent years, over 1000 liver malignancies have been treated by our group, as have lung malignancies, lymph node metastases, and other specific lesions. Follow-up is now for a long enough period to conclude reliable tumor control and survival rates, which will be published in the future.

It is our firm conviction that CT-guided HDR brachytherapy features incontrovertible advantages, particularly when treating tumors that are large and close to blood vessels; indeed the exact dosimetry that can be achieved allows protection of even adjacent structures from the effects of radiation. Accordingly, sensitive regions such as the retroperitoneal space, the mediastinal space or interloop locations are certainly accessible.

The establishment of preoperative evaluation, targeted treatments of metabolically active lesions and follow-up with MRI and PET/CT will allow the discontinuation of systemic therapy (Antoch et al. 2004; Amthauer et al. 2006). CT guidance will cease in favor of an MRI-based procedure.

References

Ahmed M, Liu Z, Afzal KS, Weeks D, Lobo SM, Kruskal JB et al (2004) Radiofrequency ablation: effect of surrounding tissue composition on coagulation necrosis in a canine tumor model. Radiology 230(3):761–767

Akeboshi M, Yamakado K, Nakatsuka A, Hataji O, Taguchi O, Takao M et al (2004) Percutaneous radiofrequency ablation of lung neoplasms: initial therapeutic response. J Vasc Interv Radiol 15(5):463–470

Amthauer H, Denecke T, Hildebrandt B, Ruhl R, Miersch A, Nicolaou A et al (2006) Evaluation of patients with liver metastases from colorectal cancer for locally ablative treatment with laser induced thermotherapy – impact of PET with F-18-fluorodeoxyglucose on therapeutic decisions. Nuklearmedizin 45(4):177–184

Antoch G, Kaiser GM, Mueller AB, Metz KA, Zhang H, Kuehl H et al (2004) Intraoperative radiation therapy in liver tissue in a pig model: monitoring with dual-modality PET/CT. Radiology 230(3):753–760

Bergk A, Wieners G, Weich V, Wiedenmann B, Berg T, Ricke J (2005) CT-guided brachytherapy of hepatocellular carcinoma in liver cirrhosis – a novel therapeutic approach. J Hepatol 42:89

de Baere T, Palussiere J, Auperin A, Hakime A, Abdel-Rehim M, Kind M et al (2006) Midterm local efficacy and survival after radiofrequency ablation of lung tumors with minimum follow-up of 1 year: prospective evaluation. Radiology 240(2):587–596

Diederich S, Hosten N (2004) Percutaneous ablation of pulmonary tumours: state-of-the-art 2004. Radiologe 44(7):658–662

Dritschilo A, Grant EG, Harter KW, Holt RW, Rustgi SN, Rodgers JE (1986) Interstitial radiation therapy for hepatic metastases: sonographic guidance for applicator placement. AJR Am J Roentgenol 147(2):275–278

Dritschilo A, Harter KW, Thomas D, Nauta R, Holt R, Lee TC et al (1988) Intraoperative radiation therapy of hepatic metastases: technical aspects and report of a pilot study. Int J Radiat Oncol Biol Phys 14(5):1007–1011

Eichler K, Mack MG, Straub R, Engelmann K, Zangos S, Woitaschek D et al (2001) Oligonodular hepatocellular carcinoma (HCC): MR-controlled laser-induced thermotherapy. Radiologe 41(10):915–922

Folprecht G, Kohne CH (2004) New therapy options in colorectal carcinoma. Ther Umsch 61(6):373–378

Hiraki T, Sakurai J, Tsuda T, Gobara H, Sano Y, Mukai T et al (2006a) Risk factors for local progression after percutaneous radiofrequency ablation of lung tumors: evaluation based on a preliminary review of 342 tumors. Cancer 107(12):2873–2880

Hiraki T, Tajiri N, Mimura H, Yasui K, Gobara H, Mukai T et al (2006b) Pneumothorax, pleural effusion, and chest tube placement after radiofrequency ablation of lung tumors: incidence and risk factors. Radiology 241(1):275–283

Holt RW, Nauta RJ, Lee TC, Heres EK, Dritschilo A, Harter KW et al (1988) Intraoperative interstitial radiation therapy for hepatic metastases from colorectal carcinomas. Am Surg 54(4):231–233

Hosten N, Stier A, Weigel C, Kirsch M, Puls R, Nerger U et al (2003) Laser-induced thermotherapy (LITT) of lung metastases: description of a miniaturized applicator, optimization, and initial treatment of patients. Rofo 175(3):393–400

Kishi K, Nakamura H, Kobayashi K, Hashimoto T, Hatao H, Oh-ishi S et al (2006) Percutaneous CT-guided radiofrequency ablation of pulmonary malignant tumors: preliminary report. Intern Med 45(2):65–72

Knappe V, Mols A (2004) Laser therapy of the lung: biophysical background. Radiologe 44(7):677–683

Lencioni R, Crocetti L, Cioni R, Mussi A, Fontanini G, Ambrogi M et al (2004) Radiofrequency ablation of lung malignancies: where do we stand? Cardiovasc Intervent Radiol 27(6):581–590

Llovet JM, Burroughs A, Bruix J (2003) Hepatocellular carcinoma. Lancet 362(9399):1907–1917

Mulier S, Ni Y, Jamart J, Ruers T, Marchal G, Michel L (2005) Local recurrence after hepatic radiofrequency coagulation: multivariate meta-analysis and review of contributing factors. Ann Surg 242(2):158–171

Nauta RJ, Heres EK, Thomas DS, Harter KW, Rodgers JE, Holt RW et al (1987) Intraoperative single-dose radiotherapy. Observations on staging and interstitial treatment of unresectable liver metastases. Arch Surg 122(12):1392–1395

Nowak AK, Chow PK, Findlay M (2004) Systemic therapy for advanced hepatocellular carcinoma: a review. Eur J Cancer 40(10):1474–1484

Pech M, Spors B, Wieners G, Warschewske G, Beck A, Cho C et al (2004) Comparison of different MRI sequences with and without application of Gd-BOPTA as follow-up after LITT. Rofo 176(4):550–555

Pech M, Mohnike K, Wieners G, Bialek E, Lopez HE, Dudek O, Fischbach F, Felix R, Wust P, Ricke J (2006) Irradiation of liver metastases: influence of imaging modality on target volume and dose-volume-histograms. (in press)

Punt CJ (2004) New options and old dilemmas in the treatment of patients with advanced colorectal cancer. Ann Oncol 15(10):1453–1459

Qian J, Feng GS, Vogl T (2003) Combined interventional therapies of hepatocellular carcinoma. World J Gastroenterol 9(9):1885–1891

Rhim H (2003) Percutaneous radiofrequency ablation therapy for patients with hepatocellular carcinoma during occlusion of hepatic blood flow: comparison with standard percutaneous radiofrequency ablation therapy. Cancer 98(2):433–434

Ricke J (2004) Interventional therapy for liver metastases. Z Gastroenterol 42(11):1321–1328

Ricke J, Wust PG, Werk M, Pech M, Beck AN, Stohlmann A (2002) CT-guided brachytherapy of liver metastasis alone or in combination with laser induced thermo therapy (LITT): Safety and efficacy. Radiology 225:447

Ricke J, Sehouli J, Hach C, Hanninen EL, Lichtenegger W, Felix R (2003) Prospective evaluation of contrast-enhanced MRI in the depiction of peritoneal spread in primary or recurrent ovarian cancer. Eur Radiol 13(5):943–949

Ricke J, Wust P, Stohlmann A, Beck A, Cho CH, Pech M et al (2004a) CT-guided brachytherapy. A novel percutaneous technique for interstitial ablation of liver malignancies. Strahlenther Onkol 180(5):274–280

Ricke J, Wust P, Stohlmann A, Beck A, Cho CH, Pech M et al (2004b) CT-guided interstitial brachytherapy of liver malignancies alone or in combination with thermal ablation: phase I–II results of a novel technique. Int J Radiat Oncol Biol Phys 58(5):1496–1505

Ricke J, Wust P, Wieners G, Beck A, Cho CH, Seidensticker M et al (2004c) Liver malignancies: CT-guided interstitial brachytherapy in patients with unfavorable lesions for thermal ablation. J Vasc Interv Radiol 15(11):1279–1286

Ricke J, Wust P, Hengst S, Wieners G, Pech M, Herzog H et al (2004d) CT-guided interstitial brachytherapy of lung malignancies. Technique and first results. Radiologe 44(7):684–686

Ricke J, Wust P, Stohlmann A, Beck A, Cho CH, Pech M et al (2004e) CT-guided brachytherapy. A novel percutaneous technique for interstitial ablation of liver metastases. Strahlenther Onkol 180(5):274–280

Ricke J, Seidensticker M, Ludemann L, Pech M, Wieners G, Hengst S et al (2005a) In vivo assessment of the tolerance dose of small liver volumes after single-fraction HDR irradiation. Int J Radiat Oncol Biol Phys 62(3):776–784

Ricke J, Wust P, Wieners G, Hengst S, Pech M, Lopez HE et al (2005b) CT-guided interstitial single-fraction brachytherapy of lung tumors: phase I results of a novel technique. Chest 127(6):2237–2242

Rose SC, Fotoohi M, Levin DL, Harrell JH (2002) Cerebral microembolization during radiofrequency ablation of lung malignancies. J Vasc Interv Radiol 13(10):1051–1054

Ruhl R, Ricke J (2006) Image-guided micro-therapy for tumor ablation: from thermal coagulation to advanced irradiation techniques. Onkologie 29(5):219–224

Sakr AA, Saleh AA, Moeaty AA, Moeaty AA (2005) The combined effect of radiofrequency and ethanol ablation in the management of large hepatocellular carcinoma. Eur J Radiol 54(3):418–425

Strehl R (2006) Finanzierungsprobleme der modernen Krebsmedizin in Deutschland. Studium Generale Vorlesung an der Eberhard-Karls-Universität Tübingen am 20.06.06

Streitparth F, Pech M, Bohmig M, Ruehl R, Peters N, Wieners G et al (2006) In vivo assessment of the gastric mucosal tolerance dose after single fraction, small volume irradiation of liver malignancies by computed tomography-guided, high-dose-rate brachytherapy. Int J Radiat Oncol Biol Phys 65(5):1479–1486

Suh RD, Wallace AB, Sheehan RE, Heinze SB, Goldin JG (2003) Unresectable pulmonary malignancies: CT-guided percutaneous radiofrequency ablation – preliminary results. Radiology 229(3):821–829

Thomas DS, Nauta RJ, Rodgers JE, Popescu GF, Nguyen H, Lee TC et al (1993) Intraoperative high-dose rate interstitial irradiation of hepatic metastases from colorectal carcinoma. Results of a phase I–II trial. Cancer 71(6):1977–1981

Vogl TJ, Straub R, Eichler K, Sollner O, Mack MG (2004a) Colorectal carcinoma metastases in liver: laser-induced interstitial thermotherapy–local tumor control rate and survival data. Radiology 230(2):450–458

Vogl TJ, Straub R, Lehnert T, Eichler K, Luder-Luhr T, Peters J et al (2004b) Percutaneous thermoablation of pulmonary metastases. Experience with the application of laser-induced thermotherapy (LITT) and radiofrequency ablation (RFA), and a literature review. Rofo 176(11):1658–1666

Vogl TJ, Fieguth HG, Eichler K, Straub R, Lehnert T, Zangos S et al (2004c) Laser-induced thermotherapy of lung metastases and primary lung tumors. Radiologe 44(7):693–699

Wieners G, Pech M, Rudzinska M, Lehmkuhl L, Wlodarczyk W, Miersch A et al (2006) CT-guided interstitial brachytherapy in the local treatment of extrahepatic, extrapulmonary secondary malignancies. Eur Radiol 16(11):2586–2593

Zangos S, Eichler K, Balzer JO, Straub R, Hammerstingl R, Herzog C et al (2007) Large-sized hepatocellular carcinoma (HCC): a neoadjuvant treatment protocol with repetitive transarterial chemoembolization (TACE) before percutaneous MR-guided laser-induced thermotherapy (LITT). Eur Radiol 17(2):553–563

Ablative Techniques (Percutaneous)

Actinic Ablative Techniques

2

2.7 Selective Internal Radiation Therapy

Thomas K. Helmberger

CONTENTS

T. K. Helmberger, MD
Professor, Department of Diagnostic and Interventional Radiology and Nuclear Medicine, Klinikum Bogenhausen, Academic Teaching Hospital of the Technical University Munich, Engelschalkinger Strasse 77, 81925 Munich, Germany

2.7.1 Background

The majority of primary and secondary malignant hepatic tumors are not suitable for surgical resection, which makes systemic chemotherapy treatments and/or local ablative therapies important components of intention-to-treat concepts or palliation. Tumor load and type of response determine the efficacy of these therapies.

Nevertheless, a considerable number of patients are either not or are no longer suitable for these therapies even when the tumor load remains confined to the liver.

Given the fact that ionizing radiation is very effective in tumor control, radiation therapy of the liver is crucial because normal hepatic parenchyma is more sensitive than tumorous tissue to radiation. The "curative" dosage for adenocarcinoma cells – the most common tumor type with respect to primary and secondary hepatic malignancies – is in the range of 70–90 Gy. Therefore, external beam radiation or interstitial brachytherapy of the liver is limited by the dilemma posed by the need for the high dosage necessary to destroy tumor tissue sufficiently whilst simultaneously protecting the normal parenchyma and adjacent anatomical structures. According to a recent dose escalation study presented by Dawson et al. (2000), the risk of substantial liver damage is low if the radiation volume is less than 20% of the total liver volume even in dosages of more than 100 Gy. However, in clinical reality commonly the tumor load does not allow the radiation beam to be limited to such volumes.

Considering these obstacles, the concept of interstitial blood-flow-derived radiation therapy was developed more than 15 years ago using two main concepts. In iodine-131 lipiodol (Stefanovic et al. 2001) embolization therapy, ^{131}I-labeled iodized oil is suspended in lipiodol (Lipiodol Ultra Fluide, Laboratoires Guerbet, Aulnay-sous-Bois, France) and the entire compound is used as in "standard" transarterial chemoembolization (TACE, see Chap. 2.5). In contrast, in droplet emulsion embolization in combination with chemotherapy, as in TACE, radioactive microparticles are used for selective internal radiotherapy (SIRT).

2.7.2 Principle of Interstitial Radiation Therapy

2.7.2.1 Radioembolization

In contrast to external beam radiation ^{90}Y microspheres represent point sources of radiation with a very limited radiation range of a few millimeters. Moreover, radioembolization in terms of SIRT combines two different therapeutic principles: (1) embolization by microparticles acting as the carrier of the radiation, resulting in microvascular occlusion, with (2) simultaneous brachytherapy by implantation of radioactive microparticles. Assuming an increased peri- and intratumoral (neo-)vascularization the microparticles will deliver a very high dose of radiation rather selectively to the tumor tissue, with reduced radiation exposure to the surrounding normal tissue.

In principle, the pathophysiological substrate is the same as in "classic" TACE: most primary and secondary malignant hepatic tumors with a diameter of more than 3 mm induce arterial neo-vascularization, which results in an arterial-dominant blood supply of 80%–100%.

Technical aspects apply to both of these therapies, as known from classic transarterial (chemo-) embolization and percutaneous catheter-directed brachytherapy with microembolization using a local-acting substance to destroy tissues.

2.7.2.2 Physical Properties of ^{90}Y Microparticles

Currently, there are two different ^{90}Y preparations available on the market: glass and resin microspheres (Tables 2.7.1, 2.7.2). In both products ^{90}Y is bound to a microparticle. Since these loaded microparticles present no pharmacological effects, rather "physico-mechanical" ones, they are considered to be medical devices in terms of a therapeutic radioactive implant and not a drug. The glass microspheres are available in USA, Canada, and recently in Europe; the resin particles are available worldwide (Gray et al. 1989; Kennedy and Salem 2003; Wollner et al. 1988).

Table 2.7.1. Properties of resin and glass microspheres loaded with ^{90}Y isotopes

	Resin	Glass
Trade name	SIRSpheres® (SIRTEX Medical, Sydney, Australia)	TheraSpheres® (MDS Nordion, Ottawa, Ontario, Canada)
Size (µm)	20–60	20–30
Embolic effect	Moderate	Minor
Specific gravity (g/dl)	1.6	3.6
Activity per particle (Bq)	50	2500
Available activity (GBq)	3	3, 5, 7, 10, 15, 20
Half-life (h)	64.2	64.2
Time to near-complete decay (2.5% residual activity) (days)	13	13
Number of microspheres per 3 GBq (70 mCi) per vial	40–80 million	~1.2–8.0 million
Material	^{90}Y bound to resin	^{90}Y in glass matrix
Solution used for suspension	Sterile water	NaCl

Table 2.7.2. Application details of resin and glass ^{90}Y microspheres

	SIRSpheres®	TheraSpheres®
Institutional review board	Supervision not required	Supervision required
Approval category	FDA, CE	FDA, CE
Indication for use	Hepatocellular carcinoma	Hepatocellular carcinoma, colorectal metastases
Dose dependent on tumor volume	Yes	No
Limiting hepatopulmonary shunt volume	20%	10%
Combination with chemotherapy	Yes	No

^{90}Y is generated by neutron bombardment of ^{89}Y in a nuclear generator. The resulting ^{90}Y is a high-energy beta emitter with an average energy of 0.9367 MeV and a maximum energy of 2.27 MeV. In biological tissue the average penetration of the emitted beta-radiation is 2.5 mm with a maximum range of up to 1.1 cm whereas 1 GBq (27 mCi) of ^{90}Y results in a total dose of 50 Gy/kg in tissue. ^{90}Y has a half-life of 64.2 hours and decays to stable zirconium-90. After 2 weeks the activity has decreased to 2.5% of the original activity.

The ^{90}Y microparticles are suspended in sterile, pyrogen-free water (SIR-Spheres®, Sirtex Medical, Sydney, Australia) or in NaCl (Thera-Spheres®, MDS Nordion, Ottawa, Ontario, Canada) ready for injection. Due to the ionic properties of the resin particles, the vendor does not permit solution with NaCl or contrast media, due to potential clotting of the particles. Due to the strong binding of ^{90}Y to resin or glass, no leach of ^{90}Y is observed. Once, the ^{90}Y activity is decayed the inactive particles stay inert and in place.

2.7.3 Indications and Contraindications

In the USA, SIRT was approved for the treatment of unresectable primary hepatic malignancies and metastases from colorectal cancer together with intrahepatic artery chemotherapy (IHAC) using floxuridine (FUDR). Nevertheless, worldwide SIRT may be used in patients with hepatic malignancies originating from various primaries, such as neuroendocrine tumors, breast, colorectal, and bronchial cancer, where the disease appears to be limited to the liver and other treatment options are no longer available.

In general, the ideal patient for SIRT has liver-dominant disease only (Table 2.7.3). Extrahepatic disease may be present, but should not determine the patient's survival. A typical example of this situation is a patient with hepatic breast cancer metastases – a rising indication beside the approved indications in HCC and colorectal cancer metastases – where often additional bone metastases are present but under clinical control by a bisphosphonate and hormone therapy for example. Nevertheless, one must always be aware that SIRT is a hepatic-directed treatment that does not affect extrahepatic disease (Fig. 2.7.1).

The decision to undertake ^{90}Y microembolization should be made following the consent of an interdisciplinary team from interventional radiology, nuclear medicine, radiotherapy, medical and surgical oncology, and transplantation medicine, since a wide variety of conditions and parameters have to be considered (Table 2.7.3).

Since possible surgical resection is a definitive exclusion criterion, the basic concept of SIRT is palliative. Furthermore, there is no commonly accepted concept making a patient eligible for SIRT and so other palliative therapies have to be taken into account. While external beam radiation is indicated and possible in only rare cases, first- and second-line chemotherapy is the standard concept in treating hepatic metastases, while TACE is applied in hepatocellular tumors. In clinical reality, many patients are referred or self-refer when many adjuvant therapies have already been performed. In consequence, the team has to re-evaluate the effects of the prior treatments, together with potential new therapy options and the recent staging of disease, incorporating also the concepts of down-staging and radiation or chemo sensitization.

While liver function can be altered by the tumor burden itself, most chemotherapies may deteriorate

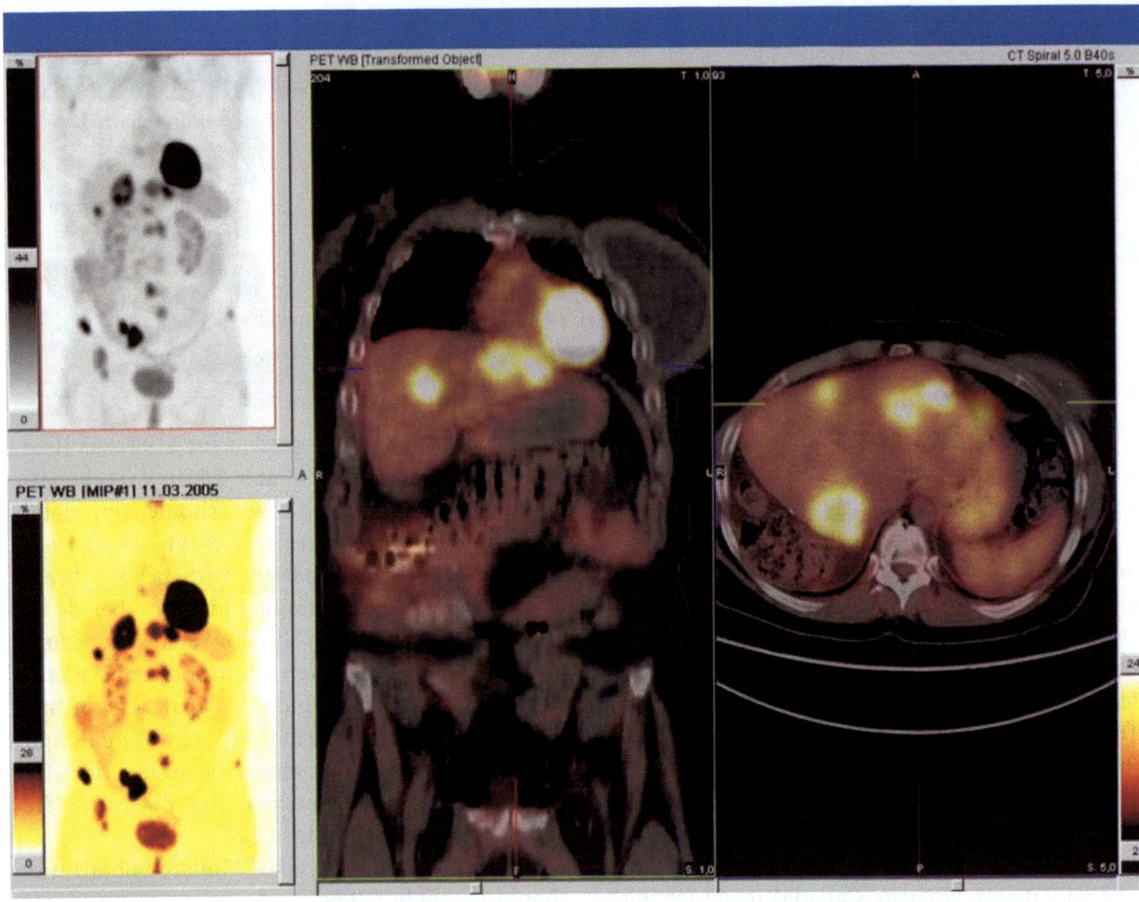

Fig. 2.7.1. Staging before planned ^{90}Y therapy in a patient with a history of breast cancer: CT-PET confirms the known hepatic metastases but also reveals multifocal lymph node metastases resulting in systemic chemotherapy

Table 2.7.3. Considerations for the use of selective internal radiotherapy (*SIRT*) in hepatic malignancies

Indication	Contraindication
• Tumors not suitable for surgical resection for cure (HCC, colorectal cancer metastases approved by the regulatory authorities, metastases from other primaries can be treated accordingly with intention-to-treat but as yet without sufficient study basis) • Tumors not suitable for local ablative therapy such as radiofrequency and laser ablation • Patient not eligible for transplantation in the case of hepatocellular carcinoma • No clinically dominant extrahepatic disease • No life-expectancy-determining concomitant disease • Life expectancy > 3 months • Sufficient performance status or Karnofsky score (ECOG PS 0–2, Karnofsky score > 60%; see Table 2.7.4) • Angiographically suitable access to the hepatic vasculature	• Disseminated, clinically dominant extrahepatic disease • Tumor volume > 50% of liver volume • Portal vein thrombosis • Lung shunting > 20% • Liver failure ± ascites (bilirubin > 2.0–3.0 ng/dl, albumin < 3 g/dl) • Reflux of hepatic arterial blood to the stomach, pancreas or bowel in preassessment angiography and MAA nuclear scan which cannot be corrected by angiographic interventional techniques • Previous external beam radiation therapy to the liver • Treatment with capecitabine within the previous 2 months, or planned treatment with capecitabine at any time following SIRT (increased risk of fatal liver failure!)

hepatic synthesis, which exposes the patient to an increased risk of hepatic failure in immediate combination with SIRT. Therefore, it is mandatory to discontinue chemotherapy 2–4 weeks before a potential SIRT. This is especially true in cases where known radio-sensitizing chemotherapeutic substances, such as 5-fluorouracil, gemcitabine or capecitabine, were utilized, which may cause fatal complications in concurrent application (Kulik et al. 2005, 2006; Lewandowski et al. 2005; Salem et al. 2005).

Besides the specific situation of the liver, the decision to use SIRT requires complete staging to exclude potential extrahepatic tumor spread, which is a contraindication to this treatment. The staging will incorporate whole-body CT, MRI or PET/PET-CT. A MRI scan of the head is necessary to exclude occult brain metastases. In general, the interval between staging and final treatment should not be longer than 6 weeks.

Table 2.7.4. Patient's performance status according to Eastern Cooperative Oncology Group (ECOG) and Karnofsky score

ECOG scale	Karnofsky score (%)	Performance status
0	100	Clinically asymptomatic, fully active
1	80–90	Symptomatic; fully ambulatory; restricted in physically strenuous activity
2	60–70	Symptomatic; ambulatory; capable of self-care; >50% of waking hours are spent out of bed
3	40–50	Symptomatic; limited self-care; spends <50% of time in bed
4	20–30	Completely disabled; no self-care; bedridden

2.7.4 Treatment Planning

Given the fact that the patient is considered eligible for SIRT in general (see above), several factors determining the eligibility for the specific treatment have to be checked:

- liver function
- type of tumor load
- vascular anatomy and specific tumor supply
- pulmonary shunting
- dose calculation

2.7.4.1 Liver Function

Regarding liver function, patients who are in general eligible for SIRT, based on the stage of their disease, must be considered able to tolerate the ^{90}Y microsphere embolization. This is because SIRT radiation may induce hepatitis, such that pre-existing liver function deterioration may become irreversible loss of liver function.

Liver function scoring systems such as Okuda and Child-Pugh classification, together with assessment of the general performance status (i.e., Karnofsky score, ECOG scale; Table 2.7.4), are essential to assess the patient's hepatic and general condition prior to SIRT (Lewandowski et al. 2005; Salem et al. 2005).

In HCC altered liver function is often determined by the underlying disease, such as hepatitis and cirrhosis, which may also settle the overall life quality and expectancy. The most reliable laboratory parameters for liver function are prothrombin time, albumin, and bilirubin, where normal values indicate a significantly better outcome in any therapy (Tateishi et al. 2005; Varela et al. 2003). Tumor markers such as alpha-fetoprotein – significantly elevated in HCC in about two-thirds of cases – and C-reactive protein may be used mainly for follow-up to assess the response (Hashimoto et al. 2005).

In contrast to HCC, increased bilirubin levels in metastatic liver disease arise more from biliary obstruction in infiltrative and end-stage disease than from chemotherapy toxicity (Goin et al. 2005).

2.7.4.2 Hepatic Tumor Load

Hepatic tumor spread can be unifocal, multifocal or diffuse, limited to single segments, lobes or bilobar multisegmental. Depending on the general stage of disease and the patient's overall performance, resection and even transplantation must be considered in HCC and sometimes in cholangiocellular carcinoma if the tumor load and growth are limited and delineated. However, in most cases of primary and secondary hepatic malignancies resection is no longer possible due to the tumor's extent and/or the secondary and tertiary tumor manifestations. If the tumor manifestation is limited by size and number local ablative techniques such as radiofrequency and laser ablation must be considered (see Chap. 2.1).

The liver's functional capacity may be determined by its basic function, depending on the underlying disease and potentially concomitant therapies that might have affected its function, furthermore by the amount of hepatic tumor mass in relation to the total liver volume and the patient's general performance status. Since SIRT id applied usually in multifocal, more or less wide spread or diffuse liver tumors even in selective and superselective administration also normal hepatic tissue will be targeted beside the tumor. Therefore, to preserve sufficient functional reserve after SIRT, the estimated or calculated hepatic tumor volume must not exceed 40%–50% of total liver volume. Radioembolization of such volumes will substantially affect residual normal liver tissue, increasing the risk of jeopardizing the liver's functional capacity. However, in clinical practice patients with such high tumor volumes are mostly no longer eligible for SIRT because of concomitant extrahepatic tumor manifestations. Thus, in our experience of about 100 cases, average tumor volume did not exceed 15% of total liver volume.

2.7.4.3 Vascular Anatomy

In principle, SIRT is based on the general vascular accessibility of the liver and the hepatic tumor load. Therefore, detailed knowledge of the hepatic vascular anatomy and the specific tumor supply is mandatory. It is particularly necessary to identify the accessory right arteries and a potential middle hepatic artery to assess the entire supply.

Pretreatment angiography must also be used to evaluate the celiac and mesenteric vascular route, including the gastroduodenal and gastric arteries, and to identify potential variants and anomalies in order to avoid aberrant and/or incomplete embolization. The latter is possible if accessory hepatic and/or tumor-feeding arteries are not recognized. In contrast, a planned SIRT must be reconsidered if the tumor manifestation is not detectable angiographically.

Reflux of microspheres during the delivery process due to altered flow dynamics may end up in aberrant embolization, which always causes severe complications such as actinic ulcerations, bleeding, cholecystitis, and pancreatitis. Unfortunately, the treatment of these complications can be only symptomatic. Therefore, aberrant particle embolization must be avoided, mainly by prophylactic selective coil embolization - a technique the interventional radiologist should be experienced in - of the gastroduodenal artery with potential variants of the supra- and retroduodenal arteries, potential gastric arteries arising from the left hepatic artery, esophageal artery, accessory phrenic and falciform artery, and sometimes also of the cystic artery (Fig. 2.7.2). Balloon occlusion techniques to direct the embolization into the target volume are in general not suitable because primarily the hypervascular flow dynamics to the tumor could be excluded. Additional negative effects might be potential vascular damage and "layering" of the microspheres, directing the particles into the descending part of the liver (Liu et al. 2005).

Based on the vascular road map the treatment plan must be tailored according to the specific vascular supply of the tumor(s) and the vessel-depen-

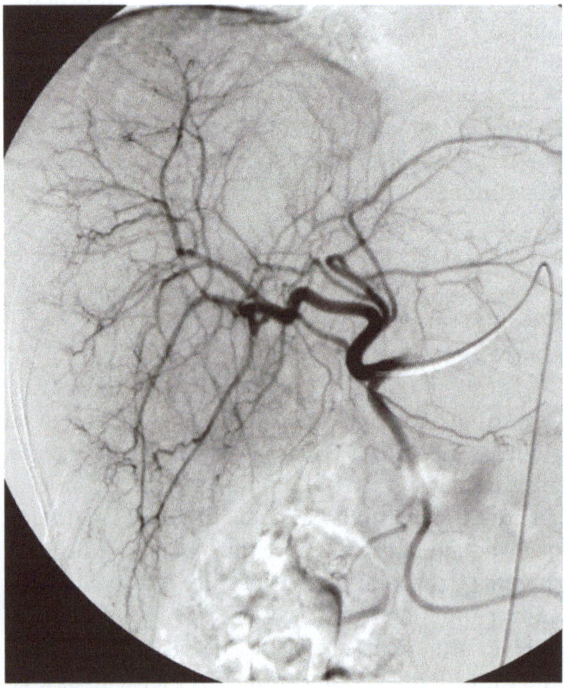

Fig. 2.7.2. Arteriography before ^{90}Y particle therapy presents no distinct tumor blushes but some vascular irregularities typical of neoangiogenesis

dent flow dynamics. This may result in subsequent particle delivery into several feeding arteries arising from the normal and variant hepatic vasculature. While calculation of the total desired dose is related to the tumor volume – calculated or estimated from cross-sectional imaging – the proportion of doses delivered to the tumor(s) has to be related to the vascular supply based on the volume of the targeted hepatic segment(s) or lobe. Therefore, it may be necessary to split the total calculated dose proportionally for delivery via all the tumor-supplying vessels. Nevertheless, these proportions are in general estimations since the tumor volume(s) calculated from cross-sectional data cannot be exactly correlated to the vascular supply volumes (for an exact correlative calculation, subsequent selective angiography of each single hepatic artery together with intra-arterial CT angiography to define each subsegment and volume would be necessary). However, in clinical practice the interventional radiologist will be able to correlate the cross-sectional with the angiographic findings and to estimate the respective dose proportions (Liu et al. 2005; Ho et al. 1996, 1997a, 1997b).

This estimation will be supported by the results of the technetium-99m macroaggregated albumin scanning (^{99m}Tc MAA scan) necessary to assess potential pulmonary shunting (see below).

2.7.4.4 Pulmonary Shunts

Radiation pneumonitis after ^{90}Y microsphere application is a severe complication with no substantial therapeutic options (Ho et al. 1996). The maximum tolerated dose to the lung is cumulatively 50 Gy, but will be much lower in patients with compromised pulmonary function, a common finding in the (mostly elderly) patient group eligible for SIRT.

While in HCC arterio-portal and arterio-venous shunting by direct tumor invasion is not uncommon, in metastases shunts are rare. Since the particle size of ^{99m}Tc MAA (30–90 µm) parallels that of the ^{90}Y microsphere, the distribution of the microspheres can be predicted by an intra-arterial MAA scan. After transcatheter injection of 4–5 mCi (148–185 MBq) ^{99m}Tc MAA into the estimated vascular territory of the tumor, intrahepatic distribution and potential pulmonary and also extrapulmonary shunting by aberrant, occult vessels can be assessed by a single photon emission CT (SPECT) gamma camera. The lung shunt fraction is calculated by the following equation:

$$\text{Lung shunt fraction} = \frac{\text{total lung counts}}{(\text{total lung counts} + \text{liver counts})}$$

Depending on the type (Table 2.7.2) of microsphere, a pulmonary shunt fraction of 10%–20% can be tolerated. Furthermore, one should be aware that evaluation of the shunt fraction can be influenced by several factors:

- degradation of ^{99m}Tc MAA during the interval between angiography and the SPECT scan can be followed by migration of smaller MAA fragments via the hepatic capillary bed to the lungs
- based on the production process of ^{99m}Tc MAA, there is a fraction of smaller MAA particles < 10 µm as well as a small fraction of free ^{99m}Tc passing to the lungs
- separation of the lung, liver, and abdominal counts depends on the exact definition of the areas of interest, which are marked manually by the nuclear medicine personnel.

2.7.5 Dosimetry and Dose Calculation

The dose calculation is based on the ratio of the tumor volume to the total liver volume, on the type of treatment (e.g., focal, lobar, whole liver), and whether resin or glass microspheres are used. To predict the distribution volume of the microspheres and to address the safety issues in terms of aberrant delivery, a pretreatment ^{99m}Tc MAA scan subsequent to the planning angiography is mandatory.

Depending on the differences regarding the loaded dose and the physical differences (Table 2.7.1) the dose calculation is different for resin and for glass ^{90}Y microspheres.

2.7.5.1 Resin ^{90}Y Microspheres

Resin ^{90}Y microspheres are delivered in V-bottomed vials containing 3 GBq in 5 ml water for injection on the day of treatment. In contrast to the glass microspheres, which may arrive a few days prior to the procedure, the total amount of the applied dose of resin ^{90}Y microspheres is customized to the tumor burden and potential lung shunting.

Following the vendor's recommendations the dose can be calculated by the body surface area method (BSA), and the empiric method. Comparing both calculation/estimation methods, the BSA calculation incorporates tumor burden and a correlation to liver mass, with liver mass increasing with BSA, while the empiric method is related only to the tumor burden.

In the author's own experience, comparing both methods the difference between the calculations varies less than 10%.

2.7.5.1.1 Body Surface Area Calculation

$$A_{\text{resin}}\ (\text{GBq}) = \text{body surface area}\ (\text{m}^2) - 0.2 + (\%\ \text{tumor involvement}/100),$$

where

A = activity.

$$\text{BSA}\ (\text{m}^2) = 0.20247 \times \text{height}\ (\text{m})^{0.725} \times \text{weight}\ (\text{kg})^{0.425}$$

2.7.5.1.2 Empiric Method

In this method the dose recommendation is based on estimation of the tumor burden:

Tumor involvement of the liver	A_{resin} (GBq)
<25%	2.0
25%–50%	2.5
50%	3.0
(>50%	no treatment)

In both methods a reduction of the total dose is recommended with respect to a potential lung shunt fraction (LSF):

LSF <10%	no reduction
LSF 10%–15%	20% reduction
LSF 15%–20%	40% reduction
LSF >20%	no treatment

2.7.5.2 Glass ^{90}Y Microspheres

In contrast to resin microspheres, the dose calculation for glass microspheres is defined by a nominal target dose (150 Gy/kg) and related to the liver mass without regard for the tumor burden, assuming a uniform distribution of the microspheres throughout the liver volume. The following formula is used for dose calculation:

$$A_{\text{glass}}\ (\text{GBq}) = D\ (\text{Gy}) \times M\ (\text{kg})/50,$$

where

A = activity (according to the calculation, the appropriate dose is ordered, with available doses of 3, 5, 7, 10, 15, and 29 GBq)

D = nominal target dose (dependent on the patient's performance status and the hepatic condition in terms of limited liver function, e.g., in cirrhosis and potential fractionation the nominal target dose will range between 80 and 150 Gy)

M = targeted liver mass [the liver volume (cm^3) estimated/calculated by CT can be converted to mass (kg) using a conversion factor of 1.03 mg/ml]

The potential disadvantage of the glass microspheres is the small amount of injectable volume containing the activity (i.e., 0.5 ml), with a variable activity of between 3 and 20 GBq that can be diluted for injection in 20–30 ml saline. This makes dose calibration easier; however, in the vast majority of the cases stasis or occlusion of the target vessels will not be reached. It remains uncertain if, at the desired dose escalation of 80–150 Gy, maintained oxygenation will improve the response. In addition, the lack of a relationship to tumor burden, the relatively low number of microspheres in comparison to the resin spheres, and the higher specific gravity may all result in inadequate tumor coverage and favor superselective administrations, such as achieved by TACE. Otherwise, infusion of the total amount of resin microspheres is not always possible due to stasis within the target vessels. Additional injection may result in reflux and aberrant sphere implantation.

With both types of spheres, residual activity after early determined delivery has to be held for apt decay.

In comparison to glass spheres, a limitation of the resin spheres may be the relatively small delivered dose, with only a rough correlation with tumor burden. However, experimental work has confirmed that a dosage of 100–300 Gy can be gained within the tumor (Kennedy et al. 2004). Even if not very realistic in clinical reality, a patient with only 1% tumor burden would get the same activity as a patient with 24% tumor burden according to the empiric method. Moreover, given a distinct tumor volume the local radiation based on the concept of point sources of radiation may be much higher in glass spheres than in resin spheres, which may be distributed more homogenously throughout the targeted volume. Nevertheless, no studies are available that compare the different concepts of dose delivery to determine which has superiority.

2.7.6 Procedure

2.7.6.1 Standard of Practice and Radiation Protection

Regulatory issues relating to the handling of ^{90}Y microsphere are controlled by the national regulatory institutions (e.g., US Nuclear Regulatory commission, European atomic regulatory commission). By definition, ^{90}Y microspheres are brachytherapy devices, permanently implanted by angiographic techniques. Dose handling and calculation are only allowed for authorized users such as nuclear medicine physicians or radiation oncologists, who have to undergo training and gain experience in the handling of radioactive materials, and receive specific training in the use and application of microspheres and specific microsphere delivery systems.

Written documentation for the dose calculation and the delivered dose is mandatory.

For dose calibration, survey, monitoring of the administration, and measuring residual activity, standard calibrators, such as a thin-window Geiger-Müller detector and a portable ionization chamber, are used.

The floor under the angiography machine must be covered with a drape protecting against potential leakage or other contaminations to the floor, and for radioprotection an acrylic Nalgene shield and a Nalgene container are needed to store contaminated material during and after the delivery of ^{90}Y microspheres, e.g., catheters and drapes.

2.7.6.2 Angiography and Particle Injection

Once the indication for SIRT has been established, and extended staging together with prior angiography with ^{99m}Tc MAA scan has confirmed the patient's eligibility for the therapy, the angiographic procedure is performed in a standard fashion. From the planning angiography the appropriate angiographic material is known and the potential coil embolization of vessels endangered by non-target embolization should have already been performed.

The celiac trunk and hepatic artery are usually catheterized by 4-F or 5-F catheters (cobra or sidewinder configuration), while the tumor-bearing target vessels should be approached by 2.7- to 3-F coaxial micro-catheters. The advantages of a micro-catheter system are the increased injection resistance, which reduces the risk of microsphere reflux, and the smaller likelihood of vascular spasms.

For both types of ^{90}Y microspheres the manufacturers provide checklists to set up the administration kits. The interdisciplinary team should have trained for this setup in advance and in general will be supported during the initial procedures by a supervisor (Figs. 2.7.3, 2.7.4).

The infusion technique has to be adjusted to the target vessels, the diameter and position of the catheter, and the type of microspheres used, to avoid back-spill of the particle suspension and secondary unintentional embolization of extrahepatic vascular territories.

SIRT may target a solitary or multiple lesions, a single or multiple segments, or one or both hepatic lobes (whole liver treatment). The treatment can be performed as a single (e.g., one lobe, whole liver) or sequential session for different parts of the liver, where the intervals between the subsequent sessions is 4–6 weeks. There is no difference between single and multiple sessions regarding safety and feasibility, although the latter have more complex logistical considerations and are more expensive.

Moreover, there are no data in patients with limited liver function supporting the concept that sequential application preserves residual hepatic function and increases life expectancy or quality.

There is limited experience of re-treatment after an intended complete treatment session. If re-treatment is therapeutically considered, a 3-month interval between the treatments would seem appropriate to minimize the risk of radiation damage and liver failure due to the recurrent radiation exposure (Liu

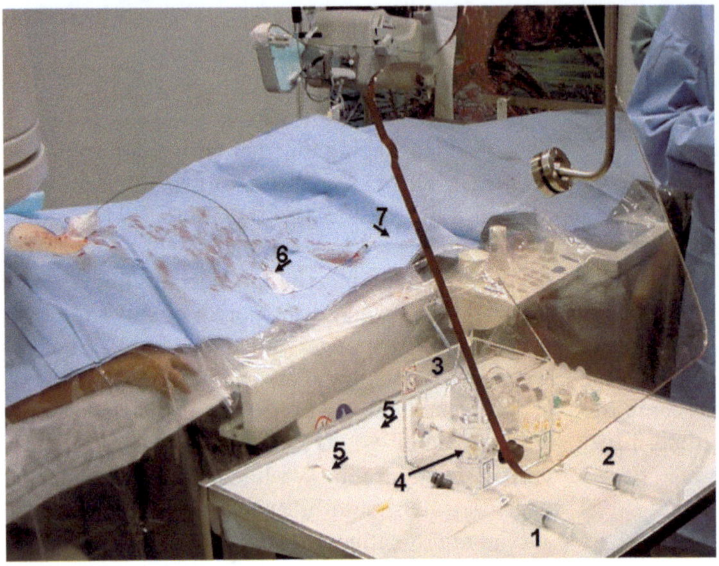

Fig. 2.7.3. Exemplary assembly of a ^{90}Y particle delivery system (SIRTEX®). (*1*, Syringe with pyrogenic free water for flushing the injection system; *2*, syringe with pyrogenic free water for push injection of the ^{90}Y particle suspension; *3*, acrylic container shielding the beta-radiation; *4*, acrylic vial containing the ^{90}Y particle suspension; *5*, connecting line; *6*, cobra 4-F guiding catheter placed in the common hepatic artery, the catheter is taped to the patient's covering rag avoiding unintentional dislocations of the catheter while the connecting line is attached; *7*, microcatheter placed coaxially via the cobra catheter into the central hepatic artery)

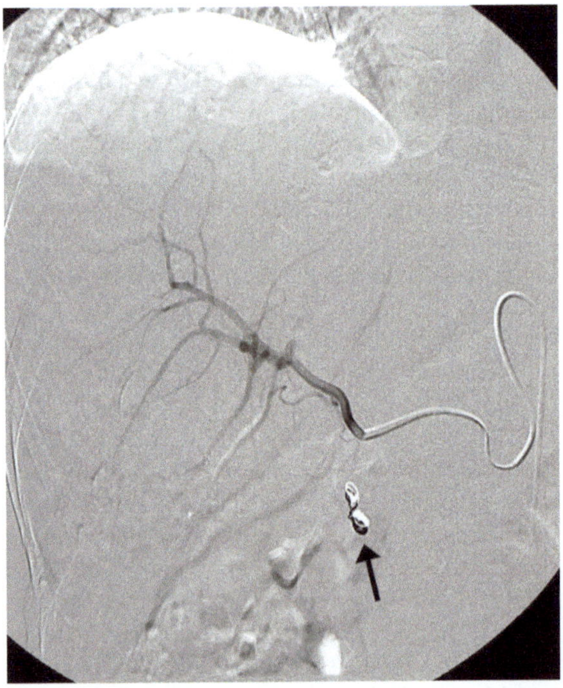

Fig. 2.7.4. Angiographic control via a microcatheter after ^{90}Y particle therapy with reduced peripheral vascularization due to microparticle embolization (compare to Fig. 2.7.2). Note the coils within the gastroduodenal artery (*arrow*) to avoid unintentional extraterritorial embolization

et al. 2004; Geschwind et al. 2004; Murthy et al. 2002).

After the injection the distribution and potential aberrant deposition of the microparticles can be displayed by planar scintigraphy or SPECT. Both detection methods can be used to obtain images of bremsstrahlung – the typical secondary gamma ray emission resulting from the interaction of the high-energy beta emission of the ^{90}Y particles with biological tissue.

2.7.6.3 Toxic Effects and Complications

As long as the patient selection procedure was appropriate and the procedure itself was performed carefully, the overall complication rate of ^{90}Y microparticle administration is low (<5%). Because of this low-risk profile many American centers perform ^{90}Y therapy on an outpatient basis.

Aberrant ^{90}Y microparticle embolization will result in inadvertent actinic effects in inappropriate vascular territories. This may lead to radiation-induced gastritis and ulcerations, duodenitis, cholecystitis, and pancreatitis, even if prophylactic antacid drugs and mucosal coating are applied, as several authors recommend (Salem and Thurston 2006). Nevertheless, these drugs may help to prevent/reduce additional enhancement of the radiation-induced inflammation. In our experience of three cases of radiation-induced duodenal ulcers, the clinical course was significantly prolonged in comparison to "classical" ulcer disease despite intensive medical supportive therapy (Fig. 2.7.5) (Salem et al. 2005; Yorke et al. 1999; Leung et al. 1995; Murthy et al. 2007).

Beside the above-mentioned "technical" complications, typical side-effects may occur in about 50%–70% of the patients treated with ^{90}Y microparticles. These effects are mainly determined by the radiation's impact on functional liver tissue and on blood components (Table 2.7.5). During the intervention, transient, self-limiting epigastric burning, back pain, chills, shaking, fever, and nausea can be experienced but symptomatic therapy is adequate. Flu-like symptoms with moderate nocturnal fever and fatigue are quite common within the first 2 weeks after therapy. These symptoms are most likely related to tumor necrosis, with the release of tumor necrosis factors, pyretic agents, and C-reactive proteins. In general, these symptoms are self-limiting and need only mild or moderate adjuvant

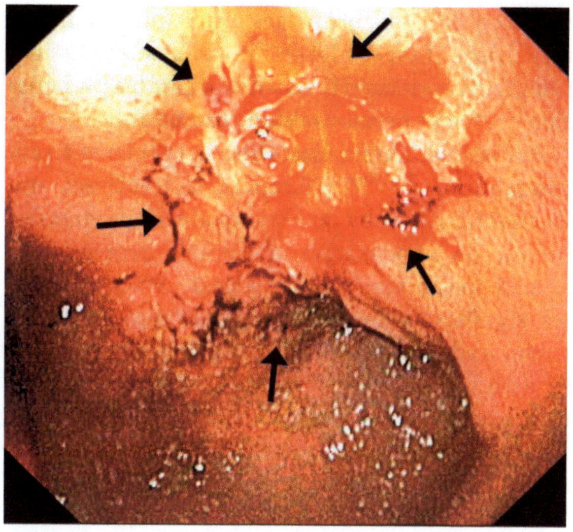

Fig. 2.7.5. Actinic, hemorrhagic, ulcerative gastritis (*arrows*) due to aberrant ^{90}Y microparticle embolization via angiographically unidentifiable collaterals, presumably from the left hepatic artery to gastric or duodenal arteries

Table 2.7.5. Grading of toxicities after ^{90}Y microparticle administration according to the South West Oncology Group (grade 5 = death; uln = upper limit of norm) according to Salem and Thurston (2006)

Toxicity	Grade				
	0	1	2	3	4
Bilirubin	< uln	< uln	< 1.5 × uln	1.5–3.0 × uln	> 3.0 × uln
Transaminase	< uln	< 2.5 × uln	2.6–5.0 × uln	5.1–20.0 × uln	> 20.0 × uln
Alkaline phosphatase	< uln	< 2.5 × uln	2.6–5.0 × uln	5.1–20.0 × uln	> 20.0 × uln
Ascites	–	Mild	Moderate	Severe, requires paracentesis	Life-threatening
Hemobilia	–	–	–	Requires stent	Life-threatening
Liver failure	–	–	–	Pre-coma	Hepatic coma
Encephalopathy	–	Mild	Moderate	Severe	Life-threatening
Pain	–	Non-narcotics	Oral narcotics	Parenteral narcotics	Uncontrollable
Flu-like symptoms	–	Mild	Moderate	Severe	Life-threatening
Nausea	–	Reasonable intake	Significantly decreased	No significant intake	
Vomiting	–	1 episode/24 h	2–5 episodes/24 h	6–10 episodes/24 h	Parenteral support
Gastritis/ulcer	No	Antacids[a]	Vigorous medical management	Requires surgery	Perforation or bleeding
Pancreatitis	–	–	–	Inflammatory, confined	Hemorrhage or necrosis
Weakness	None or no change	Subjective weakness	Mild objective weakness	Objective weakness	Paralysis

[a] Antacids or gastric coating is not able to prevent an actinic, radiation-induced ulcer; however, secondary acidic effects may be reduced by these drugs

treatment in terms of analgesia and anti-inflammatory drugs. If especially secondary gastrointestinal symptoms are related to secondary gamma ray emission caused by bremsstrahlung can be argued.

Radiation-induced liver disease (RILD) is a rare complication of ^{90}Y microparticle treatment and is characterized by an unexplained progressive hepatic decompensation of variable degrees even several weeks after the treatment. Anicteric ascites, significant elevation of transaminase and bilirubin, and complete functional deterioration can be associated complications. Histological findings from liver core biopsy samples are non-specific and do not support the concept of a manifest inflammation. Therefore, the formerly used term "radiation hepatitis" is a misnomer in this context (Lawrence et al. 1995). Predisposing factors for RILD could be primarily (borderline) reduced liver function and a reduced general performance status. High doses of corticosteroids may help to reduce edema-related symptoms in RILD, even if the pharmacological mechanisms in the absence of a true inflammation are not well understood.

Another severe complication may be radiation-induced pneumonitis due to aberrant pulmonary particle implantation via hepato-pulmonary shunts. Radiation pneumonitis may be suspected if non-productive cough together with a variably dense infiltration on a chest radiograph arise a few days after ^{90}Y microparticle treatment. There is no treatment for pneumonitis – which can take a fatal course – to justify a thorough pre-interventional work-up in order to exclude or to identify potential hepato-pulmonary shunts (Dancey et al. 2000).

2.7.7 Results

After early reports of radiolabeled particles in the 1950s and 1960s, research was discontinued in the early 1970s because the problem of radiation leaching to extrahepatic sites and the concomitant severe side-effects could not be resolved. In the late 1980s improved manufacturing techniques enabled the production of non-leaching particles, where ^{90}Y is "entrapped" in glass or resin (i.e., TheraSpheres®, SIR-Spheres®) (Gray et al. 1989; Wollner et al. 1988; Ariel 1964; Blanchard et al. 1964, 1965; Burton et al. 1989). Even though the development of the ^{90}Y microparticles for therapeutic use may be used to vividly demonstrate the joint efforts of basic science and translational research directed by the driving force of clinical need, a review of the history of this development is far beyond the scope of this chapter.

Since non-leaching ^{90}Y microparticles are available, ample study has been presented elucidating radiation effects, and safety and efficacy data.

2.7.7.1 Response and Survival

After initial phase I trials confirming its low-risk profile, there have been a substantial number of studies to gain insight into the response to, and the survival after, ^{90}Y microparticle therapy in different settings (Table 2.7.6).

For HCC most data since the 1990s have been presented for glass microspheres. With a dose range of from 50 Gy up to more than 300 Gy, response rates of up to 50% could be achieved. In a few cases even a "bridging" to liver transplantation was possible, even though the transplant had not been the original intention. Kulik et al. (2006) reported that in 66% of the patients treated, this down-staging resulted in liver transplantation, liver resection or radiofrequency ablation.

Van Hazel et al. (2004) presented very promising results in patients with colorectal cancer metastases treated with a combination of ^{90}Y microparticle embolization and 5-fluorouracil/leucovorin chemotherapy resulting in a median survival of about 30 months in 21 patients. These preliminary data compare quite favorably with the best achievable data from most recent chemotherapy regimens in combination with the administration of antiangiogenic factors. The main objective of recent studies has been to identify the best setting in which to apply ^{90}Y microparticle therapy in combination with other established therapies (Figs. 2.7.6, 2.7.7).

Table 2.7.6. Studies on treatment, using glass and resin ^{90}Y microparticle (only studies with more than 20 patients and comprehensible information about the interventional technique used were incorporated) (CEA, carcinoembyonic antigen; *CRC*, colorectal carcinoma; CT, Computed tomography; CTX, chemotherapy; *EHP*, Extrahepatic progression; *g*, glass; HAC, hepatic artery chemotherapy; *HCC*, hepatocellular carcinloma; *r*, resin; PD, *PET*, positron emission tomography; PR, progression; *RFA*, radiofrequency ablation; SD, stable disease)

Author/year	No. of patients/TU	^{90}Y therapy	Activity/dose	Survival	Response
HCC					
Dancey et al. (2000)	22 HCC	g	med. 104 Gy	12.5 months	20%
Lau et al. (2001)	82 HCC	g	268–332 Gy	4.5–21 months	
Steel et al. (2004)	28 HCC	^{90}Y vs HAC	15–150 Gy		
Carr (2004)	65 HCC	g + HAC	134 Gy	302 days (Okuda II) vs. 649 days (Okuda I)	38.4% (CT)
Geschwind et al. (2004)	80 HCC	g ± HAC, RFA ...	47–270 Gy	384 days (Okuda II) vs 628 days (Okuda I)	
Goin et al. (2005)	121HCC	g	127 Gy	108 days (high risk), 466 days (low risk)	
Kulik et al. (2006)	35 HCC	g		Median 800 days	50%
Metastases					
Gray et al. (1992)	29 CRC	r ± HAC	755–4240 MBq		70%/CEA, 45%/CT
Andrews et al. (1994)	17 CRC, 6 various mets, 1 HCC	g	50–150 Gy	60 weeks	5 PR, 11 SD, 8 PD
Gray et al. (2001)	74 CRC	HAC ± r	2000–3000 MBq		72% vs 47% (HAC alone)
Herba and Thirlwell (2002)	33 CRC	g	50–150 Gy	–	–
Van Hazel et al. (2004)	21 CRC	CTX ± r	1500–2500 MBq	14.1 months (Control) vs 29.4 months	90% (CT)
Wong et al. (2003, 2004)	27 CRC	g	139 Gy		20/27 (PET)
Popperl et al. (2005)	12 CRC, 9 various	r	1250–2500 MBq		10/13
Stubbs et al. (2006)	100 CRC	r + HAC	2000–3000 MBq	8.3 (EHP) to 12.6 months	
Kennedy et al. (2006)	243 CRC	127 g 116 r	36–150 Gy (glass) 50–85 Gy (resin)	11.0 months	35% (CT) 70% (CEA) 90% (PET)

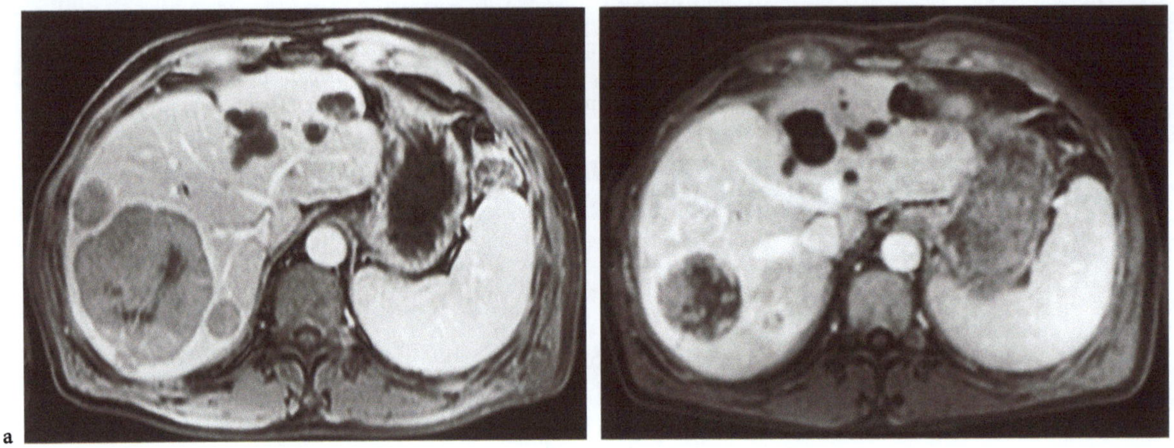

Fig. 2.7.6. a Multifocal hepatocellular carcinoma in a Child-Pugh A cirrhosis presented for ^{90}Y microparticle embolization. There is a total of five tumor nodules with a maximum diameter of 7.4 cm excluding the patient from surgical and local thermal ablative therapy (Gd-chelate enhanced T_1-weighted gradient echo). The largest nodule with two satellite nodules is presented. b The MRI control 9 months after single-session ^{90}Y embolization reveals a significant reduction in the size of the tumor nodules. One satellite nodule was no longer identifiable. While the center of the large tumor nodule is almost completely necrotic, there was persistent rim enhancement over several months with growth of the nodule

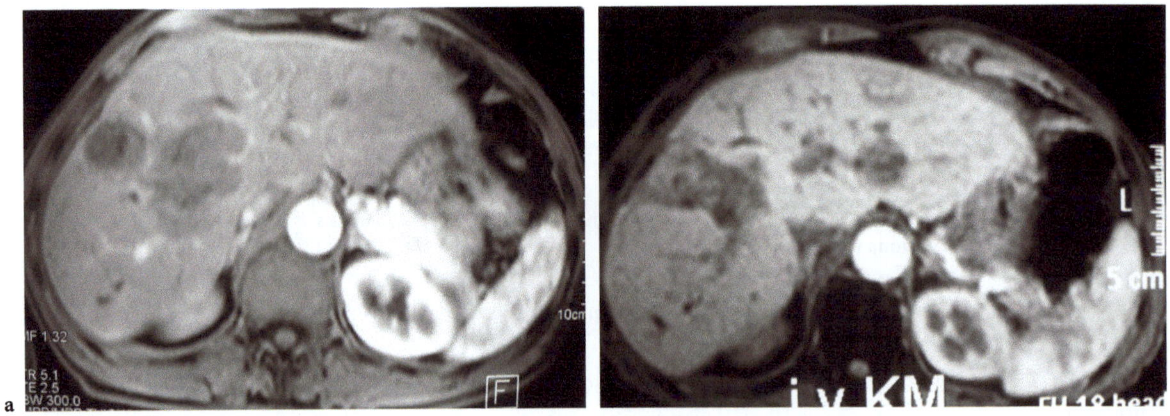

Fig. 2.7.7. a In this patient with a history of breast cancer first detected several years ago, progressive hepatic metastases developing during polychemotherapy were noted. Since re-staging confirmed no extrahepatic metastases the patient qualified for ^{90}Y therapy. b Then 12 months after ^{90}Y microparticle embolization progressive shrinkage of the metastases can be appreciated. However, at the same time new hepatic metastases were detected in the left liver lobe prompting neoadjuvant chemotherapy

2.7.8 Conclusion

Selective internal radiation therapy with ^{90}Y microparticles is a relatively new component of the armamentarium in the minimally invasive therapy of hepatic malignancies and has been reported substantially in the literature only since the late 1980s and early 1990s – similar to other minimally invasive methods such as radiofrequency or laser ablation. The potential striking benefits of local radiation dose delivery are: (1) tumoricidal effects, irrespective of tumor type, (2) much higher doses in smaller target volumes than with external-beam radiation, (3) easy adjustment to "complex" tumor distribution (i.e., multi focal, diffuse), and (4) a relatively low-risk and toxicity profile.

The key to a successful treatment with ^{90}Y microparticle embolization is adequate patient selection, and thorough treatment planning, which minimize the risk and maximize the benefit for the patient. The major factors that have to be incorporated into the treatment decisions are: (1) the patient's general condition (hepatic and renal function, overall performance status), (2) prior treatments (i.e., systemic chemotherapies, intrahepatic, transarterial therapies), (3) type of tumor presentation (i.e., focal, multifocal, diffuse), and (4) the type of extrahepatic disease, which should not determine the midterm outcome. A multidisciplinary team of surgical, medical, radiation oncology, nuclear medicine, and interventional radiology personnel is needed to gather this information to establish an appropriate treatment plan.

Most studies to date have focused mainly on the salvage treatment of HCC and colorectal cancer metastases, and have demonstrated that a significant response to the ^{90}Y treatment is possible and has comparable or superior survival rates compared to other palliative treatments. Nevertheless, the study basis is still somewhat limited, although recent studies have evaluated the ^{90}Y treatment in first-line regimens.

Outstanding issues needing to be resolved include:

- the ideal method of microsphere delivery (selective or superselective)
- the most appropriate (tumoricidal) dose and the best way of periprocedural activity monitoring
- the optimal setting of ^{90}Y microparticle therapy in combination with other therapies (e.g., in combination with first-line chemotherapy, optimized chemotherapy regimens for radiosensitization or chemosensitization, ^{90}Y treatment before liver transplantation)
- the optimal method to assess response (i.e., mismatch between imaging and metabolic response)
- the outcome-predicting factors (e.g., hepatic enzyme tests, bilirubin, tumor markers, performance status).

Therefore, ongoing trials will help to identify the proper utilization of ^{90}Y microparticle therapy as a micro-invasive therapy within the permanently growing field of chemo-, antibody, and antiangiogenic therapies.

References

Andrews JC, Walker SC, Ackermann RJ, Cotton LA, Ensminger WD, Shapiro B (1994) Hepatic radioembolization with yttrium-90 containing glass microspheres: preliminary results and clinical follow-up. J Nucl Med 35:1637–1644

Ariel IM (1964) Radioactive isotopes for adjuvant cancer therapy. Arch Surg 89:244–249

Ariel IM, Padula G (1982) Treatment of asymptomatic metastatic cancer to the liver from primary colon and rectal cancer by the intraarterial administration of chemotherapy and radioactive isotopes. J Surg Oncol 20:151–156

Blanchard RJ, Grotenhuis I, LaFave JW (1964) Treatment of experimental tumors: utilization of radioactive microspheres. Arch Surg 89:406

Blanchard RJ, LaFave JW, Kim YS (1965) Treatment of patients with advanced cancer using Y-90 microspheres. Cancer 18:375

Burton MA, Gray BN, Klemp PF, Kelleher DK, Hardy N (1989) Selective internal radiation therapy: distribution of radiation in the liver. Eur J Cancer Clin Oncol 25:1487–1491

Carr B (2004) Hepatic arterial ^{90}Yttrium glass microspheres (Therasphere) for unresectable hepatocellular carcinoma: interim safety and survival data on 65 patients. Liver Transplant 10[2, Suppl. 1]:107–110

Dancey JE, Shepherd FA, Paul K et al (2000) Treatment of nonresectable hepatocellular carcinoma with intrahepatic 90Y-microspheres. J Nucl Med 41:1673–1681

Dawson LA, McGinn CJ, Normolle D et al (2000) Escalated focal liver radiation and concurrent hepatic artery fluorodeoxyuridine for unresectable intrahepatic malignancies. J Clin Oncol 18:2210–2218

Geschwind JF, Salem R, Carr BI et al (2004) Yttrium-90 microspheres for the treatment of hepatocellular carcinoma. Gastroenterology 127:S194–S205

Goin JE, Salem R, Carr BI et al (2005) Treatment of unresectable hepatocellular carcinoma with intrahepatic yttrium 90 microspheres: factors associated with liver toxicities. J Vasc Interv Radiol 16:205–213

Gray B, Van Hazel G, Hope M et al (2001) Randomised trial of SIR-Spheres plus chemotherapy vs. chemotherapy alone for treating patients with liver metastases from primary large bowel cancer. Ann Oncol 12:1711–1720

Gray BN, Burton MA, Kelleher DK, Anderson J, Klemp P (1989) Selective internal radiation (SIR) therapy for treatment of liver metastases: measurement of response rate. J Surg Oncol 42:192–196

Gray BN, Anderson JE, Burton MA et al (1992) Regression of liver metastases following treatment with yttrium-90 microspheres. Aust N Z J Surg 62:105–110

Hashimoto K, Ikeda Y, Korenaga D et al (2005) The impact of preoperative serum C-reactive protein on the prognosis of patients with hepatocellular carcinoma. Cancer 103:1856–1864

Herba MJ, Thirlwell MP (2002) Radioembolization for hepatic metastases. Semin Oncol 29:152–159

Ho S, Lau WY, Leung TW et al (1996) Partition model for estimating radiation doses from yttrium-90 microspheres in treating hepatic tumours. Eur J Nucl Med 23:947–952

Ho S, Lau WY, Leung TW et al (1997a) Tumour-to-normal uptake ratio of 90Y microspheres in hepatic cancer assessed with 99Tcm macroaggregated albumin. Br J Radiol 70:823–828

Ho S, Lau WY, Leung TW, Chan M, Johnson PJ, Li AK (1997b) Clinical evaluation of the partition model for estimating radiation doses from yttrium-90 microspheres in the treatment of hepatic cancer. Eur J Nucl Med 24:293–298

Kennedy AS, Salem R (2003) Comparison of two ^{90}Yttrium microsphere agents for hepatic artery brachytherapy. Proceedings of the 14th International Congress on Anti-Cancer Treatment 2003, p 156

Kennedy AS, Nutting C, Coldwell D, Gaiser J, Drachenberg C (2004) Pathologic response and microdosimetry of 90Y microspheres in man: review of four explanted whole livers. Int J Radiat Oncol Biol Phys 60:1552–1563

Kennedy AS, Coldwell D, Nutting C et al (2006) Resin 90Y-microsphere brachytherapy for unresectable colorectal liver metastases: Modern USA Experience. Int J Radiat Oncol Biol Phys 65:412–425

Kulik LM, Mulcahy MF, Hunter RD, Nemcek AA Jr., Abecassis MM, Salem R (2005) Use of yttrium-90 microspheres (TheraSphere) in a patient with unresectable hepatocellular carcinoma leading to liver transplantation: a case report. Liver Transpl 11:1127–1131

Kulik LM, Atassi B, van Holsbeeck L et al (2006) Yttrium-90 microspheres (TheraSphere) treatment of unresectable hepatocellular carcinoma: downstaging to resection, RFA and bridge to transplantation. J Surg Oncol 94:572–586

Lau WY, Ho S, Leung WT, Chan M, Lee WY, Johnson PJ (2001) What determines survival duration in hepatocellular carcinoma treated with intraarterial Yttrium-90 microspheres? Hepatogastroenterology 48:338–340

Lawrence TS, Robertson JM, Anscher MS, Jirtle RL, Ensminger WD, Fajardo LF (1995) Hepatic toxicity resulting from cancer treatment. Int J Radiat Oncol Biol Phys 31:1237–1248

Leung TW, Lau WY, Ho SK et al (1995) Radiation pneumonitis after selective internal radiation treatment with intraarterial 90yttrium-microspheres for inoperable hepatic tumors. Int J Radiat Oncol Biol Phys 33:919–924

Lewandowski RJ, Thurston KG, Goin JE et al (2005) ^{90}Y microsphere (TheraSphere) treatment for unresectable colorectal cancer metastases of the liver: response to treatment at targeted doses of 135–150 Gy as measured by [18F]fluorodeoxyglucose positron emission tomography and computed tomographic imaging. J Vasc Interv Radiol 16:1641–1651

Liu DM, Salem R, Bui JT et al (2005) Angiographic considerations in patients undergoing liver-directed therapy. J Vasc Interv Radiol 16:911–935

Liu MD, Uaje MB, Al-Ghazi MS et al (2004) Use of yttrium-90 TheraSphere for the treatment of unresectable hepatocellular carcinoma. Am Surg 70:947–953

Murthy R, Kennedy AS, Coldwell D et al (2002) Technical aspects of TheraSphere (TS) infusion. J Vasc Interv Radiol 13:S2

Murthy R, Brown DB, Salem R et al (2007) Gastrointestinal complications associated with hepatic arterial Yttrium-90 microsphere therapy. J Vasc Interv Radiol 18:553–561; quiz 562

Popperl G, Helmberger T, Munzing W, Schmid R, Jacobs TF, Tatsch K (2005) Selective internal radiation therapy with SIR-Spheres in patients with nonresectable liver tumors. Cancer Biother Radiopharm 20:200–208

Salem R, Thurston KG (2006) Radioembolization with ^{90}Yttrium microspheres: a state-of-the-art brachytherapy treatment for primary and secondary liver malignancies. Part 1: Technical and methodologic considerations. J Vasc Interv Radiol 17:1251–1278

Salem R, Lewandowski RJ, Atassi B et al (2005) Treatment of unresectable hepatocellular carcinoma with use of 90Y microspheres (TheraSphere): safety, tumor response, and survival. J Vasc Interv Radiol 16:1627–1639

Steel J, Baum A, Carr B (2004) Quality of life in patients diagnosed with primary hepatocellular carcinoma: hepatic arterial infusion of Cisplatin versus 90-Yttrium microspheres (Therasphere). Psychooncology 13:73–79

Stefanovic L, Nikolic V, Obradovic M et al (2001) 131-I-lipiodol in therapy of liver carcinoma–methods and case report. Med Pregl 54:387–390

Stubbs RS, O'Brien I, Correia MM (2006) Selective internal radiation therapy with ^{90}Y microspheres for colorectal liver metastases: single-centre experience with 100 patients. ANZ J Surg 76:696–703

Tateishi R, Yoshida H, Shiina S et al (2005) Proposal of a new prognostic model for hepatocellular carcinoma: an analysis of 403 patients. Gut 54:419–425

Van Hazel G, Blackwell A, Anderson J et al (2004) Randomised phase 2 trial of SIR-Spheres plus fluorouracil/leucovorin chemotherapy versus fluorouracil/leucovorin chemotherapy alone in advanced colorectal cancer. J Surg Oncol 88:78–85

Varela M, Sala M, Llovet JM, Bruix J (2003) Review article: natural history and prognostic prediction of patients with hepatocellular carcinoma. Aliment Pharmacol Ther 17 [Suppl 2]:98–102

Wollner I, Knutsen C, Smith P et al (1988) Effects of hepatic arterial yttrium 90 glass microspheres in dogs. Cancer 61:1336–1344

Wong CY, Salem R, Qing F et al (2004) Metabolic response after intraarterial ^{90}Y-glass microsphere treatment for colorectal liver metastases: comparison of quantitative and visual analyses by 18F-FDG PET. J Nucl Med 45:1892–1897

Wong JY, Shibata S, Williams LE et al (2003) A Phase I trial of ^{90}Y-anti-carcinoembryonic antigen chimeric T84.66 radioimmunotherapy with 5-fluorouracil in patients with metastatic colorectal cancer. Clin Cancer Res 9:5842–5852

Yorke ED, Jackson A, Fox RA, Wessels BW, Gray BN (1999) Can current models explain the lack of liver complications in Y-90 microsphere therapy? Clin Cancer Res 5:3024s–3030s

Ablative Techniques (Percutaneous)

Actinic Ablative Techniques

2

2.8 Therapy with Intra-arterial Iodine-131-Lipiodol in Inoperable Hepatocellular Carcinoma

Michael Kirsch, Andreas Zinke, Gerhard Kirsch, and Norbert Hosten

CONTENTS

2.8.1 Principle

Among the palliative therapy regimens of hepatocellular carcinoma (HCC), the intra-arterial application of iodine-131-lipiodol (^{131}I-lipiodol) has been established, particularly in Asia and in French-speaking Europe (Lambert and Van de Wiele 2005). Lipiodol (Laboratoire Guerbet, France) is a poppy seed oil containing 38% iodine by weight. It was first used as an X-ray contrast medium for hepatic angiography and has been shown to be cleared less rapidly from HCC cells than normal liver tissue, when injected into the hepatic artery (Nakakuma et al. 1985; Okayasu et al. 1988).

The particular blood supply of the liver (normal tissue is fed mostly by the portal vein, HCC almost exclusively by the hepatic artery) leads to a prevalent accumulation/embolization in the tumour region.

The half-life of the substance in the tumour is about 5 days; in normal liver tissue, only 3 days. Several other mechanisms explaining this selective retention have been postulated: the presence of abnormal tumour vessels with abnormal blood flow, a lack of macrophages in the tumour and rapid active uptake of lipiodol by HCC cells through endocytosis (Bhattacharya et al. 1996). While lipiodol alone does not appear to have any significant anticancer effect, adding a radionuclide to lipiodol has proven to be an effective treatment for hepatoma (Al-Mufti et al. 1999). The iodine moiety of lipiodol can be changed to radioactive ^{131}I through an atom–atom exchange reaction. By trans-arterial application of the converted radioactive ^{131}I-lipiodol, a therapeutic dose of radiation can be delivered to the tumour, where (predominantly) the beta-ray part of the gamma- and beta-ray emitter is responsible for internal irradiation and tumour destruction. On average the HCC tissue receives 8 times the radiation of normal liver (Park et al. 1986). Furthermore, radioactivity detected in the peripheral tissue is relatively small so that systemic toxicity is minimal. A dosimetry and distribution control can be obtained by serial gamma camera scans.

2.8.2 Indication

The procedure is indicated for histologically confirmed inoperable primary HCC (also with portal vein thrombosis) and where are no possibilities for first-line treatment first-line treatment has failed. To date there have been no recommendations for its use in therapy of liver metastases.

M. Kirsch, MD, Professor; N. Hosten, MD, Professor
Department of Diagnostic Radiology and Neuroradiology, University Hospital of Greifswald, Sauerbruchstrasse, 17475 Greifswald, Germany
A. Zinke, MD, Professor; G. Kirsch, MD, Professor
Nuclear Medicine Department, University Hospital of Greifswald, Fleischmannstrasse 42, 17475 Greifswald, Germany

2.8.3
Contraindication

Absolute contraindications include: pregnancy, breast feeding, life expectancy less than 1 month, hepatic encephalopathy, tumour stage greater Okuda II and allergy to iodine-containing contrast media.

Relative contraindications include: unacceptable medical risk for isolation, unmanageable coagulation disturbance, severe reparative dysfunction, acute or severe chronic renal failure (creatinine clearance below 30 ml/min), liver cirrhosis greater than Child B, leukocytes below 1500 GPT/l, thrombocytes below 50,000 GPT/l.

2.8.4
Radiation Doses/Therapy Doses

The radiopharmaceutical is applied as a single dose maximally of 2 GBq ^{131}I-lipiodol per session. The estimated tumour-absorbed dose varies widely from a few gray to a few hundred gray (most calculated by the MIRD – Medical Internal Radiation Dose – method) but at present the correct estimation of this dose remains uncertain. Until now there has been no positive correlation between calculated dose and outcome or tumour reaction.

The radiation burden for the staff is in the range of 10–100 μSv per ^{131}I-lipiodol administration. Particular attention should be given to the hoisting and administration process of the radiopharmaceutical: it can cause a notable radiation burden to the wrist (Monsieurs et al. 2003).

The dose to nurses in the isolation ward is not different from that for other common nuclear medicine therapies and demands no specific safety precaution.

2.8.5
Pre-Therapeutic/Diagnostic Measures

Several branches of medicine are involved in making the decision to start ^{131}I-lipiodol therapy. Physicians responsible for treating these patients should have an understanding of the clinical aspects and the course of the diseases and should be familiar with other forms of therapies. Patients considered for ^{131}I-lipiodol therapy should be informed about the procedure at an appropriate interval before treatment. It should be mentioned that the therapy cannot be considered as curative. Clarification with the nuclear medicine physician and the radiologist is required. Informed written consent must be obtained from the patient.

Shortly before treatment it has to be decided whether the patent can undergo the procedure, by assessing parameters including blood count, coagulation, thyroid-stimulating hormone (TSH), liver function and the tumour marker level. A static liver scintigraphy to assess regional liver function can be helpful especially in cases of higher-grade cirrhosis. To prevent hyperthyroidism where there are latent thyroid disturbances caused by contrast media and thyroid damage caused by split-off radioiodine, the administration of potassium hypochlorite is recommended over a period of about 14 days in common dose. The patient can be prepared at the nuclear medicine facility or other medicine departments, but in most countries after ^{131}I-lipiodol administration the patient has to spend a few days in an isolation ward (nuclear medicine).

The pre-therapeutic radiological diagnostic should comprise a biphasic CT scan of the liver to assess the tumour size and the number and distribution of lesions in the liver, and to evaluate the portal vein and possible ascites or extrahepatic metastases. The arterial phase can be used by CT angiography to show variants in arterial liver supply, which are important when planning the transarterial intervention. Only if CT angiography is not diagnostic does one need a catheter angiography of the visceral arteries. The CT dataset and appropriate software allow tumour volume to be assessed. In histologically unclear cases it may be necessary to do an additional liver MRT or to take a biopsy sample.

2.8.6
Intervention Technique

In our experience the whole procedure is well tolerated by patients without a special peri-interventional drug regimen. Since ^{131}I-lipiodol may dissolve plastics it is important to use only lipiodol-resistant catheters and 3-way valves (Cook, stopcocks) to avoid leakage and contamination. For injection of the radiopharmaceutical a Luel-look syringe is recommended for safe connection to the catheter.

For planning the therapeutic injection position of the catheter a diagnostic angiography of the liver vessels (coeliac trunk/hepatic artery and superior mesenteric artery) must be performed to visualize collateral arteries to other organs and relevant intrahepatic/intratumoral arteriovenous shunts, which may contraindicate injection of the radiopharmaceutical. In the case of normal vessel anatomy, a 4-French catheter (e.g. Cobra configuration) is positioned in the main hepatic artery distal to the cystic artery for nonselective injection of ^{131}I-lipiodol. After filling a syringe with the radiopharmaceutical the physician connects it quickly to the 3-way valve and injects it under fluoroscopic control without reflux, as fast as allowed by arterial flow, followed by a saline flush over the third line of the 3-way catheter to clear the system of the radiopharmaceutical. In cases where there is an aberrant arterial blood supply, the part of the liver with the biggest tumour mass is treated in the first session and the remaining parts in the following session. Alternative possibilities, such as injecting half of the dose into each hepatic artery or using a coaxial microcatheter for more selective application, lengthen the procedure time because of the slower injection of a highly viscous oily radiopharmaceutical and in addition they raise the physician's radiation exposure.

After withdrawal of the angiography catheter an additional lead cover (1-mm-thick Pb) is put on the patient's abdomen to reduce radiation exposure originating from the patient during femoral artery compression. When the bleeding stops and the compression bandage is applied, the patient is transferred to the isolation ward of the nuclear medicine department until radiation exposure to the environment becomes low enough for the patient to be discharged.

2.8.7 Post-Therapeutic Procedure

A CT scan obtained immediately after the administration procedure can be helpful to estimate the local distribution because the applied lipiodol is clearly visible in the liver (Fig. 2.8.1). During the

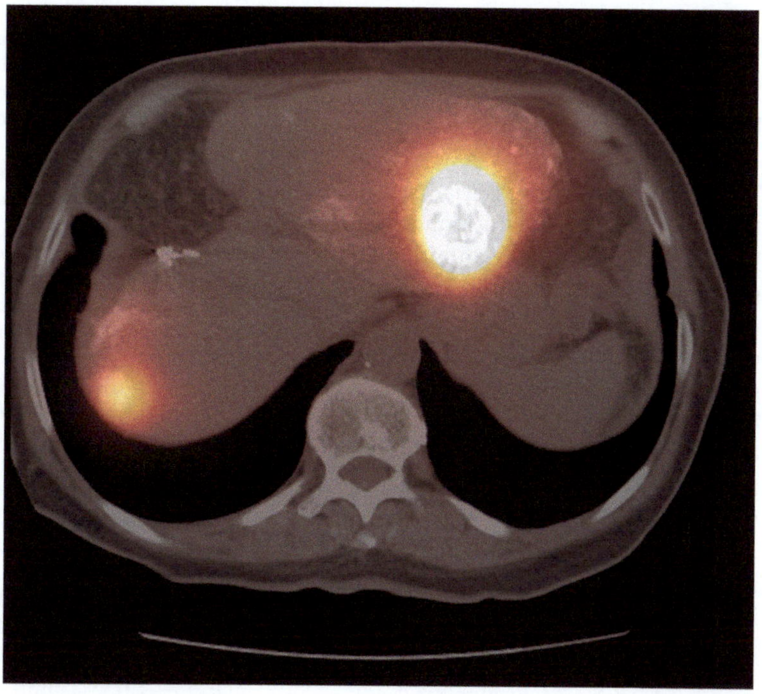

Fig. 2.8.1. Fusion image between the post-therapeutic CT scan and the ^{131}I-SPECT 24 h after ^{131}I-lipiodol application shows intensive enrichment in two major hepatocellular carcinoma focuses

stay on the isolation ward the liver values and blood counts should be taken every 2 or 3 days (a notable worsening over time is to be anticipated). At least two ^{131}I scans should be done (24 h and 72 h) for dose calculation.

An evaluation of the lung-to-liver ^{131}I ratio is necessary to estimate the likelihood of a pneumonitis caused by radiation. A first follow-up is reasonable 2 weeks after discharge (assessing blood values, looking for pneumonitis). Estimation of the treatment's success (blood values, tumour marker, CT, PET, if so static liver scintigraphy) (Fig. 2.8.2) and a decision on further ^{131}I-lipiodol treatments should be made within 3 months of the first treatment.

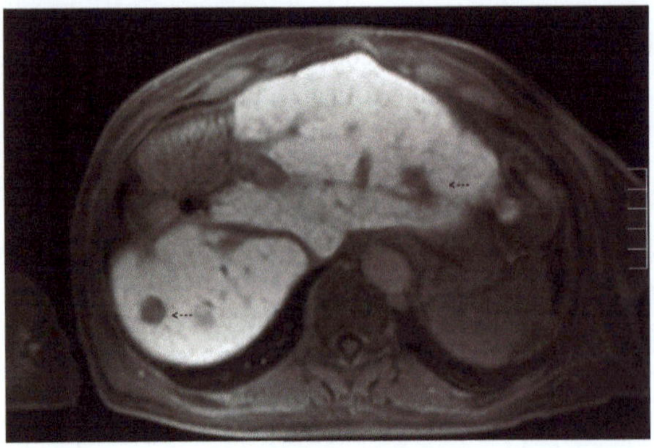

Fig. 2.8.2. Liver MRI 6 months after therapy with size reduction predominantly of the larger lesion in the left lobe of the liver

2.8.8 Therapy Course Repetition

We repeated the therapy courses in cases where there was a reasonable relationship between therapy tolerance and success, i.e. reduced or at least stable tumour volume. Repetition intervals were planned 2, 5, 8 and 12 months after the first injection and we cancelled or postponed in cases of poor performance status (Karnofsky index <60%) or if there was occurrence of extrahepatic metastases.

2.8.9 Results

Treatment with intra-arterial ^{131}I-lipiodol is well tolerated in patients with inoperable HCC, as systemic toxicity is usually minimal compared with chemoembolization (Raoul et al. 1997). Outcome and response rates in the literature are difficult to compare with our data because of the heterogeneity of patient groups. Leung et al. (1994) produced an objective response of 52% with a median survival of 6 months. The overall survival rates at 6 months, 1, 2, 3 and 4 years reported by Raoul et al. (1997) were 69%, 38%, 22%, 14% and 10%, respectively. This is in concordance with our results. Particularly in HCC patients with portal vein thrombosis, the intra-arterial injection of ^{131}I-lipiodol significantly increases survival rate, is technically feasible and is well tolerated (Raoul et al. 1994).

References

Al-Mufti RA, Pedley RB, Marshall D et al (1999) In vitro assessment of Lipiodol-targeted radiotherapy for liver and colorectal cancer cell lines. Br J Cancer 79:1665–1671

Anonymous (2003) Guidelines for ^{131}I-ethiodised oil (Lipiodol) therapy [No authors listed]. Eur J Nucl Med Mol Imaging 30:BP20–BP22

Bhattacharya S, Dhillon AP, Winslet MC et al (1996) Human liver cancer cells and endothelial cells incorporate iodised oil. Br J Cancer 73:877–881

Lambert B, Van de Wiele C (2005) Treatment of hepatocellular carcinoma by means of radiopharmaceuticals. Eur J Nucl Med Mol Imaging 32:980–989

Leung WT, Lau WY, Ho S et al (1994) Selective internal radiation therapy with intra-arterial iodine-131-Lipiodol in inoperable hepatocellular carcinoma. J Nucl Med 35:1313–1318

Monsieurs MA, Bacher K, Brans B et al (2003) Patient dosimetry for ^{131}I-lipiodol therapy. Eur J Nucl Med Mol Imaging 30:554–561

Nakakuma K, Tashiro S, Hiraoka T et al (1985) Hepatocellular carcinoma and metastatic cancer detected by iodized oil. Radiology 154:15–17

Okayasu I, Hatakeyama S, Yoshida T et al (1988) Selective and persistent deposition and gradual drainage of iodized oil, lipiodol in the hepatocellular carcinoma after injection into the feeding hepatic artery. Am J Clin Pathol 90:536–544

Park CH, Suh JH, Yoo HS et al (1986) Evaluation of intrahepatic I-131 ethiodol on a patient with hepatocellular carcinoma. Therapeutic feasibility study. Clin Nucl Med 11:514–517

Raoul JL, Guyader D, Bretagne JF et al (1994) Randomized controlled trial for hepatocellular carcinoma with portal vein thrombosis: intra-arterial iodine-131-iodized oil versus medical support. J Nucl Med 35:1782–1787

Raoul JL, Guyader D, Bretagne JF et al (1997) Prospective randomized trial of chemoembolization versus intra-arterial injection of 131I-labeled-iodized oil in the treatment of hepatocellular carcinoma. Hepatology 26:1156–1161

Ablative Techniques (Percutaneous)

Instillation Techniques

2

2.9 Instillation of Alcohol

Andreas Lubienski, Martin Simon, and Thomas K. Helmberger

CONTENTS

2.9.1 Introduction

Percutaneous alcohol instillation (PAI) continues to be performed in many centers despite gradual displacement by newer technologies such as thermoablation. It can be readily and easily performed under imaging guidance with the use of existing equipment and considerably low costs. In addition it may offer distinct advantages over other regional therapies in some situations (Livraghi et al. 1995; Lin et al. 2005).

2.9.2 Basic Principle

Animal studies have shown toxic effects of absolute alcohol at a cellular level (Festi et al. 1990). Alcohol acts according to two mechanisms: the first by means of diffusion within the neoplastic cells, which causes immediate dehydration of the cytoplasm with consequent coagulation necrosis followed by fibrous reaction; the second by means of its entry into the circulation, which induces necrosis of endothelial cells and platelet aggregation with subsequent thrombosis of the small vessels followed by ischemia of the neoplastic tissue. Neoplastic tissue such as that in hepatocellular carcinoma (HCC) is softer than the surrounding cirrhotic tissue, therefore alcohol diffuses within it easily and selectively, and hypervascularization simultaneously ensures its uniform distribution within the rich network of the neoplastic sinusoids (Livraghi et al. 1995). But it has to be stressed that the antitumoral effect of PAI is limited in HCC larger than 3 cm as a result of its inability to disrupt the intratumoral septa and the surrounding tumor capsule, thus decreasing its capacity to reach and eliminate all neoplastic cells (Llovet and Sala 2005).

2.9.3 Preprocedural Evaluation

Preprocedural evaluation should include adequate laboratory tests to rule out severe coagulopathy, acute inflammation, poor liver function (Child B and C cirrhosis) and/or other severe comorbidities. A screening for viral hepatitis should follow. Baseline serum tumor markers – alpha-fetoprotein (AFP) in patients with HCC and carcinoembryonic antigen (CEA) in metastatic patients – are helpful for monitoring the therapeutic success during follow-up. For therapy planning, assessment of the tumor extent and baseline for subsequent follow-up studies, contrast-enhanced computed tomography (CT) and magnetic resonance imaging (MRI) still play the major role,

A. Lubienski, MD; M. Simon, MD
Institut für Radiologie der Universität Lübeck, Ratzeburger Allee 160, 23538 Lübeck, Germany
T. K. Helmberger, MD
Professor, Department of Diagnostic and Interventional Radiology and Nuklear Medicine, Klinikum Bogenhausen, Engelschalkinger Strasse 77, 81925 Munich, Germany

while ultrasound is hampered by its reproducibility (VILANA et al. 2006). If there is a history of bone pain and/or the serum alkaline phosphatase is disproportionately elevated, a bone scan or whole-body MRI is necessary to rule out bone metastases (NAKANISHI et al. 2005). Informed consent is necessary 24 h prior to the procedure by the latest.

2.9.4 Technique

The equipment needed for PAI does not differ from that required for a fine-needle aspiration biopsy. In general, 20- to 22-gauge needles with endholes or a closed conical tip and several sideholes are used (LIVRAGHI 1998). Depending on the location of the tumor, usually needles 10–20 cm in length are appropriate. Depending on the tumor size an appropriate volume of 98% alcohol is required. The total volume is calculated from the radius of the tumor, using the formula for the volume of a sphere, $4/3\pi\cdot(\text{radius}+0.5\ \text{cm})^3$; 0.5 cm is added to the radius to obtain a margin. That means, for example, that a total volume of 32 ml is necessary to cover a tumor of 3 cm in diameter [$V=4/3\pi\cdot(1.5\ \text{cm}+0.5\ \text{cm})^3$]. Tumors up to 3 cm are easily treated in a single session. Since the toxic dose of ethanol is 0.8–1.0 cm^3/kg, tumors 4 cm and larger will usually require multiple treatment sessions (LEE et al. 1995). The injected volume per session/per tumor varies between 2 ml and 10 ml with a recommended maximum volume of 30–40 ml per single session treatment. Usually tumors smaller than 2 cm are treated in 3–4 sessions; tumors of 2–3.5 cm, in 8–12 sessions. Multisession treatment is performed with two to four treatment sessions per week. In contrast, single-session treatment uses volumes of more than 40 ml up to more than 200 ml per session. Single-session treatment offers the advantage that bigger tumors can be treated much faster and, therefore, the "treatment logistics" are more acceptable for the patient. The disadvantage is that general anesthesia is recommended in order to have optimal treatment conditions and to provide appropriate pain relief for the patient.

Care has to be taken to avoid direct injection of ethanol into the hepatic veins, because a sudden and high concentration of ethanol in terms of a bolus may lead to prolonged hypoxemia with cardiopulmonary arrest (LIVRAGHI 1998). LIVRAGHI et al. (1998) reported a significantly higher rate of mortality (0.1% versus 4.6%) while performing single-session treatment using alcohol volumes of more than 200 ml, with the patient under general anesthetic. However, results of single-session PAI are based on uncontrolled trials and when critically compared with recent data about the natural history and prognosis of untreated nonsurgical HCC the benefits of the procedure are not evident (LENCIONI and CROCETTI 2005).

The patient is placed in a supine position and an intravenous access line for sedation, analgesia and emergent medication is established using an intravenous cannula placed in a cubital vein. Prophylactic antibiotics are usually not necessary. For image guidance ultrasound, CT or MRI can be used (ADAM et al. 1997). The major advantage of ultrasound monitoring is the real-time visualization of alcohol diffusion, since microbubbles contained in the injected alcohol are markedly echogenic just after injection. In the late course of alcohol injection under ultrasound guidance, a dense echogenic cloud forms with distal acoustic shadowing, which makes it difficult to evaluate whether the alcohol has diffused through the entire tumor or not. According to the literature, ultrasound is reported to be the guiding method of choice (EBARA et al. 2005). Since ultrasound is a real-time, multiplanar technique and can be performed in the operating room it seems to be the most appropriate guiding tool. Nevertheless it should be mentioned that, due to its physicochemical properties, alcohol injection/diffusion can also readily be visualized by CT and MRI. Both techniques are more "panoramic" than ultrasound and allow optimal targeting of almost all hepatic tumors in all anatomical localizations. In particular, MR-guided PAI is advantageous in locations unfavorable for CT guidance or in patients in whom iodized contrast media are contraindicated. CT fluoroscopy allows for real-time monitoring of alcohol diffusion with the disadvantage of repeated radiation exposure, especially to the interventionalist (KATAOKA et al. 2006). Absolute alcohol has low attenuation values on CT (~–240 HU) so that an admixture of contrast material is not necessary for CT visualization. On MRI it is suggested to use an inversion-recovery spin-echo sequence with an inversion time of 250 ms and an echo time of 150 ms in combination with water saturation pulses, which effectively suppresses the tissue water signal from human liver while obtaining a high signal from the alcohol (ALEXANDER et al. 1996). Although CT (SHANKAR et al. 2004) and MRI (KIM et al. 2005)

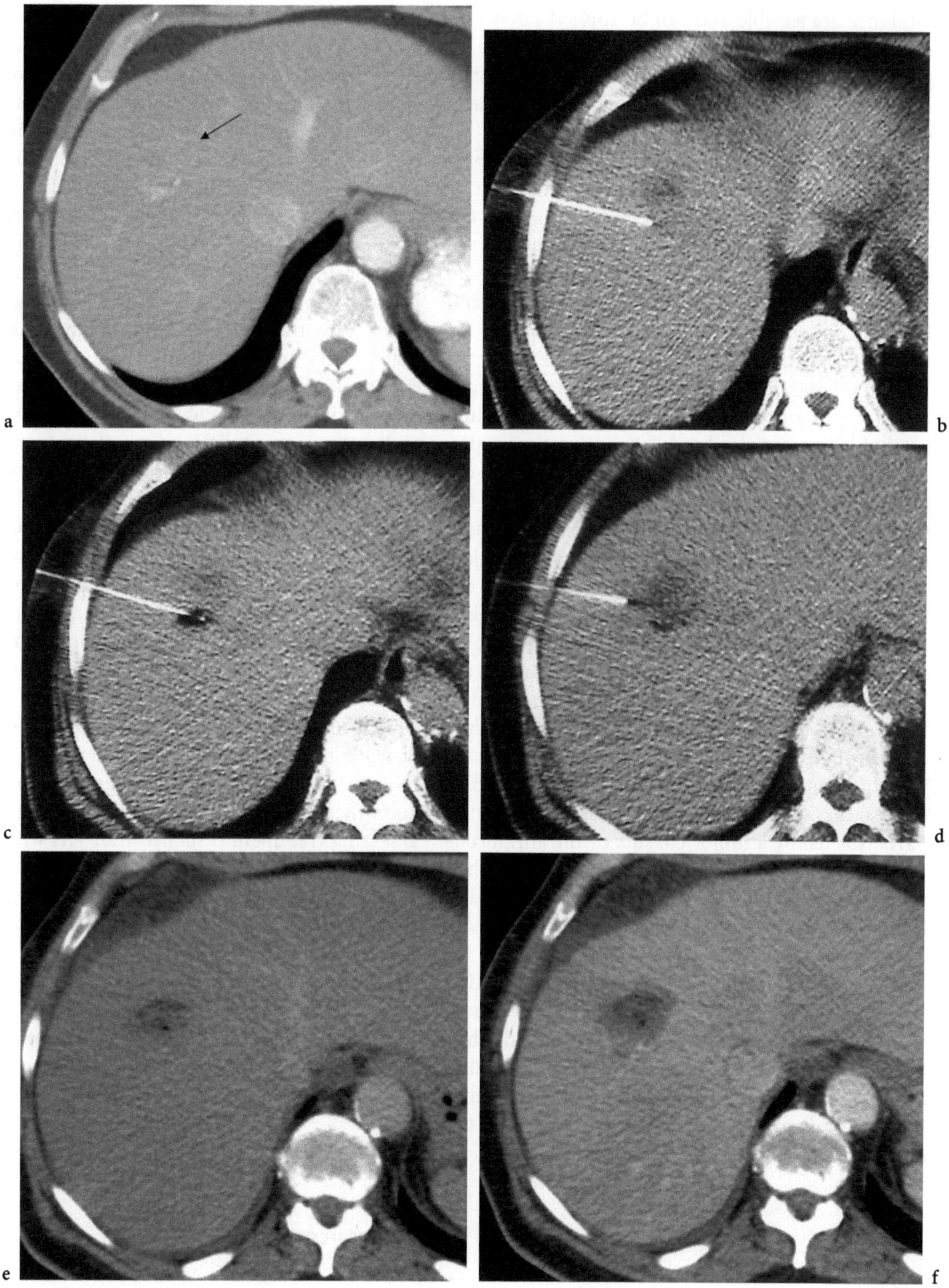

Fig. 2.9.1. a Hepatocellular carcinoma (3.8 cm in diameter) in liver segment 8 with only slight contrast enhancement in the arterial phase. **b** Needle placement under CT guidance into the dorsal part of the tumor. **c** CT directly after ethanol injection into the dorsal part of the tumor. The ethanol "pools" at the injection site. **d** CT after completion of percutaneous alcohol instillation (*PAI*) (60 ml of alcohol) with the tumor completely saturated with ethanol and the needle still in place in order to allow the alcohol to diffuse. **e, f** CT in the arterial (**e**) and the portovenous phase (**f**) directly after completion of PAI. No tumor enhancement can be seen in the arterial phase. The portovenous phase demarcates the homogenous saturation of the tumor with ethanol

guidance are feasible and can be applied safely and effectively, they do not play an important role in guiding PAI. In most centers, ultrasound guidance is still the guiding method of choice (Lencioni and Crocetti 2005).

After localization of the tumor using the preferred guidance method (Fig. 2.9.1a), the skin is prepped and draped. Then local anesthesia from the entry point of the needle into the skin down to the liver capsule is administered. For local anesthesia, common local anesthetics such as mepivacaine can be used; for sedation, midazolam or fentanyl; for analgesia, piritramid. Subsequently, the tumor is punctured, passing the needle to the distal margin of the tumor without crossing the tumor. Absolute alcohol is injected slowly while rotating the needle. Ethanol usually spreads within a radius of 1–3 cm around the tip of the needle to the periphery of the tumor (Livraghi 1998) (Fig. 2.9.1b). Real-time imaging during the procedure allows for controlled injection. The needle is gradually withdrawn towards the proximal edge of the tumor (Fig. 2.9.1b–d). Injection is stopped when most of the alcohol leaks outside the tumor or when diffusion is not clearly seen. The needle is repositioned if alcohol is observed to flow into a blood vessel, bile duct, or into the liver outside of the tumor. The alcohol should be injected into different portions of the tumor even close to its edge so that viable tumor tissue does not remain in parts isolated by a tumor capsule or intratumorous septae (Fig. 2.9.1b, c). The treatment is ended when the alcohol saturation of the tumor is considered to be total. This is given when the entire tumor appears hyperechoic on ultrasound or hypodense on CT (Livraghi et al. 1995) (Fig. 2.9.1d). After completing the injection, the needle is left in place for 1–2 min to allow the alcohol to diffuse further (Fig. 2.9.1d), then the needle is aspirated firmly during withdrawal to minimize leakage, since alcohol reflux may cause pain. Additional passes may be required to treat the entire tumor volume.

2.9.5 Follow-Up Imaging

Monitoring of therapy effectiveness is deemed to be a major issue in interventional tumor therapy. Recent studies have shown that achievement of a complete response to HCC ablation therapies is associated with improved survival in both Child-Pugh A and B patients (Sana et al. 2004). Thus, evaluation of treatment efficacy is highly important not only to ensure that patients have no complications but also to promptly identify treatment failure and decide the need to complete treatment. CT or MRI evaluation of response to therapy is delayed to 1 month, as earlier assessments may be flawed by the presence of vascular abnormalities related to the treatment itself, just reflecting inflammatory changes or microscopic fistulae (Bruix et al. 2001). In ideal conditions, treatment evaluation would be done immediately after applying therapy and imply a minimal burden for patients and physicians, but so far no diagnostic tool is able to detect residual tumor foci with enough sensitivity and specificity immediately after treatment. At 1 month ultrasound combined with specific contrast media is able to achieve the same results of MRI and CT but is still hampered concerning its reproducibility (Nakanishi et al. 2005). Dynamic contrast-enhanced CT and MRI play the major role in follow-up imaging after PAI. In most centers, follow-up scans are performed at 3-month intervals and are often combined with measurement of serum tumor markers such as AFP and CEA (Lencioni et al. 1997). Complete coagulation necrosis corresponds to a hypoattenuated area and fails to enhance after contrast injection on both CT and MRI (Bruix et al. 2001). It has been shown that assessing treatment response after PAI with MRI is nonspecific, with marked variations in signal characteristics (Clark and Soulen 2002). Any increase in lesion size or irregularity or residual enhancement should be carefully interpreted in terms of residual tumor foci or recurrent tumors. Biopsies of ablated areas in order to prove complete necrosis are generally unreliable and therefore not recommended (Solbiati et al. 2001). It is mandatory to look for evidence of both intra- and extrahepatic spread.

References

Adam G, Neuerburg J, Bucker A, Glowinski A, Vorwerk D, Stargardt A, Van Vaals JJ, Guenther RW (1997) Interventional magnetic resonance. Initial clinical experience with a 1.5-tesla magnetic resonance system combined with c-arm fluoroscopy. Invest Radiol 32:191–197

Alexander AL, Barrette TR, Unger EC (1996) Magnetic resonance guidance of percutaneous ethanol injection in liver. Acad Radiol 3:18–25

Bruix J, Sherman M, Llovet JM Beaugrand M, Lencioni R, Burroughs AK, Christensen E, Pagliaro L, Colombo M, Rodes J, EASL Panel of Experts on HCC (2001) Clinical Management of Hepatocellular carcinoma: conclusions of the Barcelona-2000 EASL Conference. J Hepatol 35:421–430

Clark TWI, Soulen MC (2002) Chemical ablation of hepatocellular carcinoma. J Vasc Interv Radiol 13:S245–S252

Ebara M, Okabe S, Kita K, Sugiura N, Fukuda H, Yoshikawa M, Kondo F, Saisho H (2005) Percutaneous ethanol injection for small hepatocellular carcinoma: therapeutic efficacy based on 20-year observation. J Hepatol 43:458–464

Festi D, Monti F, Casanova S, Livraghi T, Frabboni R, Roversi CA, Bertoli D, Borelli G, Mazzella G, Bazzoli F et al (1990) Morphological and biochemical effects of intrahepatic alcohol injection in the rabbit. J Gastroenterol Hepatol 5:402–406

Kataoka ML, Raptopoulos VD, Lin P-JP, Siewert B, Goldberg SN, Kruskal JB (2006) Multiple-image in-room CT imaging guidance for interventional procedures. Radiology 239:863–868

Kim YJ, Raman SS, Yu NC, Lu DS (2005) MR-guided percutaneous ethanol injection for hepatocellular carcinoma in a 0.2 T open MR system. J Magn Reson Imaging 22:566–571

Lee MJ, Mueller PR, Dawson SL, Gazelle SG, Hahn PF, Goldberg MA, Boland GW (1995) Percutaneous ethanol injection for the treatment of hepatic tumors: indications, mechanism of action, technique, and efficacy. Am J Roentgenol 164:215–220

Lencioni R, Crocetti L (2005) A critical appraisal of the literature on local ablative therapies for hepatocellular carcinoma. Clin Liver Dis 9:301–314

Lencioni R, Pinto F, Armillotta N, Bassi AM, Moretti M, Di Giulio M, Marchi S, Uliana M, Della Capanna S, Lencioni M, Bartolozzi C (1997) Long-term results of percutaneous ethanol injection therapy for hepatocellular carcinoma in cirrhosis: a European experience. Eur Radiol 7:514–519

Lin SM, Lin CJ, Lin CC, Hsu CW, Chen YC (2005) Randomised controlled trial comparing percutaneous radiofrequency thermal ablation, percutaneous ethanol injection, and percutaneous acetic acid injection to treat hepatocellular carcinoma of 3cm or less. Gut 54:1151–1156

Livraghi T (1998) Percutaneous ethanol injection in the treatment of hepatocellular carcinoma in cirrhosis. Hepatogastroenterology 45:1248–1253

Livraghi T, Giorgio A, Marin G, Salmi A, Sio I de, Bolondi L, Pompili M, Brunello F, Lazzaroni S, Torzilli G, Zucchi A (1995) Hepatocellular carcinoma and cirrhosis in 746 patients: long-term results of percutaneous ethanol injection. Radiology 197:101–108

Livraghi T, Benedini V, Lazzaroni S, Meloni F, Torzilli G, Vettori C (1998) Long term results of single session percutaneous ethanol injection in patients with large hepatocellular carcinoma. Cancer 83:48–57

Llovet JM, Sala M (2005) Non-surgical therapies of hepatocellular carcinoma. Eur J Gastroenterol Hepatol 17:505–513

Nakanishi K, Kobayashi M, Takahashi S, Nakata S, Kyakuno M, Nakaguchi K, Nakamura H (2005) Whole body MRI for detecting metastatic bone tumor: comparison with bone scintigrams. Magn Reson Med Sci 4:11–17

Sana M, Llovet JM, Vilana R, Bianchi L, Solé M, Ayuso C, Brú C, Bruix J (2004) Initial response to percutaneous ablation predicts survival in patients with hepatocellular carcinoma. Hepatology 40:1352–1360

Shankar S, van Sonnenberg E, Morrison PR, Tuncali K, Silverman SG (2004) Combined radiofrequency and alcohol injection for percutaneous hepatic tumor ablation. Am J Roentgenol 183:1425–1429

Solbiati L, Ierace T, Tonolini M, Osti V, Cova L (2001) Radiofrequency thermal ablation of hepatic metastases. Eur J Ultrasound 13:149–158

Vilana R, Bianchi L, Varela M, Nicolau C, Sanchez M, Ayuso C, Garcia M, Sala M, Llovet JM, Bruix J, Brú C, BCLC Group (2006) Is microbubble-enhanced ultrasonography sufficient for assessment of response to percutaneous treatment in patients with early hepatocellular carcinoma? Eur Radiol 16:2454–2462

Ablative Techniques (Percutaneous)

2

Instillation Techniques

2.10 Instillation of Bone Cement

Ralf-Thorsten Hoffmann, Tobias F. Jakobs, Christoph Trumm, Thomas K. Helmberger, and Maximilian F. Reiser

CONTENTS

2.10.1 Introduction

The first percutaneous vertebroplasty was performed in 1984 by the interventional neuroradiologists Galibert and Deramond and reported first in the literature in 1987 for the treatment of an aggressive hemangioma of a vertebral body (Galibert et al. 1987). Since then, vertebral augmentation with an injection of a mixture of polymethylmethacrylate (PMMA) and a contrast agent has been widely accepted as an option to treat vertebral body compression fractures due to different underlying pathologies, such as hemangioma, multiple myeloma, osteolytic metastases, and primary or secondary osteoporosis (Kobayashi et al. 2005; Larsson 2002). The other option for treating an osteoporotic compression fracture of a vertebral body is to use an inflatable balloon to restore the height of the vertebral body – so-called kyphoplasty. One of the postulated effects is that kyphoplasty is able to reduce the resulting kyphotic deformity and stabilizes its effect by a cement injection; it was first described by Reiley in the early 1990s (Mathis et al. 2004). Vertebroplasty and kyphoplasty differ mainly only in the underlying technique, where vertebroplasty involves the injection of liquid PMMA into the closed space of a collapsed vertebral body, and kyphoplasty involves the creation of a cavity in the centrum of the vertebral body followed by filling with cement. Osteoplasty – the injection of cement into other bones besides vertebral bodies – plays a minor role compared to kyphoplasty and vertebroplasty and is especially used as an adjunct to surgical stabilization and in osteolytic bone metastases in a palliative situation.

2.10.2 Bone Cement

The material used during augmentation of a fractured vertebral body, an osteolytic bone or as an adjunct to surgical treatment requires specific mechanical and biological features to support the spinal column or the osteolytic bone. Normally the filler materials are injected into load-bearing parts of the body; therefore, it has to withstand complex dynamic and static loading patterns. Furthermore, due to the method of percutaneous approach to the bone, the cement used has to be easy to prepare and has to have applicable flow characteristics and polymerization time. Due to the underlying different techniques the cement has to have different characteristics. While during vertebroplasty the ideal material should have a longer semi-liquid

R.-T. Hoffmann, MD; T. F. Jakobs, MD;
Christoph Trumm, MD; M. F. Reiser, MD, Professor
Department of Cinical Radiology, University Hospitals – Grosshadern, Ludwig-Maximilians-University of Munich, Marchioninistrasse 15, 81377 Munich, Germany
T. K. Helmberger, MD
Professor, Department of Diagnostic and Interventional Radiology and Nuclear Medicine, Klinikum Bogenhausen, Engelschalkinger Strasse 77, 81925 Munich, Germany

phase and a very short set time, the ideal material for kyphoplasty should have a shorter liquid phase and a longer paste-like phase. Today, PMMA is the filler material of choice due to its properties as an inert, biomechanical proper and cost-effective substance, while other bone substitutes such as ceramic bone cements and composite material are still under development. PMMA bone cement has a long history in the fixation of the components of joint replacement, and – less frequently – for the stabilization or fixation of pathological fractures and has been reported as early as in the 1960s (Charnley 1964). Since this publication, PMMA has been increasingly accepted for a wide variety of applications. PMMA is inert and shows good biocompatibility over long-term follow-up (Lieberman et al. 2005). Moreover, PMMA has additional advantages including the familiarity, the ease of handling, good biomechanical strength and stiffness, and cost-effectiveness. Disadvantages of PMMA are the lack of biological potential to remodel or integrate into the surrounding bone, an excessive inherent stiffness, high polymerization temperature, and potential monomer toxicity. Radio-opacity is the most important feature of cement because it is necessary to gain good visualization of the cement during injection and, therefore, an early and easy detection of leaks. The older-generation cements were not sufficiently radio-opaque for good visualization during percutaneous vertebroplasty and, therefore, barium sulfate, tungsten, or tantalum had to be mixed in the cement to increase the visibility under radiological control. However, the disadvantage of this addition was that it interfered with the polymerization of the cement and changed its chemical properties. With the advent of the cements newly developed especially for vertebroplasty these problems have been overcome. The new generation of cements are intrinsically radio-opaque. Although good clinical results have been reported in several series of both vertebroplasty and kyphoplasty procedures (Cortet et al. 1999; Gangi et al. 1994; Ledlie and Renfro 2003) it remains unclear whether the pain relief is due to the mechanical stabilization, chemical toxicity, or thermal necrosis of surrounding tissues and nerve endings (Lieberman et al. 2005).

2.10.3 Vertebroplasty

2.10.3.1 Technique

The various methods of performing percutaneous vertebroplasty described in literature differ only slightly and have evolved on the basis of the European (Cotten et al. 1998; Deramond et al. 1998) and American (Jensen et al. 1997; Jensen and Dion 2000) experiences. The differences in technique, patient selection, cement used, and visualization of the intervention are minor and are dependent on the products and equipment available. Furthermore, the operators' training and personal experience have a major influence on the quality of the results after the therapy. Since there are continuous changes in methods and indications, it is highly recommended to review the guidelines of interventional societies such as CIRSE (Cardiovascular and Interventional Radiological Society of Europe) or SIR (Society of Interventional Radiology) on a regular basis – for example recently published by Gangi et al. ("Quality assurance guidelines for percutaneous vertebroplasty"; Gangi et al. 2006) for CIRSE.

A crucial topic in performing a vertebroplasty is to decide the best radiological method for visualizing needle placement and cement application. All authors agree that complications are more likely to occur when visualization of needle placement or cement injection is poor (Laredo and Hamze 2004). Therefore, operators should use the highest quality fluoroscopy available to them and avoid poor-quality imaging systems. Although vertebroplasty can be performed using a single-plane unit, biplane monitoring or CT with the possibility of creating fluoroscopic images decreases procedural time and enables accurate visualization of the injection. In cases of osteolytic metastases or treatment of cervical or upper thoracic vertebrae, needle placement is easier and less risky using CT guidance or CT fluoroscopy (Gangi et al. 1994). Regardless of the modality used for needle placement, the injection of PMMA should always be performed with direct fluoroscopic control.

The procedure itself can be performed under local anesthesia, conscious sedation (Mathis and Wong 2003) or under general anesthesia (White 2002) depending on the patient and their ability to cooperate. For conscious sedation different medication are used – in our institution we mostly prefer a combination of midazolam and piritramide and a mandatory monitoring of vital signs using at least pulse oximetry. Using conscious sedation does not remove the need for adequate local anesthesia. Intraprocedural intravenous antibiotics are suggested by many authors (Gangi et al. 2006; Kallmes and Jensen 2003) and should be mandatory, especially in immunocompromised patients.

For the treatment of the thoracic and lumbar spine the patient is positioned in a prone position and the skin overlying the vertebral body is cleaned and draped under strict sterile conditions and local anesthetic is administered to the skin and the subcutaneous tissue including the periosteum. The access route depends on the region of the spine that has to be treated. Vertebroplasty can be performed by a unipedicular or bipedicular approach, but most authors think that the unipedicular approach is adequate (Peh and Gilula 2003; Peh and Gilula 2005) to gain sufficient cement distribution. The transpedicular route is preferred in lumbar vertebrae (Figs. 2.10.1a, 2.10.2a) while intercostovertebral access (Figs. 2.10.1b, 2.10.2b) is useful in the thoracic spine when the pedicle is too small or destroyed by metastases. The posterolateral approach (Figs. 2.10.1c, 2.10.2c) is an alternative in the lumbar vertebrae but is only used if the pedicles are destroyed. In the cervical spine, the patient has to be in a supine position and an anterolateral approach is commonly used (Figs. 2.10.1d, 2.10.2d). Special care has to be taken to avoid the carotid–jugular complex and the vertebral arteries during insertion of the trocar. Under fluoroscopic guidance, the needle positioning is done using a light-weight surgical hammer, as it provides better control compared to other methods. Use of CT and CT fluoroscopy allows precise positioning of the needle tip. In contrast to authors of early reports (Cotten et

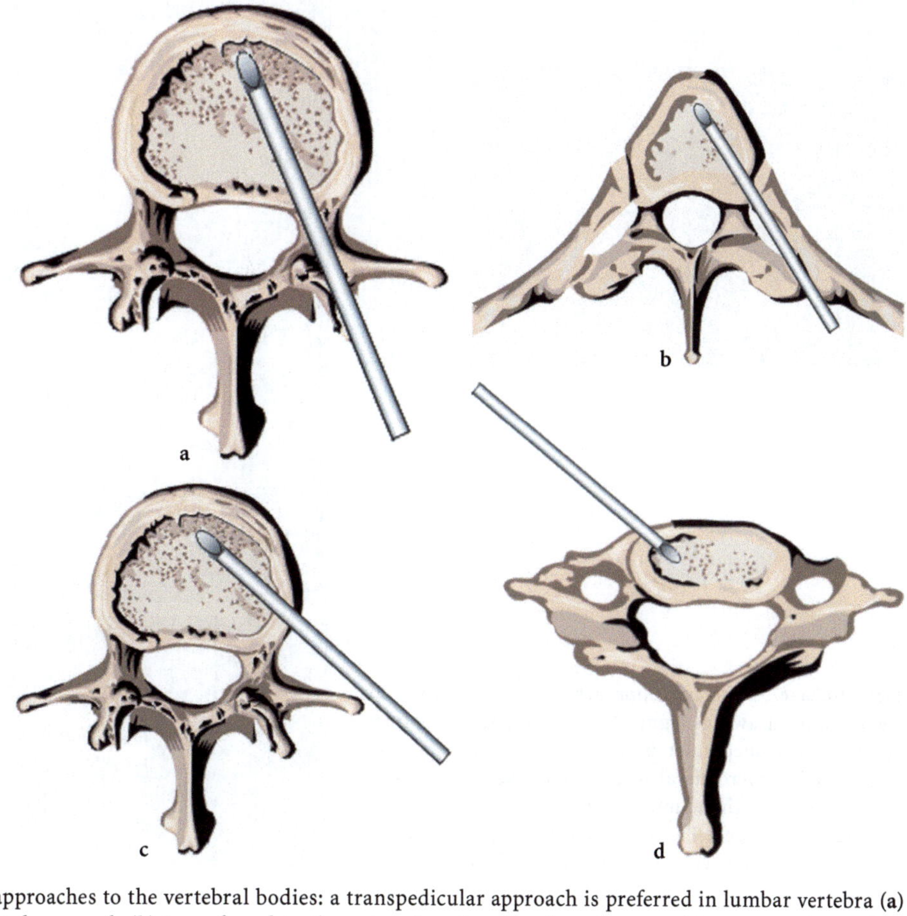

Fig. 2.10.1a–d. Different approaches to the vertebral bodies: a transpedicular approach is preferred in lumbar vertebra (**a**) while an intercostovertebral approach (**b**) is preferred in thoracic spine. A posterolateral access (**c**) route can be used in lumbar vertebral bodies, if the pedicles are destroyed or this access route is complicated by surgical implanted material. In cervical vertebrae an anterolateral approach (**d**) is chosen – special care has to be taken not to harm the carotid–jugular complex

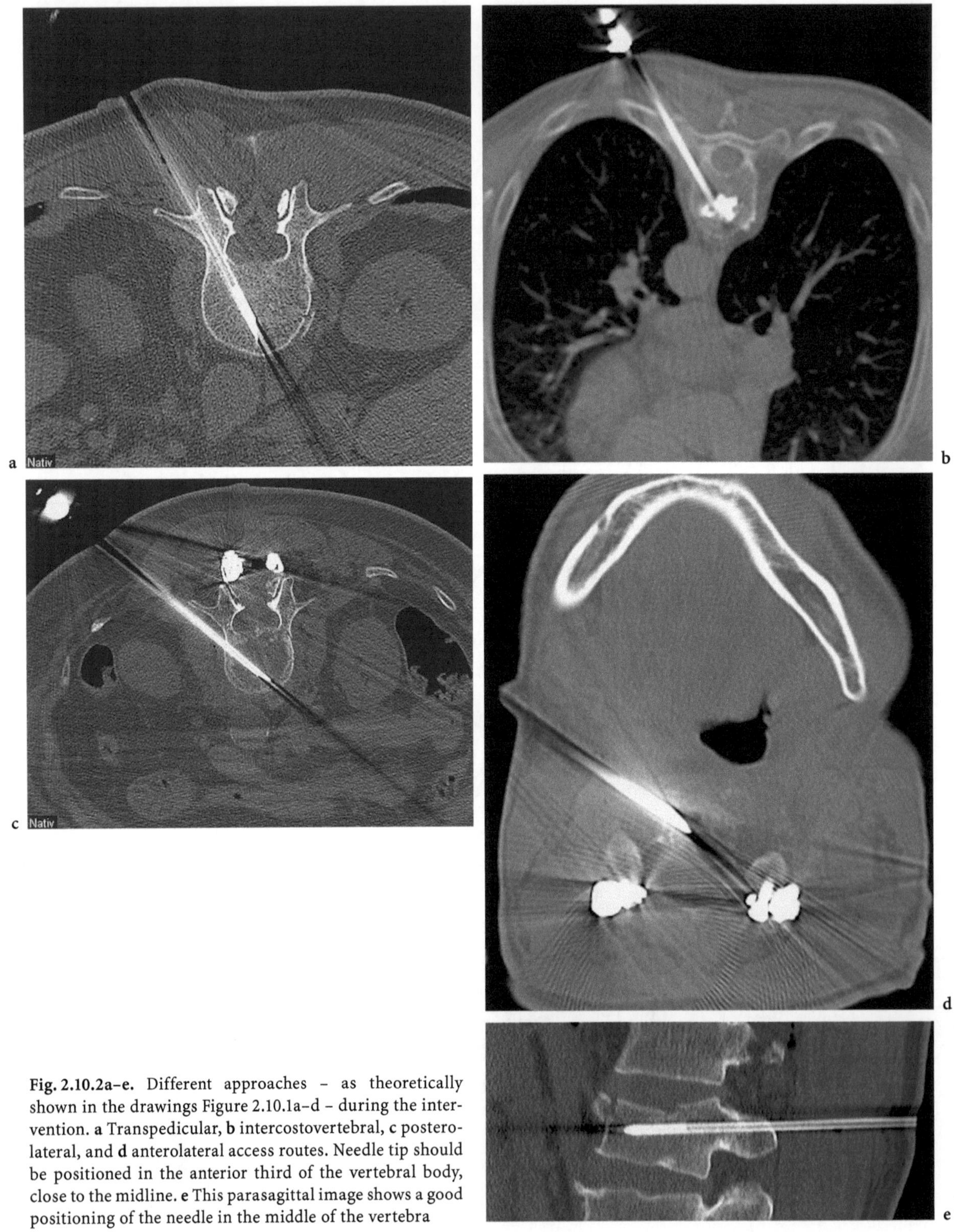

Fig. 2.10.2a–e. Different approaches – as theoretically shown in the drawings Figure 2.10.1a–d – during the intervention. **a** Transpedicular, **b** intercostovertebral, **c** posterolateral, and **d** anterolateral access routes. Needle tip should be positioned in the anterior third of the vertebral body, close to the midline. **e** This parasagittal image shows a good positioning of the needle in the middle of the vertebra

al. 1998; Deramond et al. 1997; Galibert et al. 1987) it has been shown that the positioning of the needle in the anterior third of the vertebral body close to the midline enables sufficient filling of the central portion of the vertebral body and therefore there is no need for a contralateral access (Fig. 2.10.2e) (Kim et al. 2002). To our knowledge, there are no studies on comparison of performance among needle types that might guide selection. The selection of the needle depends only on the operator. Due to the large choice of needle length and diameters, shapes of needle and mandrin and the possibility of connecting syringes or pressure syringes to the needle, every operator has to choose one manufacturer which pleases his or her requirements best. We recommend not using too many different systems because mistakes occur, most often due to unfamiliarity in handling a new system. Important attributes include the shape of the tip of the mandrin and the cannula, as well as the type of handle. While many needle cannulas have a square distal shape, some cannulas available have a beveled distal end (for example Cook, Optimed) that allows one to direct cement in a given direction. Furthermore, 10-cm-long needles can be used in most patients but 15-cm-long needles are utilized when treating lower lumbar vertebral bodies or corpulent patients. In addition, an advantage in using needles with larger diameters (e.g., 10 gauge) is that the cement can be much more viscous during injection and can therefore be administered for longer compared to needles with a smaller diameter (e.g. 15 gauge). However, in the cervical spine a needle with a smaller diameter should be favored. After optimal positioning of the needle, the stylet has to be removed from the needle and the cement can be prepared according to the manufacturer's instructions. Most manufacturers recommend a closed mixing system providing a homogenous mixing, to avoid cement contamination and inclusion of air bubbles in cement, which can reduce its strength (Mathis and Wong 2003). During the first 30–60 s, the cement has a fluid-like consistency (Gangi et al. 2006). After 60 s the PMMA becomes more like tooth-paste. During the tooth-paste-like polymerization phase the cement is injected to reduce the risk of extravasation into the surrounding tissue or venous plexus. The administration of the cement should be performed using a pressure syringe from a dedicated injection set (Optimed; Allegiance; Cook; Stryker) or several small (1–2 ml) Luer lock syringes. The injection sets allow aspiration of a larger amount of cement (up to 10 ml) and direct injection of cement in a continuous flow, with minimal effort. Although the use of the injection sets increases the expense of the procedure, it is safer than free-hand injection. The injection of the cement has to be carefully controlled either under lateral and ap fluoroscopy or CT fluoroscopy to avoid cement leakage harming the patient. Special care has to be taken if the cement starts to leak out into the peridural space, since this can cause severe neurological deficits. The risk of cement leakage is particularly high at the beginning of cement injection. The operator should be very careful during the injection of the first amount of cement. The administration of the PMMA has to be stopped immediately if the mixture starts to leak out from the vertebral body into the surrounding tissue, especially into the discal space. However, waiting for 30–60 s can often resolve this problem because the cement hardens and seals the leak. If the leak persists, needle position and bevel direction should be changed. If cement is still pouring into the surrounding structures, the injection has to be stopped and the needle removed. However, if the vertebroplasty cannot be completed due to an uncorrectable leakage of the cement, the vertebroplasty could be immediately repeated using the contralateral pedicle as the access path for complete filling of the vertebral body. The cement injection can be stopped when the anterior two-thirds of the vertebral body are filled and the cement is homogenously distributed between both endplates (Fig. 2.10.3). The mandrin of the needle has to be replaced under fluoroscopic control to rule out any unwanted cement distribution along the access pathway before the cement begins to set and the needle is then carefully removed (Gangi et al. 2006). The effective working time after mixing the PMMA at room temperature is approximately 8–10 min before it starts to harden (Gangi et al. 2006). However, some new cements have longer setting times and the setting time can be prolonged if the cement is cooled before mixing (Chavali et al. 2003). The volume of the cement needed for a good result regarding stiffness and reduction of complaints by the patients has never been systematically studied. However, the risk of extraosseous extravasation increases in good correlation with an increasing amount of cement administered. To reduce these risks, we tend to give only a relatively small amount of cement. In patients with osteoporosis or hemangiomas, 2.5–4 ml of cement provides good filling of the vertebra and achieves both consolidation and pain relief. In metastatic disease, where the aim of vertebroplasty is relief of excruciating pain, smaller volumes (1.5–2.5 ml) are usually sufficient.

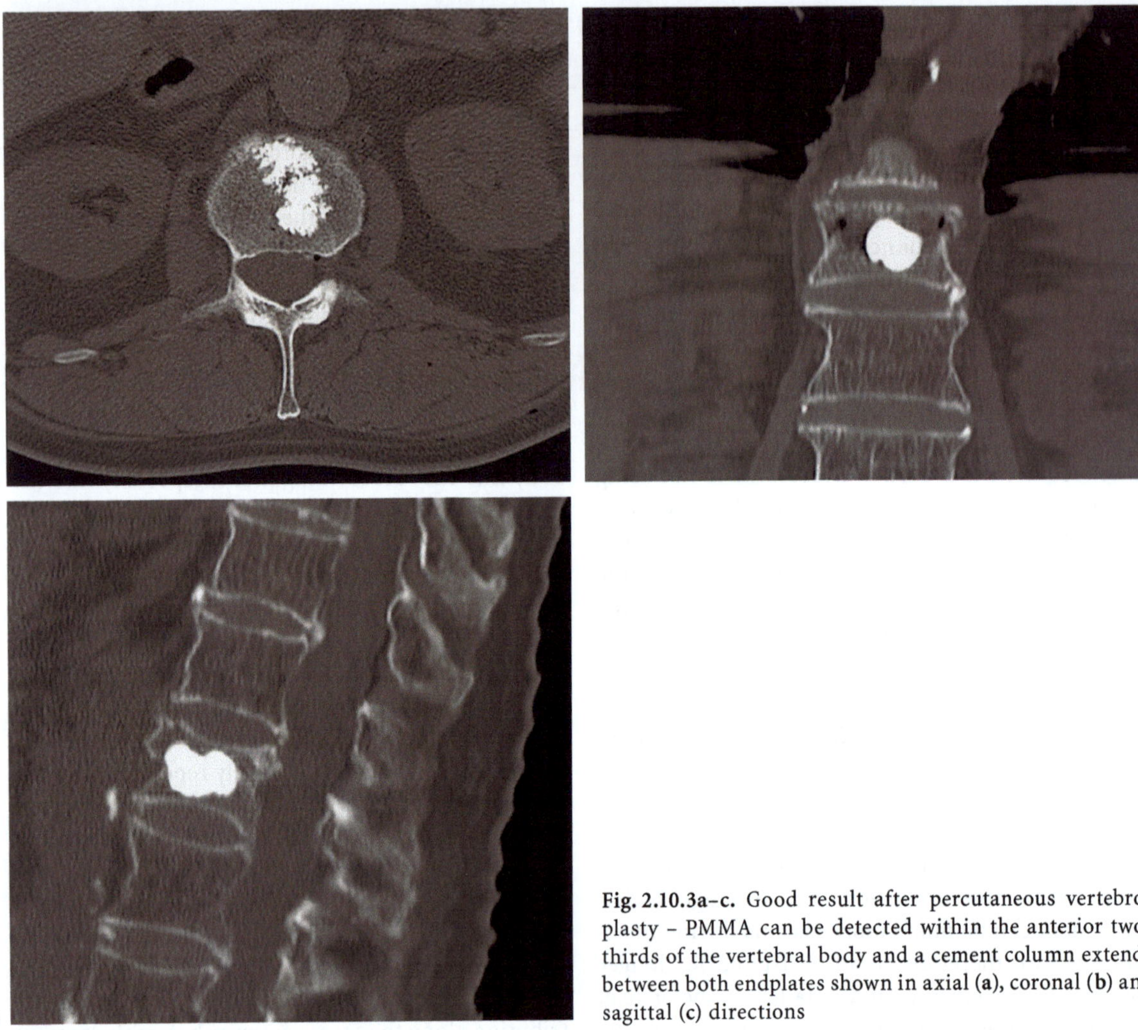

a b c

Fig. 2.10.3a–c. Good result after percutaneous vertebroplasty – PMMA can be detected within the anterior two-thirds of the vertebral body and a cement column extends between both endplates shown in axial (**a**), coronal (**b**) and sagittal (**c**) directions

2.10.3.2 Venography

Angiographic evaluation of the vertebral venous system (venography) prior to the vertebroplasty or kyphoplasty has been advocated for the identification of potential routes of venous cement extravasation during the procedure. The need for venography is still a controversial issue (Mathis et al. 2001). In our opinion there are more major drawbacks than advantages. Pooling of contrast agent in the vertebra to be treated makes the following cement administration under fluoroscopy more difficult, whereas the injection of an iodinated contrast agent carries the risk of potentially severe allergic reaction. Furthermore, the viscosity of the cement is completely different from those of iodinated contrast media, making it difficult to compare a potential venous efflux after contrast with the behavior of cement during injection. Therefore, for routine cases, it is not generally performed and according to several authors it could be recommended for hypervascularized lesions with a high blood flow (Deramond et al. 1998; Vasconcelos et al. 2002).

2.10.3.3 Complications

The major risk of vertebroplasty is cement extravasation. Extravasation rates are described to be as high as 40% in the treatment of osteoporotic fractures, and even higher with osteolytic fractures (Lieberman and Reinhardt 2003). The risk of extravasation increases with a low viscosity and large amount of cement. However, cement may leak into a wide variety of anatomical compartments, including the spinal canal (Fig. 2.10.4), intervertebral disc (Fig. 2.10.5), needle tract (Fig. 2.10.6), paravertebral soft tissue, epidural veins (Fig. 2.10.7), prevertebral veins, but even cement extravasation into the vena cava, lungs and heart has been described (BAUMANN et al. 2006; FREITAG et al. 2006; KIM et al. 2005; MACTAGGART et al. 2006). However, studies have proven that cement extravasations in the surrounding soft tissue have – at least in the short term – no clinical relevance (HEINI et al. 2000). The clinical impact of a cement extravasation depends only on its localization and size. Especially in epidural or foraminal extravasation, nerve root compression and radiculopathy is the major risk, occurring only in less than 1% of patients (NUSSBAUM et al. 2004), but making neurosurgical intervention and decompression of the spinal cord or nerve route often mandatory. Extravasation of PMMA into perivertebral veins can cause cement embolism to the lungs, leading – in the worst case – to death due to sudden right heart failure caused by a massive cement embolism (PADOVANI et al. 1999). Extravasation of cement into adjacent discs or paravertebral tissue is quite common and reported to occur in up to 65% (CORTET et al. 1999), however a leakage of the cement most often produces no symptoms and therefore has little clinical significance. However, in patients suffering from osteoporotic frac-

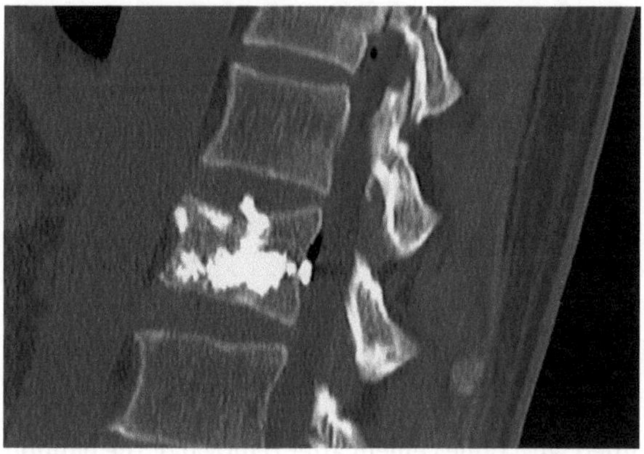

Fig. 2.10.4. A small amount of cement extravasation can be found in both the spinal canal and the intervertebral disc space. Patient did not suffer from any clinical symptoms due to the leakage

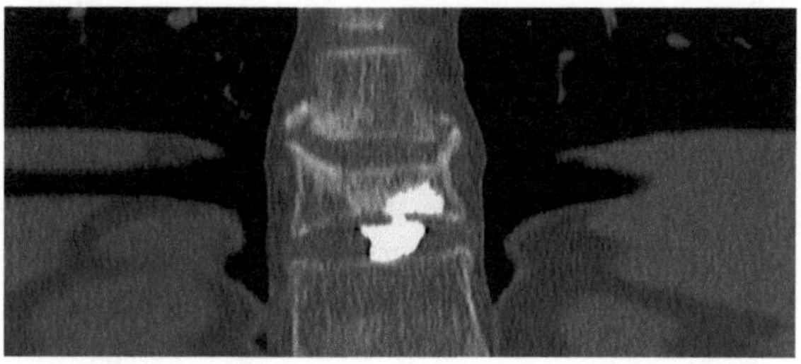

Fig. 2.10.5. Huge amount of cement within the intervertebral space after vertebroplasty. Especially in patients suffering from osteoporosis a fracture of the adjacent vertebra is more likely to occur

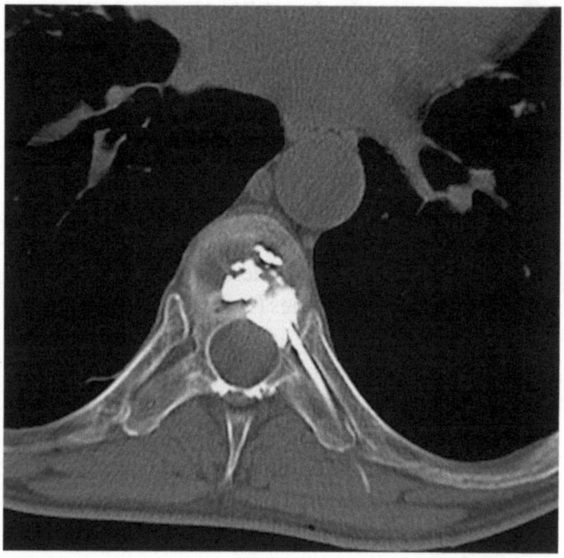

Fig. 2.10.6. Repositioning of the mandrin was impossible due to an already hardened PMMA – cement causing this cement antenna along the needle tract

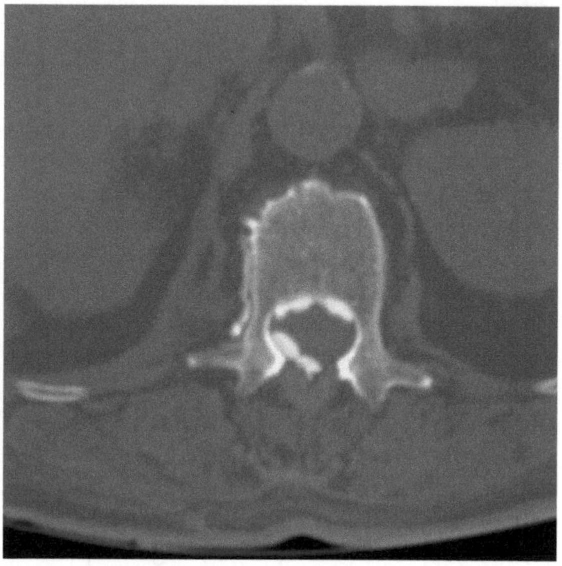

Fig. 2.10.7. PMMA in the epidural venous plexus caused by too early an administration of relative liquid cement after vertebroplasty of an osteolytic vertebra – patient had no neurological symptoms

tures treated with vertebroplasty, a new fracture of the adjacent vertebra occurs significantly more often, especially if cement leakage is found within the intervertebral disc (TROUT et al. 2006; UPPIN et al. 2003). Other complications after vertebroplasty are produced by the specific features of the PMMA (CUNIN et al. 2000). One of its maybe dangerous properties is the high polymerization temperature (86–107°C within the cement core) (LEESON and LIPPITT 1993) with the ability to cause thermal damage to adjacent tissue, including the spinal cord and nerve roots (DERAMOND et al. 1999) and furthermore leading to an inflammatory reaction and transitory exacerbation of pain. It has been established that cement monomer is arrhythmogenic and cardiotoxic at the volumes used during hip surgery. Absorption of monomer during the injection can induce hypotension by virtue of its cardiotoxic and arrhythmogenic properties (LIEBERMAN et al. 2005). Taking into account the amount of cement used in vertebroplasty compared to hip surgery, it seems to be appropriate to do no more than two to three heights per session.

However, the risk of major complications after percutaneous vertebroplasty is only below 1% making vertebroplasty a very safe treatment option (HOCHMUTH et al. 2006).

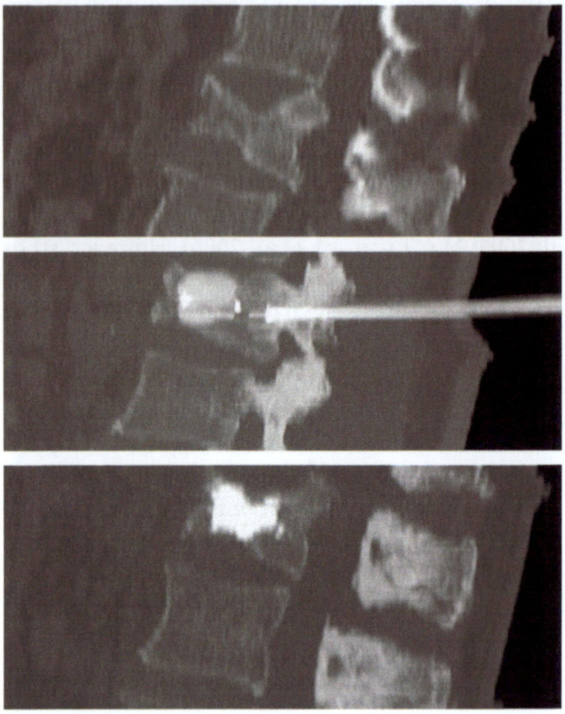

Fig. 2.10.8a–c. **a** Patient suffering from an osteoporotic fracture of his 1st lumbar vertebra. **b** Balloon kyphoplasty was performed to increase the height of the fractured vertebra. After kyphoplasty good cement distribution within the preformed cavity with a marginal benefit regarding height was achieved (images courtesy of Christof Weber, Munich)

2.10.4 Kyphoplasty

Kyphoplasty, developed in the 1990s, is a combination of vertebroplasty with balloon angioplasty (LIEBERMAN et al. 2001) and relies on the same vertebral stabilization principal used in percutaneous vertebroplasty, and the introduction of bone cement into a comprised vertebra (Fig. 2.10.8). Even biomechanical data comparing vertebroplasty and kyphoplasty show similar results (MATHIS et al. 2004). Therefore, the technique, cement, and possible complications are very similar to those for vertebroplasty as described above. After the insertion of a cannula in the used manner, an inflatable balloon tamp is induced into the compressed vertebral body, with the intent of elevating or expanding the fractured vertebra towards its original height. After positioning the balloon via a working cannula under the collapsed end plate, the balloon is filled under fluoroscopy until maximum fracture reduction is achieved. Furthermore, the filling of the balloon creates a cavity within the vertebral body and pushes bone to the edge of the cavity, thereby sealing fissures and cracks. The cavity is filled with bone cement after removal of the balloon tamp. The cement is injected into the preformed cavity at a more viscous phase than with classical vertebroplasty. The lower pressure during cement application, the preformed cavity with a compacted wall and the higher cement viscosity reduce the risk of extravasation compared to vertebroplasty (KRAUSS et al. 2006; LIEBERMAN and REINHARDT 2003; PHILLIPS et al. 2002). However, due to the normally clinically irrelevant extravasation of cement into paravertebral tissue, there is doubt whether this is a real advantage over vertebroplasty. By reducing and fixing the fracture in this manner, kyphoplasty is said to restore lost height and sagittal alignment as well as restore the normal load transmission patterns from vertebra to vertebra. However, some authors describe a restoration of height in 82% (compared to 93% after kyphoplasty) of vertebral bodies during vertebroplasty, only due to the positioning of the patient in a prone position causing a hyperextension of the affected spinal segment (HIWATASHI et al. 2003, 2005). However, the cost of the material used for kyphoplasty is at least five times the cost for vertebroplasty.

2.10.5 Osteoplasty

Percutaneous injection of PMMA for malignant osteolyses, including destruction of long bones (Fig. 2.10.9), acetabular osteolyses (Fig. 2.10.10), and other osteolyses within the pelvis is an exclusively palliative procedure (COTTEN et al. 1995, 1999). Due to its palliative character, it should be offered only to patients unable to tolerate surgery. PMMA provides early and reliable pain reduction due to the heat during hardening, chemical effects, and stabilization of microfractures. It also provides bone strengthening; consequently, PMMA injection is indicated if an increase of mobility for a patient suffering from an osteolysis in a weight-bearing part of the skeleton should be achieved. The injection of PMMA can be performed in connection with radiation therapy to immediately resolve pain for the patient, stabilize their bones and so enable them to be mobile during therapy (HIERHOLZER et al. 2003). However, no studies can be found in the literature,

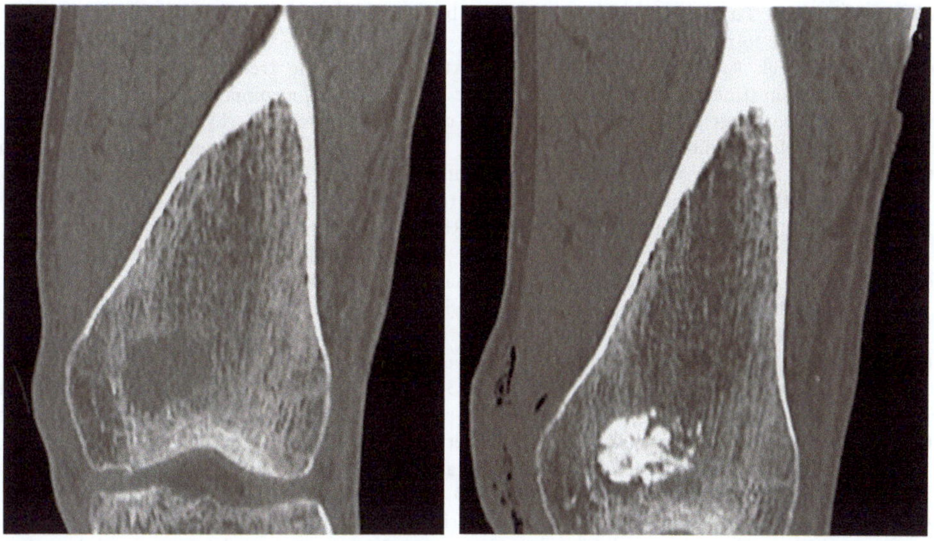

a b

Fig. 2.10.9a,b. Patient suffering from pain due to an osteolytic metastasis of a renal cell carcinoma within his femur. After osteoplasty pain was significantly reduced

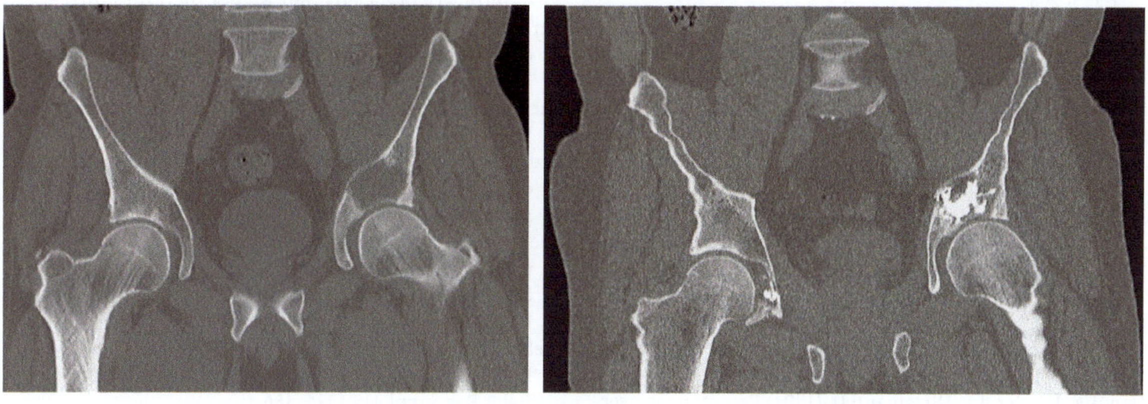

a b

Fig. 2.10.10a,b. Osteolysis in the left acetabulum causing severe pain. After osteoplasty pain was reduced and patient was allowed to get up – due to the stabilizing effect no fracture occurred except case reports or reports on a small number of patients, proving the possibility of strengthening any bone other than vertebrae and, due to its palliative character, no long-term data are available. Therefore, the osteoplasty should only be performed after an interdisciplinary consensus between surgeons, orthopedic surgeons, colleagues from internal medicine and interventional radiologists.

References

Baumann A, Tauss J, Baumann G et al (2006) Cement embolization into the vena cava and pulmonal arteries after vertebroplasty: interdisciplinary management. Eur J Vasc Endovasc Surg 31(5):558–561

Charnley J (1964) The bonding of prostheses to bone by cement. J Bone Joint Surg Br 46:518–529

Chavali R, Resijek R, Knight SK et al (2003) Extending polymerization time of polymethylmethacrylate cement in percutaneous vertebroplasty with ice bath cooling. AJNR Am J Neuroradiol 24:545–546

Cortet B, Cotten A, Boutry N et al (1999) Percutaneous vertebroplasty in the treatment of osteoporotic vertebral compression fractures: an open prospective study. J Rheumatol 26:2222–2228

Cotten A, Deprez X, Migaud H et al (1995) Malignant acetabular osteolyses: percutaneous injection of acrylic bone cement. Radiology 197:307–310

Cotten A, Boutry N, Cortet B et al (1998) Percutaneous vertebroplasty: state of the art. Radiographics 18:311–320; discussion 320–313

Cotten A, Demondion X, Boutry N et al (1999) Therapeutic percutaneous injections in the treatment of malignant acetabular osteolyses. Radiographics 19:647–653

Cunin G, Boissonnet H, Petite H et al (2000) Experimental vertebroplasty using osteoconductive granular material. Spine 25:1070–1076

Deramond H, Depriester C, Toussaint P et al (1997) Percutaneous vertebroplasty. Semin Musculoskelet Radiol 1:285–296

Deramond H, Depriester C, Galibert P et al (1998) Percutaneous vertebroplasty with polymethylmethacrylate. Technique, indications, and results. Radiol Clin North Am 36:533–546

Deramond H, Wright NT, Belkoff SM (1999) Temperature elevation caused by bone cement polymerization during vertebroplasty. Bone 25:17S–21S

Freitag M, Gottschalk A, Schuster M et al (2006) Pulmonary embolism caused by polymethylmethacrylate during percutaneous vertebroplasty in orthopaedic surgery. Acta Anaesthesiol Scand 50:248–251

Galibert P, Deramond H, Rosat P et al (1987) [Preliminary note on the treatment of vertebral angioma by percutaneous acrylic vertebroplasty.] Neurochirurgie 33:166–168

Gangi A, Kastler BA, Dietemann JL (1994) Percutaneous vertebroplasty guided by a combination of CT and fluoroscopy. AJNR Am J Neuroradiol 15:83–86

Gangi A, Sabharwal T, Irani FG et al (2006) Quality assurance guidelines for percutaneous vertebroplasty. Cardiovasc Intervent Radiol 29:173–178

Heini PF, Walchli B, Berlemann U (2000) Percutaneous transpedicular vertebroplasty with PMMA: operative technique and early results. A prospective study for the treatment of osteoporotic compression fractures. Eur Spine J 9:445–450

Hierholzer J, Anselmetti G, Fuchs H et al (2003) Percutaneous osteoplasty as a treatment for painful malignant bone lesions of the pelvis and femur. J Vasc Interv Radiol 14:773–777

Hiwatashi A, Moritani T, Numaguchi Y et al (2003) Increase in vertebral body height after vertebroplasty. AJNR Am J Neuroradiol 24:185–189

Hiwatashi A, Sidhu R, Lee RK et al (2005) Kyphoplasty versus vertebroplasty to increase vertebral body height: a cadaveric study. Radiology 237:1115–1119

Hochmuth K, Proschek D, Schwarz W et al (2006) Percutaneous vertebroplasty in the therapy of osteoporotic vertebral compression fractures: a critical review. Eur Radiol 1–7

Jensen ME, Dion JE (2000) Percutaneous vertebroplasty in the treatment of osteoporotic compression fractures. Neuroimaging Clin N Am 10:547–568

Jensen ME, Evans AJ, Mathis JM et al (1997) Percutaneous polymethylmethacrylate vertebroplasty in the treatment of osteoporotic vertebral body compression fractures: technical aspects. AJNR Am J Neuroradiol 18:1897–1904

Kallmes DF, Jensen ME (2003) Percutaneous vertebroplasty. Radiology 229:27–36

Kim AK, Jensen ME, Dion JE et al (2002) Unilateral transpedicular percutaneous vertebroplasty: initial experience. Radiology 222:737–741

Kim SY, Seo JB, Do KH et al (2005) Cardiac perforation caused by acrylic cement: a rare complication of percutaneous vertebroplasty. AJR Am J Roentgenol 185:1245–1247

Kobayashi K, Shimoyama K, Nakamura K et al (2005) Percutaneous vertebroplasty immediately relieves pain of osteoporotic vertebral compression fractures and prevents prolonged immobilization of patients. Eur Radiol 15:360–367

Krauss M, Hirschfelder H, Tomandl B et al (2006) Kyphosis reduction and the rate of cement leaks after vertebroplasty of intravertebral clefts. Eur Radiol 16(5):1015–1021

Laredo JD, Hamze B (2004) Complications of percutaneous vertebroplasty and their prevention. Skeletal Radiol 33:493–505

Larsson S (2002) Treatment of osteoporotic fractures. Scand J Surg 91:140–146

Ledlie JT, Renfro M (2003) Balloon kyphoplasty: one-year outcomes in vertebral body height restoration, chronic pain, and activity levels. J Neurosurg 98:36–42

Leeson MC, Lippitt SB (1993) Thermal aspects of the use of polymethylmethacrylate in large metaphyseal defects in bone. A clinical review and laboratory study. Clin Orthop Relat Res 295:239–245

Lieberman I, Reinhardt MK (2003) Vertebroplasty and kyphoplasty for osteolytic vertebral collapse. Clin Orthop Relat Res Suppl 415:S176–186

Lieberman IH, Dudeney S, Reinhardt MK et al (2001) Initial outcome and efficacy of «kyphoplasty» in the treatment of painful osteoporotic vertebral compression fractures. Spine 26:1631–1638

Lieberman IH, Togawa D, Kayanja MM (2005) Vertebroplasty and kyphoplasty: filler materials. Spine J 5:305S–316S

MacTaggart JN, Pipinos II, Johanning JM et al (2006) Acrylic cement pulmonary embolus masquerading as an embolized central venous catheter fragment. J Vasc Surg 43:180–183

Mathis JM, Wong W (2003) Percutaneous vertebroplasty: technical considerations. J Vasc Interv Radiol 14:953–960

Mathis JM, Barr JD, Belkoff SM et al (2001) Percutaneous vertebroplasty: a developing standard of care for vertebral compression fractures. AJNR Am J Neuroradiol 22:373–381

Mathis JM, Ortiz AO, Zoarski GH (2004) Vertebroplasty versus kyphoplasty: a comparison and contrast. AJNR Am J Neuroradiol 25:840–845

Nussbaum DA, Gailloud P, Murphy K (2004) A review of complications associated with vertebroplasty and kyphoplasty as reported to the Food and Drug Administration medical device related web site. J Vasc Interv Radiol 15:1185–1192

Padovani B, Kasriel O, Brunner P et al (1999) Pulmonary embolism caused by acrylic cement: a rare complication of percutaneous vertebroplasty. AJNR Am J Neuroradiol 20:375–377

Peh WC, Gilula LA (2003) Percutaneous vertebroplasty: indications, contraindications, and technique. Br J Radiol 76:69–75

Peh WC, Gilula LA (2005) Percutaneous vertebroplasty: an update. Semin Ultrasound CT MR 26:52–64

Phillips FM, Todd Wetzel F, Lieberman I et al (2002) An in vivo comparison of the potential for extravertebral cement leak after vertebroplasty and kyphoplasty. Spine 27:2173–2178; discussion 2178–2179

Trout AT, Kallmes DF, Kaufmann TJ (2006) New fractures after vertebroplasty: adjacent fractures occur significantly sooner. AJNR Am J Neuroradiol 27:217–223

Uppin AA, Hirsch JA, Centenera LV et al (2003) Occurrence of new vertebral body fracture after percutaneous vertebroplasty in patients with osteoporosis. Radiology 226:119–124

Vasconcelos C, Gailloud P, Beauchamp NJ et al (2002) Is percutaneous vertebroplasty without pretreatment venography safe? Evaluation of 205 consecutives procedures. AJNR Am J Neuroradiol 23:913–917

White SM (2002) Anaesthesia for percutaneous vertebroplasty. Anaesthesia 57:1229–1230

Clinical Indications

Liver

Primary Tumors

3.1 Transarterial Chemoembolization (TACE) and Combined Therapies

Stephan Zangos, Katrin Eichler, Martin G. Mack, and Thomas J. Vogl

CONTENTS

3.1.1 Basics

Surgical procedures are a standard treatment of primary and secondary malignant hepatic tumors. However, surgery is only a therapeutic option in 15% of hepatocellular carcinoma (HCC) cases and only overall 5-year survival rates of 25%–40% are reported (Nagasue et al. 1993). On this account new forms of treatments with the aim of an improved survival are needed, such as several promising minimally invasive treatment techniques which may replace or augment surgical resection. These include amongst others new minimally invasive ablative treatment techniques such as laser-induced thermotherapy (LITT), radiofrequency ablation (RF), microwave ablation or cryoablation. The survival rates of these procedures seem to be favorably comparable with those of hepatic surgery (Allgaier et al. 1998; Curley et al. 2000; Dwerryhouse et al. 1998; Finlay et al. 2000; Goldberg et al. 2000; Lencioni et al. 2003; Livraghi 2001; Shibata et al. 2002a; Shiina et al. 2002; Solbiati et al. 2001; Vogl et al. 2002a).

Currently, these minimally invasive techniques are limited by the size and location of the liver tumors. The maximum size of the ablation lesion is up to 5 cm for most techniques. With the use of liquid-cooled applicator systems and improved application techniques coagulation necrosis of up to 6–8 cm can be created (Vogl et al. 2003). For reduction of tumor relapse a safety margin of 1 cm to the tumor border is necessary. On this account the maximum tumor size is between 4 and 6 cm in diameter for the lesions treatable with LITT.

Nevertheless, the majority of patients with liver tumors present at the time of diagnosis with unresectable hepatic disease due to multicentricity, large tumor size, poor hepatic function or severe co-morbidity. In these patients local ablative treatments are not promising either and the degree of hepatic tumor manifestation is a life-threatening prognostic factor (Fiorentini et al. 2000). Thus, new therapeutic options for the treatment of huge malignant hepatic tumors aimed at decreasing the risk of recidivism and improving survival are needed.

Transarterial chemoembolization (TACE) is widely used as a palliative non-surgical therapeutic option for the treatment of unresectable HCC, enabled by the fact that liver tumors are almost exclusively supplied by the hepatic artery (Allgaier et al. 1998; Bruix et al. 2004; Tellez et al. 1998; Vogl et al. 2000, 2003; Zangos et al. 2001). TACE interrupts the blood supply to the tumor, resulting in better tumor growth control. However, TACE is only a palliative treatment modality and tumor necrosis can usually be found in variable degrees

S. Zangos, MD; K. Eichler, MD; M. G. Mack, MD, PD; T. J. Vogl, MD, Professor
Institute for Diagnostic and Interventional Radiology, University Hospital, Johann Wolfgang Goethe University, Theodor-Stern-Kai 7, 60590 Frankfurt am Main, Germany

after effective TACE (Vogl et al. 2002b; Zangos et al. 2001). Tumor cells may remain viable after TACE treatment and complete tumor necrosis occurs only in 16.9% of patients (Fan et al. 1998).

After experimental distal occlusion of the hepatic arteries in rats necrotic areas were observed. However, these necroses were bypassed by vessels similar to the capillarized sinusoids observed in the cirrhotic liver in humans. These vessels acted as sinusoidal shunts in the embolized territories (Tancredi et al. 1999) and were the reason for the resulting viable tumor cells after TACE treatment (Fan et al. 1998). Based on these results, the antitumor effect of TACE showed a mean partial response rate of 26.9%, while the mean complete response rate was only 6% (Camma et al. 2002). To improve the therapeutic results for large liver tumors and increase the survival rates, it is still necessary to eliminate the remaining viable tumor cells at the tumor–host interface.

As a result, tumor ablation is still a necessary component in the treatment of huge tumors as a possible local curative therapy after effective TACE treatment. Neoadjuvant TACE before local ablative treatments might improve the resectability rate of huge liver tumors and diminish the frequency of tumor recurrence after tumor treatment.

Fan et al. ascertained that TACE treatment can provide a chance for tumor resection in those patients with initially judged unresectable HCCs. Liver resection should be performed when the tumor has shrunk to a resectable situation after TACE, even when the alpha-fetoprotein (AFP) level has returned to normal (Fan et al. 1998). This principle can also be used by the combination of TACE with local ablative treatments. This technique seems to be promising for large liver tumors and the first results showed that sequential ablation of a large liver tumor after effective TACE treatment can result in a possible local curative outcome (Fan et al. 1998; Vogl et al. 2003).

During local ablative techniques, such as laser treatment, hepatic perfusion is the major factor limiting the size of the produced coagulation areas. Several studies have shown the reduced sizes of the coagulation areas by hepatic inflow (Verhoef et al. 2003; Wacker et al. 2001) and preservation of viable cells surrounding larger vessels after local ablation. These cells probably survive as a result of the cooling effect provided by the blood flow and increase the risk of tumor recidivism (Matthewson et al. 1987; Whelan et al. 1995).

The combination of TACE with local ablative techniques reduces the blood flow during the ablation resulting in complete ablation of the tumor cells (Vogl et al. 2003). The principles of combined interventional therapies in large liver tumors are to destroy the tumor completely without increasing the side-effects, whilst maintaining the patient's liver function and immunity.

Subsequently we present our results of a combined neoadjuvant treatment protocol and review the current status of combined interventional therapies for unresectable liver tumors.

3.1.1.1 Neoadjuvant TACE – Frankfurt Protocol (TACE Followed by LITT)

A total of 48 patients (10 females and 38 males ranging in age from 50.1 to 81.2 years; mean age 67.7 years) with unresectable primary liver tumors were treated with repetitive 195 TACE cycles in neoadjuvant intention.

Neoadjuvant TACE treatment was limited to patients with no more than five HCCs and no extrahepatic spread. In addition two of the five tumors were allowed to have a diameter of between 50 mm and 80 mm, the other lesions had to be smaller than 50 mm. The other exclusion criteria were similar to the criteria of palliative TACE. The patients should be in a good performance status without neoplastic ascites, high serum bilirubin level (>3 mg%), poor hepatic synthesis (serum albumin <2.0 mg/dl) or renal failure (serum creatinine >2 mg%).

Treatment response was defined as a shrinking of the target lesions to a diameter of less than 50 mm after the TACE treatment courses, documented with unenhanced MR images. Stable disease was defined as no significant change in size during the TACE treatment courses. Progressive disease was defined as an increase in size of a target lesion during TACE or newly developed lesions in the liver.

The TACE treatments were performed after exclusion of contraindications as already described. In our treatment protocol we administered three courses of chemoembolization at individual 4-week intervals. The first course of TACE was directed to embolize the area of the largest liver tumors. In the second course we embolized the other lesions and then the large lesions again in the third course. The embolization suspension containing a maximum of 10 mg/m^2 mitomycin C (Medac, Hamburg, Germany) as a chemotherapeutic agent and a maximum of 15 ml lipiodol, an iodized oil (Guerbet, Sulzbach,

Germany), followed by injection of 200–450 mg microspheres (Spherex, Pharmacia and Upjohn, Erlangen, Germany) for vascular occlusion was applied slowly under fluoroscopic control until stasis of blood flow was observed. Generally, the patients tolerated the TACE procedure well and all patients were discharged on the same day after TACE treatment. No fatal or major complications related to the TACE treatment were observed.

The MRI scans after the final course of TACE demonstrated in 32 patients (66.7%) a decrease in size of the treated lesions, forming the basis for performing MR-guided LITT for ablation of liver tumors (Fig. 3.1.1). In other patients post-interventional imaging after the third course of TACE showed a stable disease in 12 (25.0%) patients and a progressive disease in 4 (8.3%) patients. MR-guided LITT using a neodymium yttrium-aluminum-garnet (Nd: YAG) laser in the same technique as described before was performed 4–6 weeks after the last TACE cycle. Sixty-nine LITT treatment sessions were performed with a mean of 1.9 LITT procedures. Based on the size and topographical relationship of the liver tumors, a minimum of two applicator systems and a maximum of five applicator systems (mean 3.2 applicators) were positioned per MR-guided LITT. The cumulative survival time of the patients with HCC treated with the combined protocol was 36.0 months (95% confidence interval 29.3–42.6 months) after the first treatment (Fig. 3.1.2).

During and immediately after laser treatments, no major complications occurred. In 15 patients minor complications such as pain, pleural effusion or subcapsular hematoma were noted with MR imaging 24 h after LITT treatment. Follow-up in the other patients treated with the combined protocol

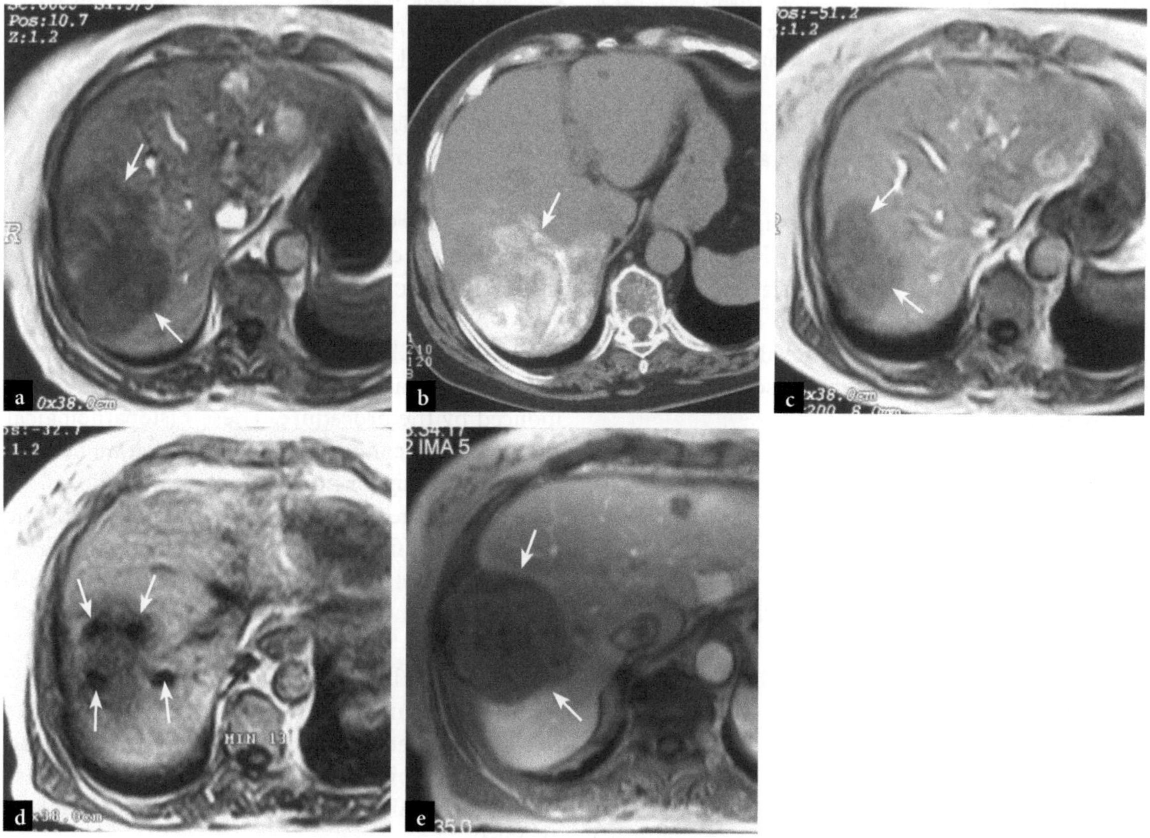

Fig. 3.1.1a–e. Unenhanced transverse GRE T_1-weighted MR images (TE/TR = 140/12, flip angle 80°) demonstrate a 65 × 45 mm HCC (*arrows*) in the right liver lobe with irregular borders before treatment (**a**). Unenhanced transverse CT scan obtained after the first TACE course shows high intratumoral lipiodol retention (*arrows*, **b**). Unenhanced transverse T_1-weighted GRE MR scan shows a decreasing of the residual lesion (*arrows*) after the third transarterial chemoembolization (*TACE*) treatment (**c**). Five weeks after the last TACE course laser ablation was performed, introducing four laser catheters (*arrowhead*). MR imaging during the ablation shows a decreasing of the signal as a sign of temperature development (**d**). Gd-DTPA-enhanced transverse T_1-weighted MR scan following 24 h after laser-induced thermotherapy (*LITT*) documents the induced necrosis (*arrows*)

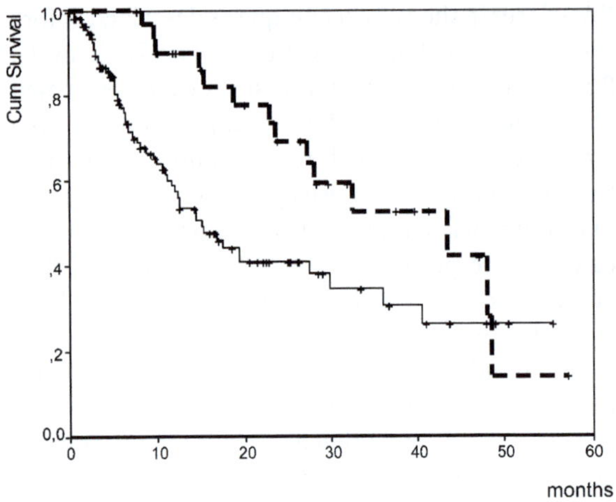

Fig. 3.1.2. Survival data calculated by the Kaplan–Meier method for patients with hepatocellular carcinoma (*HCC*) treated only with (-) TACE ($n=123$) or patients ($n=32$) treated with (---) the combined treatment protocol (TACE followed by LITT). The mean survival of patients with TACE treatment was 25.0 months and significant lower than the median survival of 36.0 months in patients treated with the combined protocol

did not show any long-term sequelae or worsening of the liver function.

In summary our results showed that the combined treatment protocol (TACE followed by MR-guided LITT) appears to be a safe and effective treatment of large unresectable liver tumors (Fig. 3.1.3). The combination of TACE and LITT results in significant increased survival rates in comparison to the results of TACE alone.

3.1.2 Combined Interventional Therapies

Recently various reports of promising results after combining TACE with local ablative treatment therapies have been published. TACE combined with other local ablative treatment options such as MR-guided LITT or radiofrequency (RF) ablation have shown increased effectiveness. With the combined protocol better results were observed than with either of these therapies alone (Bartolozzi et al. 1995; Ishida et al. 2002; Lencioni et al. 1998; Rossi et al. 2000; Takamura et al. 2001; Trevisani et al. 2001; Vogl et al. 2003). At the time of writing, the majority of the publications discuss the combined treatment in patients with HCC.

3.1.2.1 Combination of TACE and PEI

Percutaneous ethanol injection (PEI) is a well-tolerated and effective treatment in patients with HCC. PEI showed a high anti-tumoral efficacy in nodules smaller than 3 cm with a complete response rate in 80% (Bruix et al. 2001). Nevertheless, the high recurrence rate in patients with HCC after PEI, especially in those with high levels of AFP and those without peritumoral capsule or with large lesions and cirrhosis, decreases the long-term prognosis.

In contrast to this, patients with inoperable HCCs treated by the combination of TACE and PEI have a clear survival benefit versus patients treated only with repeated TACE (Allgaier et al. 1998; Bartolozzi et al. 1995; Dohmen et al. 2001). Lubienski et al. (2004) showed that the combination of TACE and PEI is an effective and safe method in the palliative treatment of large HCC. In this study 6-,12-, and 36-month survival rates for TACE monotherapy of 61%, 21%, and 4% in comparison to 77%, 55%, and 22% for combined TACE and PEI were observed.

A favorable outcome of this combined therapy can be expected in patients with solitary and encapsulated HCC (low Okuda stage, AFP level < 100 ng/ml), compensatory cirrhosis, and absence of portal vein thrombosis (Acunas and Rozanes 1999; Lencioni et al. 1998).

Hereby TACE results in disruption of the intratumoral septa as a result of the necrotic phenomena induced by the procedure. These histopathological changes allow complete ethanol infiltration in large tumors, with higher intratumoral ethanol doses.

Moreover, treatment with PEI is facilitated by the TACE-derived fibrous wall around the lesion, which favors better retention of the injected ethanol within the tumor (Kirchhoff et al. 1998; Lencioni et al. 1998).

Similar results were shown by Chen et al. (2004) for the combination of TACE with percutaneous injection of chemical agents and acetic acids instead PEI. This combination is also efficacious at increasing the survival rate of patients with HCC (Chen et al. 2004).

3.1.2.2 Combination of TACE and Radiation

To this day radiotherapy has not played a significant role in treating liver tumors because of the poor

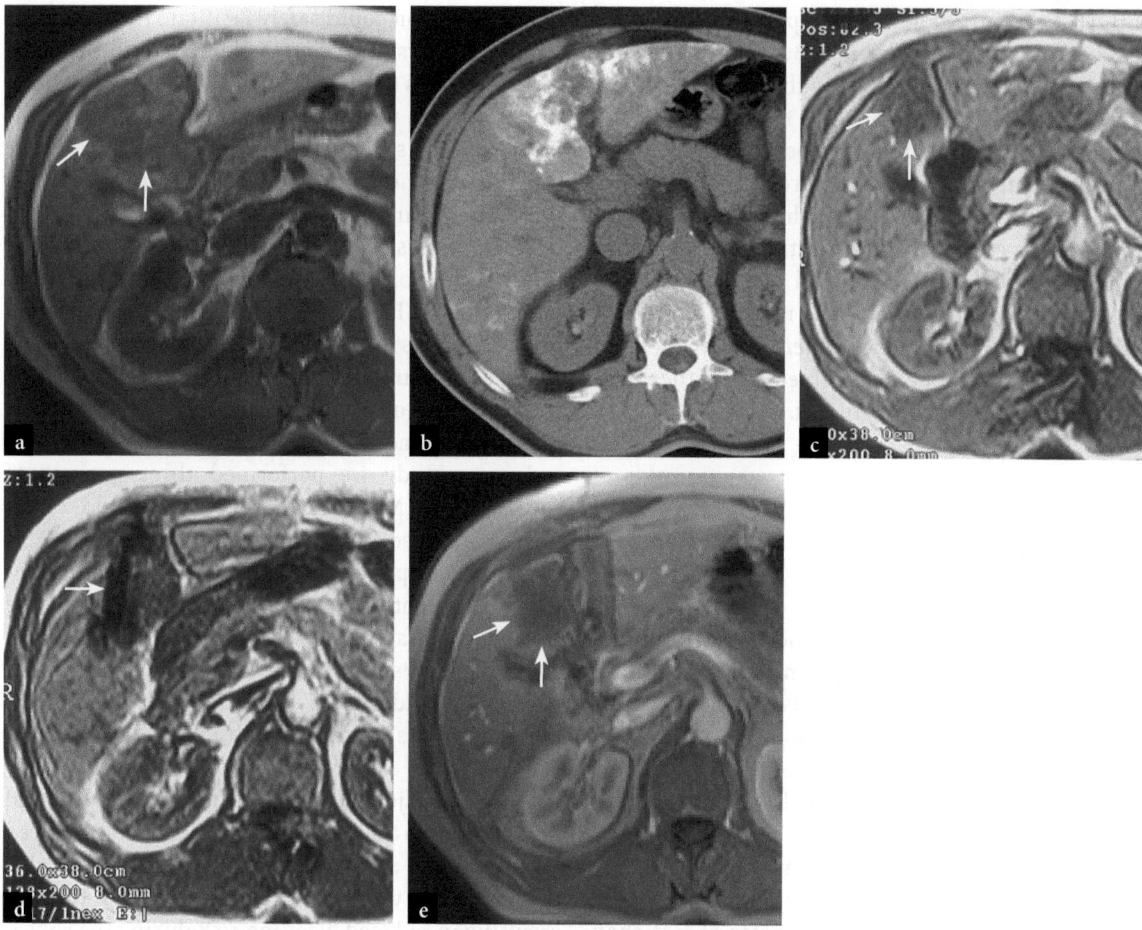

Fig. 3.1.3a–e. Transverse GRE T_1-weighted MR image shows a large liver tumor in segment 4b (*arrows*, **a**). Unenhanced CT after the first TACE course documented high intratumoral lipiodol retention (**b**). After the third course of TACE a 50% decrease in tumor volume (*arrows*) could be observed (**c**), followed by MR-guided LITT after 4 weeks. Unenhanced MR images documented the position of one laser applicator (*arrow*) to the residual tumor (**d**). Contrast-enhanced transverse MR scan 24 h after LITT demonstrates the ablated volume (*arrows*), characterized by a low signal intensity surrounded by a hyperintense rim (**e**)

radiation tolerance of the liver and the benefit of radiotherapy is still uncertain (Guo et al. 2003). Delivering the highest irradiation dose within the tolerance of the liver is the key to improving the long-term effect. The combination of TACE with radiotherapy may remedy the limitation of each technique alone and have synergistic effects. Tumor shrinkage after TACE allows the use of smaller irradiation fields, which permits higher tumor doses and improves radiation tolerance of normal liver tissue. Matsuura et al. (1998) reported the 2-year survival of 36.4% for 22 patients with HCC treated with radiotherapy alone or with combination of TACE and radiation therapy. Seong et al. (1999) treated 30 patients with local radiotherapy starting within 7–10 days following TACE. They indicated their median survival to be 17 months and 2-year survival to be 33.3%. The combination of TACE with radiotherapy for large unresectable HCC showed a higher response rate than that in the TACE alone group (47.4% vs 28.1%). The 1-year survival rate in the TACE plus irradiation group was 64.0% and significantly higher than for those given TACE alone, at 39.9% (Guo et al. (2003).

In patients with large unresectable HCC who failed with TACE, local RT induced a substantial tumor response of 66.7%, with a 3-year survival rate of 21.4% and a median survival time of 14 months (Seong et al. 2000).

The combination of embolization and internal radiation with intra-arterial injection of radioactive lipiodol has shown promising results in patients with HCC. Raoul et al. (1997) reported that overall survival rates at 6 months, 1, 2, 3, and 4 years were 69%, 38%, 22%, 14% and 10%, in the ^{131}I-labeled lipiodol group and 66%, 42%, 22%, 3%, and 0% in the chemoembolization group, respectively. In terms of patient survival and tumor response, radioactive ^{131}I-labeled lipiodol and chemoembolization were equally effective in the treatment of HCC, but tolerance to ^{131}I-labeled lipiodol was significantly better. Whether this therapeutic method can really increase the survival rate of patients suffering from liver cancer should be determined by further prospective and comparative studies.

3.1.2.3 Combination of TACE and Thermal Ablation (LITT / RF)

Thermal ablation techniques, such as MR-guided LITT or radiofrequency, are promising in situ ablation techniques for malignant liver tumors. However, clinical use of thermal ablative techniques is still limited because of the size of the inducible coagulation necroses. This results in insufficient tumor destruction in large liver tumors. Curley and Izzo (2002) suggested that radiofrequency ablation is a safe, well-tolerated, effective treatment for unresectable hepatic malignancies of less than 6.0 cm in diameter. Depending on the application technique LITT can create an area of coagulation necrosis up to 6–8 cm (Vogl et al. 2003). Additional, hepatic perfusion affects the size of the coagulation areas produced during thermal ablation. Consequently experimental studies found also that temporary interruption of blood flow to the liver significantly increases the size of the coagulated area during the laser treatment (Albrecht et al. 1998; Heisterkamp et al. 1997; Wacker et al. 2001). The combination of TACE and radiofrequency ablation increased the extent of induced coagulation compared to radiofrequency alone (Buscarini et al. 1999; Bloomston et al. 2002; Kitamoto et al. 2003). Yamakado et al. (2004) achieved complete necrosis in all HCC lesions regardless of tumor size or morphology after combination of radiofrequency ablation within 2 weeks after single chemoembolization. Laser coagulation for treating liver tumors should preferably be performed by application routes that permit temporary interruption of hepatic perfusion (Albrecht et al. 1998). Likewise temporary hepatic vein or portal branch occlusion during radiofrequency ablation could safely facilitate the treatment of large tumors or tumors in contact with the walls of large vessels (de Baere et al. 2002). Nevertheless, this study also showed a limitation of the therapeutic effect of this combined therapy. One-third of the treated large nonnodular lesions recurred beyond tumor-free margins.

Nevertheless, the combination of radiofrequency thermal ablation and TACE allows an effective treatment of larger HCCs resulting in improved survival rates (Bloomston et al. 2002; Buscarini et al. 1999). Mean survival was months longer after TACE with radiofrequency ablation compared with TACE alone, at 11.4 months.

In our study we performed three courses of TACE before MR-guided LITT. We could document a decrease of the tumor volume after TACE in two-thirds of patients with HCC treated with neoadjuvant intention, such that safe ablation of the treated tumors could be achieved (Zangos et al. 2004). These results indicate that neoadjuvant TACE before MR-guided LITT can extend the use of ablative techniques in patients with large liver tumors (Fig. 3.1.4).

With neoadjuvant TACE tumor shrinkage could be achieved, so that safe laser ablation with a reduced risk of tumor recidivism was possible. TACE also decreases the vascularization of the liver tumors, resulting in reduced bleeding risk during the subsequent procedure. During the 3-month TACE course more detailed insight about the biological data of the tumor and possible multifocal manifestation could be acquired. Small lesions, which could not be detected with other imaging modalities, could be detected and treated during TACE treatments. Therefore, the risk of new lesions developing immediately after LITT might be reduced.

3.1.2.4 Combination of TACE and Microwave Coagulation

Microwave ablation is the most recent development in the field of tumor ablation. The technique allows for flexible approaches to treatment, including percutaneous, laparoscopic, and open surgical access (Simon et al. 2005).

Nevertheless, the indication of percutaneous microwave coagulation therapy as an alternative to hepatic resection should be limited to cases of a well-differentiated HCC tumor smaller than 2 cm up

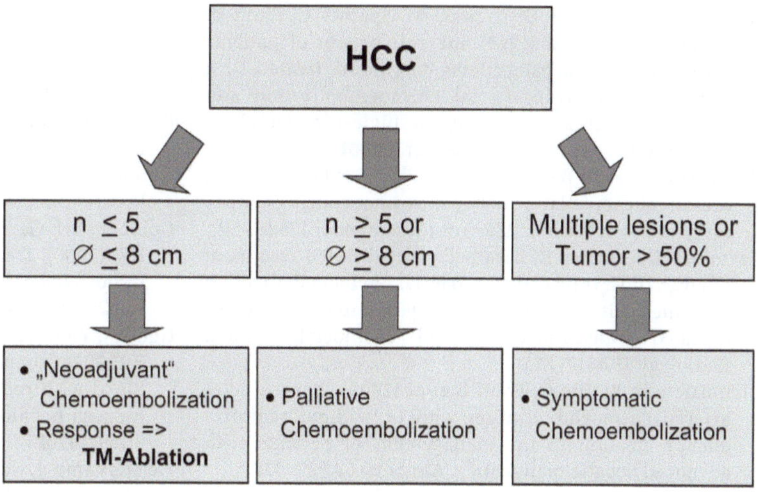

Fig. 3.1.4. Flow chart of different treatment options in patients with HCC using chemoembolization

to 3 cm in diameter without combination of TACE or multiple insertions of electrodes (Imamoto et al. 2001; Liang et al. 2004). At present, there are no published studies concerning the clinical value of the combination of TACE with microwave ablation.

Ishikawa et al. (2000) suggested that microwave coagulation therapy can destroy the peripheral part of the tumor that might remain viable after transarterial embolization (TAE), but combination therapy with TAE was preferable, especially when a viable part existed within tumors.

Hepatic outflow obstruction by balloon occlusion of the hepatic vein and combination with hepatic artery block can cause larger areas of coagulation with microwave coagulation therapy (Hiraki and Kanazawa 2005; Shibata et al. 2002b). However, clinical trials are required to define the role of this combined therapy in the treatment of liver tumors.

3.1.2.5 Combination of TACE and Cryotherapy

Cryosurgery may permit successful ablation of hepatic tumors but can be complicated by postoperative hemorrhage and is also associated with a significant risk of recurrence (Clavien et al. 2002). The combination of cryotherapy and TACE might be beneficial. TACE may reduce the risk of hemorrhage after cryosurgery but can increase the risk of hepatic failure in patients with poor hepatic function.

Qian et al. (2003) proposed that percutaneous cryoablation combined with TACE is a treatment of choice for liver carcinoma. It is minimally invasive, safe and effective for those patients with liver cancer unsuitable for surgery.

3.1.3 Conclusion

The combination of TACE with local ablative techniques is more effective than TACE or ablation alone. This multimodal therapy is a promising treatment option for patients with large unresectable HCCs. While an increased survival could be documented for the patients who were treated with combined protocols, the issue of the effectiveness of TACE in treating huge unresectable liver tumors remains unanswered. To establish an optimal therapy schedule, controlled randomized studies comparing the different methods and defining the value of the combined treatments are necessary.

References

Acunas B, Rozanes I (1999) Hepatocellular carcinoma: treatment with transcatheter arterial chemoembolization. Eur J Radiol 32:86–89

Albrecht D, Germer CT, Isbert C, Ritz JP, Roggan A, Muller G, Buhr HJ (1998) Interstitial laser coagulation: evaluation of the effect of normal liver blood perfusion and the application mode on lesion size. Lasers Surg Med 23:40–47

Allgaier HP, Deibert P, Olschewski M, Spamer C, Blum U, Gerok W, Blum HE (1998) Survival benefit of patients with inoperable hepatocellular carcinoma treated by a combination of transarterial chemoembolization and percutaneous ethanol injection – a single-center analysis including 132 patients. Int J Cancer 79:601–605

de Baere T, Bessoud B, Dromain C et al (2002) Percutaneous radiofrequency ablation of hepatic tumors during temporary venous occlusion. AJR Am J Roentgenol 178:53–59

Bartolozzi C, Lencioni R, Caramella D et al (1995) Treatment of large HCC: transcatheter arterial chemoembolization combined with percutaneous ethanol injection versus repeated transcatheter arterial chemoembolization. Radiology 197:812–818

Bloomston M, Binitie O, Fraiji E et al (2002) Transcatheter arterial chemoembolization with or without radiofrequency ablation in the management of patients with advanced hepatic malignancy. Am Surg 68:827–831

Bruix J, Sherman M, Llovet J et al (2001) Clinical management of hepatocellular carcinoma. Conclusions of the Barcelona-2000 EASL conference. European Association for the Study of the Liver. J Hepatol 35:421–430

Bruix J, Sala M, Llovet J (2004) Chemoembolization for hepatocellular carcinoma. Gastroenterology 127:S179–S188

Buscarini L, Buscarini E, Di Stasi M, Quaretti P, Zangrandi A (1999) Percutaneous radiofrequency thermal ablation combined with transcatheter arterial embolization in the treatment of large hepatocellular carcinoma. Ultraschall Med 20:47–53

Camma C, Schepis F, Orlando A, Albanese M, Shahied L, Trevisani F, Andreone P, Craxi A, Cottone M (2002) Transarterial chemoembolization for unresectable hepatocellular carcinoma: meta-analysis of randomized controlled trials. Radiology 224:47–54

Chen HB, Huang Y, Dai DL, Zhang X, Huang ZW, Zhang QK, Wang HH, Zhang JS, Pan G (2004) Therapeutic effect of transcatheter arterial chemoembolization and percutaneous injection of acetic acids on primary liver cancer. Hepatobiliary Pancreat Dis Int 3:55–57

Clavien PA, Kang KJ, Selzner N, Morse MA, Suhocki PV (2002) Cryosurgery after chemoembolization for hepatocellular carcinoma in patients with cirrhosis. J Gastrointest Surg 6:95–101

Curley SA, Izzo F (2002) Radiofrequency ablation of primary and metastatic hepatic malignancies. Int J Clin Oncol 7:72–81

Curley SA, Izzo F, Ellis LM, Nicolas Vauthey J, Vallone P (2000) Radiofrequency ablation of hepatocellular cancer in 110 patients with cirrhosis. Ann Surg 232:381–391

Dohmen K, Shirahama M, Shigematsu H, Miyamoto Y, Torii Y, Irie K, Ishibashi H (2001) Transcatheter arterial chemoembolization therapy combined with percutaneous ethanol injection for unresectable large hepatocellular carcinoma: an evaluation of the local therapeutic effect and survival rate. Hepatogastroenterology 48:1409–1415

Dwerryhouse SJ, Seifert JK, McCall JL, Iqbal J, Ross WB, Morris DL (1998) Hepatic resection with cryotherapy to involved or inadequate resection margin (edge freeze) for metastases from colorectal cancer. Br J Surg 85:185–187

Fan J, Tang ZY, Yu YQ, Wu ZQ, Ma ZC, Zhou XD, Zhou J, Qiu SJ, Lu JZ (1998) Improved survival with resection after transcatheter arterial chemoembolization (TACE) for unresectable hepatocellular carcinoma. Dig Surg 15:674–678

Finlay IG, Seifert JK, Stewart GJ, Morris DL (2000) Resection with cryotherapy of colorectal hepatic metastases has the same survival as hepatic resection alone. Eur J Surg Oncol 26:199–202

Fiorentini G, Poddie DB, Giorgi UD et al (2000) Global approach to hepatic metastases from colorectal cancer: indication and outcome of intra-arterial chemotherapy and other hepatic-directed treatments. Med Oncol 17:163–173

Goldberg SN, Gazelle GS, Compton CC, Mueller PR, Tanabe KK (2000) Treatment of intrahepatic malignancy with radiofrequency ablation: radiologic-pathologic correlation. Cancer 88:2452–2463

Guo WJ, Yu EX, Liu LM, Li J, Chen Z, Lin JH, Meng ZQ, Feng Y (2003) Comparison between chemoembolization combined with radiotherapy and chemoembolization alone for large hepatocellular carcinoma. World J Gastroenterol 9:1697–1701

Heisterkamp J, van Hillegersberg R, Mulder PG, Sinofsky EL, Ijzermans JN (1997) Importance of eliminating portal flow to produce large intrahepatic lesions with interstitial laser coagulation. Br J Surg 84:1245–1248

Hiraki T, Kanazawa S (2005) Hepatic outflow obstruction created by balloon occlusion of the hepatic vein: induced hepatic hemodynamic changes and the thherapeutic applications of hepatic venous occlusion with a balloon catheter in interventional radiology. Acta Med Okayama 59:171–178

Ishida T, Murakami T, Shibata T, Inoue Y, Takamura M, Niinobu T, Sato T, Nakamura H (2002) Percutaneous microwave tumor coagulation for hepatocellular carcinomas with interruption of segmental hepatic blood flow. J Vasc Interv Radiol 13:185–191

Ishikawa M, Ikeyama S, Sasaki K et al (2000) Intraoperative microwave coagulation therapy for large hepatic tumors. J Hepatobiliary Pancreat Surg 7:587–591

Itamoto T, Katayama K, Fukuda S et al (2001) Percutaneous microwave coagulation therapy for primary or recurrent hepatocellular carcinoma: long-term results. Hepatogastroenterology 48:1401–1405

Kirchhoff T, Chavan A, Galanski M (1998) Transarterial chemoembolization and percutaneous ethanol injection therapy in patients with hepatocellular carcinoma [comment]. Eur J Gastroenterol Hepatol 10:907–909

Kitamoto M, Imagawa M, Yamada H et al (2003) Radiofrequency ablation in the treatment of small hepatocellular carcinomas: comparison of the radiofrequency effect with and without chemoembolization. AJR Am J Roentgenol 181:997–1003

Lencioni R, Paolicchi A, Moretti M et al (1998) Combined transcatheter arterial chemoembolization and percutaneous ethanol injection for the treatment of large hepatocellular carcinoma: local therapeutic effect and long-term survival rate. Eur Radiol 8:439–444

Lencioni RA, Allgaier HP, Cioni D et al (2003) Small hepatocellular carcinoma in cirrhosis: randomized comparison of radio-frequency thermal ablation versus percutaneous ethanol injection. Radiology 228:235–240

Liang JD, Yang PM, Huang GT, Lee HS, Chen CH, Liang PC, Sheu JC, Chen DS (2004) Percutaneous microwave coagulation therapy under ultrasound guidance for small hepatocellular carcinoma. J Formos Med Assoc 103:908–913

Livraghi T (2001) Guidelines for treatment of liver cancer. Eur J Ultrasound 13:167–176

Lubienski A, Bitsch RG, Schemmer P, Grenacher L, Dux M, Kauffmann GW (2004) Long-term results of interventional treatment of large unresectable hepatocellular carcinoma (HCC): significant survival benefit from combined transcatheter arterial chemoembolization (TACE) and percutaneous ethanol injection (PEI) compared to TACE monotherapy. Rofo 176:1794–1802

Matsuura M, Nakajima N, Arai K, Ito K (1998) The usefulness of radiation therapy for hepatocellular carcinoma. Hepatogastroenterology 45:791–796

Matthewson K, Coleridge-Smith P, O'Sullivan JP, Northfield TC, Bown SG (1987) Biological effects of intrahepatic neodymium:yttrium-aluminum-garnet laser photocoagulation in rats. Gastroenterology 93:550–557

Nagasue N, Kohno H, Chang YC et al (1993) Liver resection for hepatocellular carcinoma. Results of 229 consecutive patients during 11 years. Ann Surg 217:375–384

Qian GJ, Chen H, Wu MC (2003) Percutaneous cryoablation after chemoembolization of liver carcinoma: report of 34 cases. Hepatobiliary Pancreat Dis Int 2:520–524

Raoul JL, Guyader D, Bretagne JF, Heautot JF, Duvauferrier R, Bourguet P, Bekhechi D, Deugnier YM, Gosselin M (1997) Prospective randomized trial of chemoembolization versus intra-arterial injection of ^{131}I-labeled-iodized oil in the treatment of hepatocellular carcinoma. Hepatology 26:1156–1161

Rossi S, Garbagnati F, Lencioni R et al (2000) Percutaneous radio-frequency thermal ablation of nonresectable hepatocellular carcinoma after occlusion of tumor blood supply. Radiology 217:119–126

Seong J, Keum KC, Han KH, Lee DY, Lee JT, Chon CY, Moon YM, Suh CO, Kim GE (1999) Combined transcatheter arterial chemoembolization and local radiotherapy of unresectable hepatocellular carcinoma. Int J Radiat Oncol Biol Phys 43:393–397

Seong J, Park HC, Han KH et al (2000) Local radiotherapy for unresectable hepatocellular carcinoma patients who failed with transcatheter arterial chemoembolization. Int J Radiat Oncol Biol Phys 47:1331–1335

Shibata T, Iimuro Y, Yamamoto Y, Maetani Y, Ametani F, Itoh K, Konishi J (2002a) Small hepatocellular carcinoma: comparison of radio-frequency ablation and percutaneous microwave coagulation therapy. Radiology 223:331–337

Shibata T, Morita T, Okuyama M, Kitada M, Shimano T, Ishida T (2002b) Comparison of percutaneous microwave coagulation area under interruption of hepatic arterial blood flow with that under hepatic arterial and venous blood flow for hepatocellular carcinoma. Gan To Kagaku Ryoho 29:2146–2148

Shiina S, Teratani T, Obi S, Hamamura K, Koike Y, Omata M (2002) Nonsurgical treatment of hepatocellular carcinoma: from percutaneous ethanol injection therapy and percutaneous microwave coagulation therapy to radiofrequency ablation. Oncology 62:64–68

Simon CJ, Dupuy DE, Mayo-Smith WW (2005) Microwave ablation: principles and applications. Radiographics 25 [Suppl 1]:S69–S83

Solbiati L, Livraghi T, Goldberg SN, Ierace T, Meloni F, Dellanoce M, Cova L, Halpern EF, Gazelle GS (2001) Percutaneous radio-frequency ablation of hepatic metastases from colorectal cancer: long-term results in 117 patients. Radiology 221:159–166

Takamura M, Murakami T, Shibata T et al (2001) Microwave coagulation therapy with interruption of hepatic blood in- or outflow: an experimental study. J Vasc Interv Radiol 12:619–622

Tancredi T, McCuskey PA, Kan Z, Wallace S (1999) Changes in rat liver microcirculation after experimental hepatic arterial embolization: comparison of different embolic agents. Radiology 211:177–181

Tellez C, Benson AB 3rd, Lyster MT, Talamonti M, Shaw J, Braun MA, Nemcek AA Jr, Vogelzang RL (1998) Phase II trial of chemoembolization for the treatment of metastatic colorectal carcinoma to the liver and review of the literature. Cancer 82:1250–1259

Trevisani F, De Notariis S, Rossi C, Bernardi M (2001) Randomized control trials on chemoembolization for hepatocellular carcinoma: is there room for new studies? J Clin Gastroenterol 32:383–389

Verhoef C, Kuiper JW, Heisterkamp J et al (2003) Interstitial laser coagulation with temporary hepatic artery occlusion for patients with cirrhosis and irresectable hepatoma. Br J Surg 90:950–955

Vogl TJ, Trapp M, Schroeder H, Mack M, Schuster A, Schmitt J, Neuhaus P, Felix R (2000) Transarterial chemoembolization for hepatocellular carcinoma: volumetric and morphologic CT criteria for assessment of prognosis and therapeutic success – results from a liver transplantation center. Radiology 214:349–357

Vogl TJ, Straub R, Eichler K, Woitaschek D, Mack MG (2002a) Malignant liver tumors treated with MR imaging-guided laser-induced thermotherapy: experience with complications in 899 patients (2,520 lesions). Radiology 225:367–377

Vogl TJ, Zangos S, Balzer JO, Thalhammer A, Mack MG (2002b) Transarterial chemoembolization of liver metastases: Indication, technique, results. Rofo Fortschr Geb Rontgenstr Neuen Bildgeb Verfahr 174:675–683

Vogl TJ, Mack MG, Balzer JO, Engelmann K, Straub R, Eichler K, Woitaschek D, Zangos S (2003) Liver metastases: neoadjuvant downsizing with transarterial chemoembolization before laser-induced thermotherapy. Radiology 229:457–464

Wacker FK, Reither K, Ritz JP, Roggan A, Germer CT, Wolf KJ (2001) MR-guided interstitial laser-induced thermotherapy of hepatic metastasis combined with arterial blood flow reduction: technique and first clinical results in an open MR system. J Magn Reson Imaging 13:31–36

Whelan WM, Wyman DR, Wilson BC (1995) Investigations of large vessel cooling during interstitial laser heating. Med Phys 22:105–115

Yamakado K, Nakatsuka A, Akeboshi M, Shiraki K, Nakano T, Takeda K (2004) Combination therapy with radiofrequency ablation and transcatheter chemoembolization for the treatment of hepatocellular carcinoma: short-term recurrences and survival. Oncol Rep 11:105–109

Zangos S, Mack MG, Straub R, Engelmann K, Eichler K, Balzer J, Vogl TJ (2001) Transarterial chemoembolization (TACE) of liver metastases. A palliative therapeutic approach. Radiologe 41:84–90

Zangos S, Mack MG, Balzer JO et al (2004) Neoadjuvant transarterial chemoembolization (TACE) before percutaneous laser-induced thermotherapy (LITT): results in large-sized primary and secondary liver tumors. Medical Laser Application 19:98–108

Liver

Primary Tumors

3.2 Percutaneous Alcohol Instillation

Andreas Lubienski, Martin Simon, and Thomas K. Helmberger

CONTENTS

3.2.1 Introduction

As yet there is no general consensus on a common rational therapeutic approach to hepatocellular carcinoma (HCC). Therefore, treatment strategies for HCC vary throughout the world due to geographical differences in the incidence and presentation of the disease and the treatment options available. Several treatment guidelines have been published by the European Association for the Study of the Liver (EASL) (Bruix et al. 2001), with the Barcelona Clinic Liver Cancer (BCLC) staging recommendation being the most accepted (Fig. 3.2.1) (Mor et al. 1998; Sala et al. 2004). It links tumoral stage with treatment strategy, and is aimed at incorporating an estimation of the prognosis and potential treatment advancements in a single unified proposal (Sala et al. 2004). According to these guidelines percutaneous alcohol instillation (PAI) has a place in the treatment strategy of HCC, generally as a second choice when surgical techniques are precluded, such as in patients with early-stage tumors; nevertheless, in some centers in Italy and Japan PAI is used as a first-line treatment option (Llovet et al. 2003). The role of PAI as the percutaneous treatment of choice for early-stage HCC is challenged by other local ablative techniques. Over the last two decades, several percutaneous ablation techniques for thermal tumor destruction have been developed and clinically tested (Ebara et al. 2005; Llovet 2005). This was particularly driven by several specific shortcomings of PAI. It has been shown that neoplastic dissemination by means of tumor satellites occurs at very early stages in HCC, first near the boundaries of the tumor, later within the anatomic segments and, finally, beyond them. Even tumors of as little as 2 cm in diameter present local metastases less than 10 mm distant to the primary in about 10% of cases, and microscopic portal invasion in up to 25% of cases (Kojiro 2004); hence the rationale to produce a 1-cm safety margin surrounding the tumor. Radiofrequency (RF) ablation but not PAI can provide this safety margin, which may reduce late treatment failures. The limited antitumoral effect of PAI in HCC larger than 3 cm is due to its inability to disrupt the intratumoral septa, thus decreasing its capacity to reach and eliminate all neoplastic cells (Lencioni and Llovet 2005).

A. Lubienski, MD; M. Simon, MD
Institut für Radiologie der Universität Lübeck, Ratzeburger Allee 160, 23538 Lübeck, Germany
T. K. Helmberger, MD
Professor, Department of Diagnostic and Interventional Radiology and Nuclear Medicine, Klinikum Bogenhausen, Engelschalkinger Strasse 77, 81925 Munich, Germany

3.2.2 Patient Selection

Patient selection is very crucial for successful treatment with PAI. It should be based upon tumor localization, size, proximity to large vessels, bleeding risk, respiratory motion, pathway of probe, and last but not least the physician's experience. Tumors must be accessible under image guidance. Patients classified

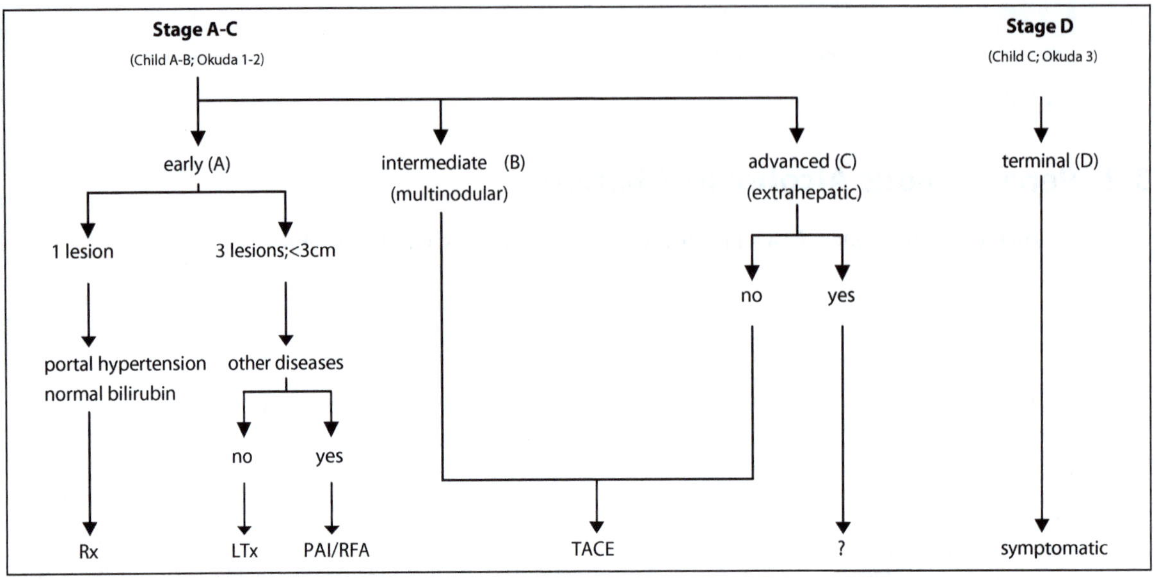

Fig. 3.2.1. Barcelona Clinic Liver Cancer (BCLC): stage-dependent treatment of HCC. (*HCC* Hepatocellular carcinoma, *LTx* liver transplantation, *Rx* liver resection)

as stage A according to the Barcelona Clinic Liver Cancer Staging Classification (Fig. 3.2.1), who are not candidates for surgery, qualify for percutaneous ablation (Bruix et al. 2001). Thus, the best candidates for PAI are those with Child A cirrhosis and small tumors (≤3 cm), who are expected to achieve complete responses and whose cancer is confined to the liver, but is nonetheless unresectable because of the distribution of disease or the severity of underlying cirrhosis (Ebara et al. 2005). Treatment of patients with larger tumours (3–5 cm), multiple tumours (three nodules <3 cm) and advanced liver failure (Child B) has to be decided on each patient's individual basis. From a practical point of view, in most centers the cut-off rate for the number of hepatic tumors to be treated is limited to four to five. In general, despite a few absolute contraindications such as systemic tumor progression, severe coagulopathy (Quick <35%, platelets <40,000/µl), Child C cirrhosis with refractory ascites, and limited life expectancy, there are no real limitations for PAI (Ebara et al. 2005; Lencioni et al. 2003).

3.2.3 Results

The efficacy of PAI in the treatment of early-stage HCC with low complication rates (morbidity 1.7%) and a negligible rate of treatment-related deaths (mortality 0.1%) has been shown in numerous studies, with complete response rates in 80% of tumors smaller than 3 cm in diameter, but only in 50% of tumors of 3–5 cm in size (Lencioni and Crocetti 2005; Livraghi et al. 1995). Histopathology revealed complete coagulation necrosis after PAI in about 70% of tumors smaller than 3 cm in diameter and no damage to healthy tissue at a distance from the treated tumor (Shiina et al. 1991). The 5-year survival ranged between 48% and 78% (Table 3.2.1) (Arii et al. 2000; Ebara et al. 2005; Lencioni et al. 1997; Livraghi et al. 1995, 2004; Omata et al. 2004; Sakamoto and Hirohashi 1998). Because injected alcohol damages cancer cells immediately (Shiina et al. 1991), seeding of cancer cells is unlikely to occur. Nevertheless, seeding is reported to be present in <0.01% to 0.6% (Di Stasi et al. 1997; Livraghi et al. 1995). Based on these results, in most centers PAI has an accepted role in the treatment strategy of small HCC, generally as a second choice when surgical techniques are precluded, such as in patients with early-stage tumors (Llovet et al. 2003).

Recent long-term data – 20 years of follow-up – by Ebara et al. (2005) confirmed in a single-center study of 270 patients that PAI is able to achieve local tumor destruction with no mortality or life-threatening complications. This group could also demonstrate that PAI – when administered as first-line treatment to patients with Child A cirrhosis and small HCCs – may achieve a 5-year survival as high as 65%. In

Table 3.2.1. Long-term outcome of PAI in the treatment of HCC

Author	Year	No. of patients, *n*	Selection criteria	Five-year survival (%)
Livraghi et al.	1995	169	Child A, single <3 cm	48
Lencioni et al.	1997	70	Child A, single <3 cm	63
Sakamoto and Hirohashi	1998	88	Single <2 cm	71
Arii et al.	2000	767	Stage I, single <2 cm	54
Livraghi et al.	2004	210	Early HCC	49
Omata et al.	2004	144	Single <2 cm	70
Ebara et al.	2005	270	Three nodules <3 cm	60
		96	Child A, <2 cm	78

addition Ebara et al. (2005) showed that Child A patients with a solitary tumor ≤2 cm in diameter are different regarding long-term outcomes. Patients with such small tumors not only had the best overall survival, but also showed significantly fewer tumor recurrences, occurring remotely from the treated nodule, than patients bearing a 2- to 3-cm HCC. This was confirmed by a recent study by Sala et al. (2004) showing that patients with a solitary HCC 2 cm or less in diameter treated with percutaneous ablation are more likely to achieve a sustained complete response in the long term. Independent predictors of survival are initial complete response, Child–Pugh score, number or size of nodules, and base-line AFP levels (Sala et al. 2004). In contrast to the above-mentioned studies, the major limitation of PAI, besides the uncertainty of tumor ablation and the long treatment time, is still the high local recurrence rate, which may reach 33% in tumors smaller than 3 cm and 43% in tumors exceeding 3 cm (Khan et al. 2000; Koda et al. 2000). It should be stressed that a recent study suggests RFA to be superior to PAI with 80% versus 90% of complete response rates. This could be achieved in a substantially lower number of treatment sessions (Livraghi et al. 1999). A similar study was conducted by Ikeda et al. (2001), who treated a series of 119 patients with solitary HCC less than 3 cm in diameter with either RFA ($n=23$) or PAI ($n=96$). Complete tumor response after RFA was 100%, and after PAI 94% was achieved in 1.5 versus 4 treatment sessions. Lencioni et al. (2003) presented in a prospective randomized comparison of RFA and PAI overall 1- and 2-year survival rates of 100% and 98% compared to 96% and 88%, which was not statistically significant. However, 1- and 2-year local recurrence-free survival was significantly higher (98% and 96% versus 83% and 62%). RF treatment was confirmed as an independent prognostic factor for local-recurrence-free survival by multivariate analysis. Recently, additional randomized studies comparing RF ablation and PAI for the first-line treatment of early-stage HCC have been published (Table 3.2.2). Survival advantages favoring RFA over PAI were identified in the study by Shiina et al. (2005) including 232 Japanese patients, with 4-year survival being 74% versus 57% ($P=0.02$). Two additional randomized controlled trials from Lin et al. (2004, 2005) reported survival advantages in the subgroup analysis of tumors larger than 2 cm, favoring RFA compared with either percutaneous ethanol or acetic acid injection. All four randomized trials showed that RF ablation had a greater local anticancer effect than PAI, leading to a better local control of the disease. However, the main drawback of RFA is its higher rate of adverse events compared with PAI, as it was described in one RCT (Lin et al. 2005). Therefore, the present data are not yet robust enough to definitively establish RF ablation as superior to PAI in the treatment of small tumors, although RF ablation appears to be the preferred percutaneous therapy for patients with early-stage HCC on the basis of more consistent local tumor control.

3.2.4 Combined Interventional Treatments

In order to reduce the risk of recurrent tumors and to enhance overall survival, combined treatment options including PAI have been evaluated for HCC. It has been demonstrated that transarterial chemoembolization (TACE) combined with alcohol injection has the potential to prolong survival compared to TACE alone in small HCC (Koda et al. 2001) and even in nodules with a mean size of 7 cm (Lubienski et al. 2004). Most recent data suggested PAI to be an important modulator of tissue properties prior to or

Table 3.2.2. Randomized controlled studies for the evaluation of percutaneous alcohol instillation (*PAI*) in HCC

Author Treatment	Patients	Tumor (≤2/>2 cm)	Complete necrosis (%)	Survival in years (%)			Local recurrence
				1	2	4	Overall recurrence
Huang et al. (2005)	76	45/31					
PAI	38			100	100	92	47%
Resection	38			97	91	88	39%
Lin et al. (2005)	187	111/76					2-year
RFA	62		96	93	81		14%
PAI	62		88	88	66		34%
Acetic acid	63		92	90	67		31%
Shiina et al. (2005)	232	102/130					2-year
RFA	118		100	97	91	74	2%
PAI	114		100	92	81	57	11%
Lin et al. (2004)	157	47/110					2-year
RFA	52		96	90	82		18%
PAI	52		88	85	61		45%
High dose PAI	53		92	88	63		33%
Lencioni et al. (2003)	102						2-year LRFS
RFA	52		91	100	98		4%
PAI	50		82	96	88		38%

directly during RFA for HCC. Tissue modulation for example with high-percent alcohol lowers the boiling point of the tissue resulting in reduced ablation times. Kurokohchi et al. (2005) showed that injection of alcohol prior to RFA therapy may equally enhance the volume of coagulated necrosis in three dimensions to the same extent regardless of the type of RFA instruments. More importantly and interestingly this group demonstrated that the volume and diameter of areas of coagulated necrosis were significantly larger in PAI-RFA than in RFA alone, although the total energy requirement was comparable between the groups. Thus, the energy needed for coagulation per unit volume was significantly lower in PAI-RFA than in RFA alone. The degree of enhancement of coagulated necrosis was higher between the groups classified according to the amount of injected alcohol than between those classified according to the amount of total energy requirement. Furthermore, the volume of coagulated necrosis showed a stronger correlation with the amount of alcohol injected than with the total energy requirement ($r=0.71$ versus 0.47) respectively. The results clearly indicate that less energy is required when combining PAI and RFA to induce comparable ablation areas than when using RFA alone. In addition, due to intrinsic antitumoral effects, PAI may lower recurrence rates when combined with RFA (Kurokohchi et al. 2005).

3.2.5 Conclusion

PAI will continue to play a role in the treatment of HCC, especially in patients where RFA cannot be applied. In addition, PAI will probably be an important part in combined interventional treatment strategies, whereas its final role in such strategies is not definitely established due to the lack of study evidence.

References

Arii S, Yamaoka Y, Futugawa S, Inoue K, Kobayashi K, Kojiro M, Makuuchi M, Nakamura Y, Okita K, Yamada R (2000) Results of surgical and nonsurgical treatment for small-sized hepatocellular carcinomas: a retrospective and nationwide survey in Japan. Hepatology 32:1224–1229

Bruix J, Sherman M, Llovet JM, Beaugrand M, Lencioni R, Burroughs AK, Christensen E, Pagliaro L, Colombo M, Rodés J, for the EASL Panel of Experts on HCC (2001) Clinical management of hepatocellular carcinoma. Conclusions of the Barcelona-2000 EASL Conference. J Hepatol 35:421–430

Di Stasi M, Buscarini L, Livraghi T, Giorgio A, Salmi A, De Sio I, Brunello F, Solmi L, Caturelli E, Magnolfi F, Caremani M, Filice C (1997) Percutaneous ethanol injection in the treatment of hepatocellular carcinoma. A multi-

center survey of evaluation practices and complication rates. Scand J Gastroenterol 32:1168–1173
Ebara M, Okabe S, Kita K, Sugiura N, Fukuda H, Yoshikawa M, Kondo F, Saisho H (2005) Percutaneous ethanol injection for small hepatocellular carcinoma: therapeutic efficacy based on 20-year observation. J Hepatol 43:377–380
Huang GT, Lee PH, Tsang YM, Lai MY, Yang PM, Hu RH, Chen PJ, Kao JH, Sheu JC (2005) Percutaneous ethanol injection versus surgical resection for the treatment of small hepatocellular carcinoma: a prospective study. Ann Surg 242:36–42
Ikeda M, Okada S, Ueno H, Okusaka T, Kuriyama H (2001) Radiofrequency ablation and percutaneous ethanol injection in patients with small hepatocellular carcinoma: a comparative study. Jpn J Clin Oncol 31:322–326
Khan KN, Yatsuhashi H, Yamasaki K, Yamasaki M, Inoue O, Koga M, Yano M (2000) Prospective analysis of risk factors for early intrahepatic recurrence of hepatocellular carcinoma following ethanol injection. J Hepatol 32:269–278
Koda M, Murawaki Y, Mitsuda A, Ohyama K, Horie Y, Suou T, Kawasaki H, Ikawa S (2000) Predictive factors for intrahepatic recurrence after percutaneous ethanol injection therapy for small hepatocellular carcinoma. Cancer 88:529–537
Koda M, Murawaki Y, Mitsuda A, Oyama K, Okamoto K, Idobe Y, Suou T, Kawasaki H (2001) Combination therapy with transcatheter arterial chemoembolization and percutaneous ethanol injection compared with percutaneous ethanol injection alone for patients with small hepatocellular carcinoma: a randomized control study. Cancer 92:1516–1524
Kojiro M (2004) Focus on dysplastic nodules and early hepatocellular carcinoma: an eastern point of view. Liver Transpl 10:S3–S8
Kurokohchi K, Watanabe S, Masaki T, Hosomi N, Miyauchi Y, Himoto T, Kimura Y, Nakai S, Deguchi A, Yoneyama H, Yoshida S, Kuriyama S (2005) Comparison between combination therapy of percutaneous ethanol injection and radiofrequency ablation and radiofrequency ablation alone for patients with hepatocellular carcinoma. World J Gastroenterol 11:1426–1432
Lencioni R, Crocetti L (2005) A critical appraisal of the literature on local ablative therapies for hepatocellular carcinoma. Clin Liver Dis 9:301–314
Lencioni R, Llovet JM (2005) Percutaneous ethanol injection for hepatocellular carcinoma: alive or dead? J Hepatol 43:377–380
Lencioni R, Pinto F, Armillotta N, Bassi AM, Moretti M, Di Giulio M, Marchi S, Uliana M, Della Capanna S, Lencioni M, Bartolozzi C (1997) Long-term results of percutaneous ethanol injection therapy for hepatocellular carcinoma in cirrhosis: a European experience. Eur Radiol 7:514–519
Lencioni RA, Allgaier HP, Cioni D, Olschewski M, Deibert P, Crocetti L, Frings H, Laubenberger J, Zuber I, Blum HE (2003) Small hepatocellular carcinoma in cirrhosis: randomized comparison of radio-frequency thermal ablation versus percutaneous ethanol injection. Radiology 228:235–240
Lin SM, Lin CJ, Lin CC, Hsu CW, Chen YC (2004) Radiofrequency ablation improves prognosis compared with ethanol injection for hepatocellular carcinoma ≤4 cm. Gastroenterology 127:1714–1723
Lin SM, Lin CJ, Lin CC, Hsu CW, ChenYC (2005) Randomized controlled trial comparing percutaneous radiofrequency thermal ablation, percutaneous ethanol injection, and percutaneous acetic acid injection to treat hepatocellular carcinoma of 3cm or less. Gut 54:1151–1156
Livraghi T, Giorgio A, Marin G, Salmi A, de Sio I, Bolondi L, Pompili M, Brunello F, Lazzaroni S, Torzilli G, Zucchi AL (1995) Hepatocellular carcinoma and cirrhosis in 746 patients: long-term results of percutaneous ethanol injection. Radiology 197:101–108
Livraghi T, Goldberg SN, Lazzaroni S, Meloni F, Solbiati L, Gazelle GS (1999) Small hepatocellular carcinoma: treatment with radio-frequency ablation versus ethanol injection. Radiology 210:655–661
Livraghi T, Meloni F, Morabito A, Vettori C (2004) Multimodal image-guided tailored therapy of early and intermediate hepatocellular carcinoma: long-term survival in the experience of a single radiologic referral center. Liver Transpl 10:S98–S106
Llovet JM (2005) Updated treatment approach to hepatocellular carcinoma. J Gastroenterol 40:225–235
Llovet JM, Burroughs A, Bruix J (2003) Hepatocellular carcinoma. Lancet 362:1907–1917
Lubienski A, Bitsch RG, Schemmer P, Grenacher L, Düx M, Kauffmann GW (2004) Long-term results of interventional treatment of large unresectable hepatocellular carcinoma (HCC): significant survival benefit from combined transcatheter arterial chemoembolization (TACE) and percutaneous ethanol injection (PEI) compared to TACE monotherapy. Fortschr Röntgenstr 176:1794–1802
Mor E, Kaspa RT, Sheiner P, Schwartz M (1998) Treatment of hepatocellular carcinoma associated with cirrhosis in the era of liver transplantation. Ann Intern Med 129:643–653
Omata M, Tateishi R, Yoshida H, Shiina S (2004) Treatment of hepatocellular carcinoma by percutaneous tumor ablation methods: ethanol injection therapy and radiofrequency ablation. Gastroenterology 127:S159–S166
Sakamoto M, Hirohashi S (1998) Natural history and prognosis of adenomatous hyperplasia and early hepatocellular carcinoma: multi-institutional analysis of 53 nodules followed up for more than 6 months and 141 patients with single early hepatocellular carcinoma treated by surgical resection or percutaneous ethanol injection. Jpn J Clin Oncol 28:604–608
Sala M, Llovet JM, Vilana R, Bianchi L, Sole M, Ayuso C, Brú C, Bruix J, Barcelona Clinic Liver Cancer Group (2004) Initial response to percutaneous ablation predicts survival in patients with hepatocellular carcinoma. Hepatology 40:1352–1360
Shiina S, Tagawa K, Unuma T, Takanashi R, Yoshiura K, Komatsu Y, Hata Y, Niwa Y, Shiratori Y, Terano A, Sugimoto T (1991) Percutaneous ethanol injection therapy for hepatocellular carcinoma: a histopathologic study. Cancer 68:1524–1530
Shiina S, Teratani T, Obi S, Sato S, Tateishi R, Fujishima T, Ishikawa T, Koike Y, Yoshida H, Kawabe T, Omata M (2005) A randomized controlled trial of radiofrequency ablation with ethanol injection for small hepatocellular carcinoma. Gastroenterology 129:122–130

Liver

3

Primary Tumors

3.3 Radiofrequency Ablation (RFA)

Tobias F. Jakobs, Ralf-Thorsten Hoffmann, Thomas K. Helmberger, and Maximilian F. Reiser

CONTENTS

3.3.1 Introduction

A diagnosis of hepatocellular carcinoma (HCC) implies a poor prognosis. HCC is the cause of 250,000 deaths worldwide each year. Early HCC is typically clinically silent, and the disease is often well advanced at the first manifestation. Since the introduction of surveillance in patients at high risk of developing HCC, the diagnosis of small HCC has increased, especially in endemic areas such as in parts of Asia. Without treatment, there is a 5-year survival rate of less than 5% (Llovet et al. 1999b; Ulner 2000). According to the World Health Organization, by the year 2010, HCC will have surpassed lung cancer as the foremost cause of cancer mortality. The increasing incidence may be related to the widespread transmission of viral hepatitis, specifically of types B and C, during the 1970s and early 1980s, when illicit use of intravenous narcotics, needle sharing, unsafe sexual activity, and transfusion of unsafe blood and blood products were common practices (Bruix et al. 2001). Patients with liver cirrhosis are at greatest risk for developing HCC and should be monitored every 6 months to detect the tumor at an asymptomatic stage (Bruix and Llovet 2002). The Barcelona-Clinic Liver Cancer (BCLC) group has developed a system that stratifies patients into four categories based on performance status, severity of liver dysfunction caused by the underlying cirrhosis, and the kind of tumor involvement, thus simultaneously setting prognosis and guiding treatment (Llovet et al. 1999a). In the BCLC staging classification, patients who have early-stage HCC, who have a good performance status, Child-Pugh class A or B cirrhosis and an asymptomatic single tumor smaller than 5 cm or as many as three lesions, each smaller than 3 cm are referred to radiofrequency ablation (RFA) (Fig. 3.3.1) (Llovet et al. 1999a).

These patients should be considered for any of the available radical treatment options, such as surgical resection, liver transplantation, or percutaneous techniques of tumor ablation (Bruix et al. 2001). However, surgical resection is only suitable for 9%–27% of patients with HCC because of their poor hepatic reserve due to the underlying chronic liver disease with significant portal hypertension and abnormal bilirubin levels or multifocal distribution of tumor nodules (Bruix and Llovet 2002; Fan et al. 1995; Lai et al. 1995; Liver Cancer Study Group of Japan 1990; Llovet et al. 1999a). Orthotopic liver transplantation (OLT) is a strategy that can treat both HCC and liver dysfunction, and indeed has shown excellent survival in patients at an early stage of the cancer (Llovet et al. 1999c; Mazzaferro et al. 1996). However, with an increasing demand for donor organs but a limited supply,

T. F. Jakobs, MD; R.-T. Hoffmann, MD;
M. F. Reiser, MD, Professor
Department of Clinical Radiology, University Hospitals - Grosshadern, Ludwig-Maximilians-University of Munich, Marchioninistrasse 15, 81377 Munich, Germany
T. K. Helmberger, MD
Professor, Department of Diagnostic and Interventional Radiology and Nuclear Medicine, Klinikum Bogenhausen, Engelschalkinger Strasse 77, 81925 Munich, Germany

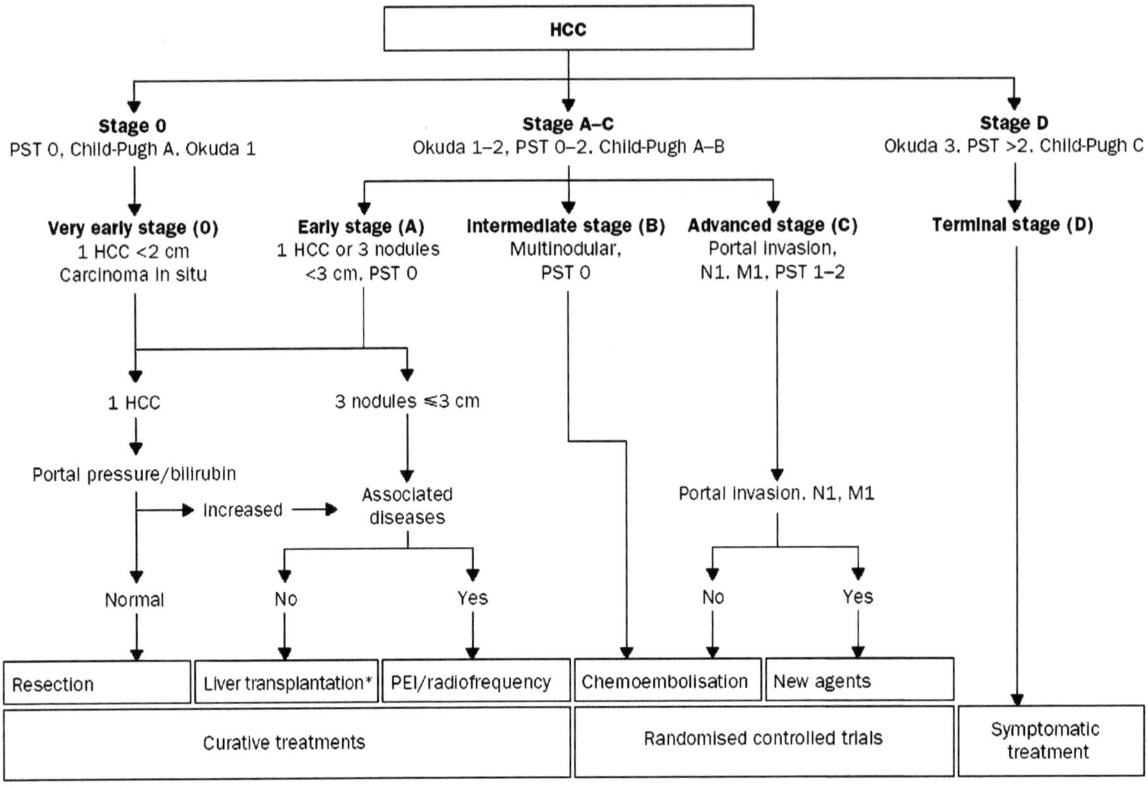

Fig. 3.3.1. This flowchart illustrates the algorithm used for selecting the appropriate treatment option for patients with hepatocellular carcinoma (*HCC*) including surgical resection, transplantation, radiofrequency ablation (*RFA*), transarterial chemoembolization (*TACE*), new agents such as selective internal radiation therapy (*SIRT*), systemic therapy and best supportive care. RFA is offered to patients with early-stage HCC with a single tumor smaller than 5 cm or as many as three lesions, each smaller than 3 cm, good performance status and evidence for neither vascular invasion nor extrahepatic tumor spread based on clinical and imaging findings. (*M* Metastases, *N* nodules, *PEI* percutaneous ethanol injection, *PST* performance status test.) *Cadaveric liver transplantation or living donor liver transplantation With permission from Llovet et al. (2003) *Lancet* 362:1907–1917

the waiting time for an OLT is now longer then 1 year in Europe and the United States (Llovet et al. 1999c; Sarasin et al. 1998). Living donor liver transplantation is still at an early stage of clinical application (Bruix and Llovet 2002). Regarding these issues, percutaneous ablation plays a major role in the management of early-stage HCC (Lencioni et al. 2004, 2005; Tateishi et al. 2005b).

Various percutaneous, locoregional therapeutic modalities have been developed and tested clinically over recent years for the treatment of HCC. These include intratumoral injection of ethanol or acetic acid and thermal ablation with RF, laser, microwaves, or cryosurgery. Percutaneous ethanol injection (PEI), more frequently performed in the past, is considered to be effective for the treatment of relatively small-sized, encapsulated early-stage HCC and therefore may achieve 5-year survival rates of 32%–47% (Lencioni et al. 1995; Livraghi et al. 1995). The major limitation of PEI is the high local recurrence rate that may reach up to 43% (Koda et al. 2000).

RFA has emerged as the most powerful alternative method for percutaneous ablation (Gadaleta et al. 2004; Gillams 2003, 2005; Goldberg and Ahmed 2002; Raut et al. 2005) and is rapidly gaining importance worldwide as the percutaneous treatment of choice for patients with early-stage tumors. A tumor nodule ≤3 cm in diameter can be ablated with a single application of RFA (Goldberg et al. 1996). The predictability of the ablation area is one of the major advantages of RFA compared with PEI. The treatment efficacy and complication rate have been described in numerous studies (Moreno Planas et al. 2005; Chen et al. 2005).

Patients who have a more advanced, multi-nodular HCC with neither evidence of vascular invasion nor extrahepatic spread are classified as having intermediate-stage HCC according to the BCLC staging system (Llovet et al. 1999a). Transarterial chemoembolization (TACE) is an accepted and worldwide-used palliative treatment option for patients with intermediate-stage HCC (Bruix et al. 1998; Llovet et al. 2002, 2003). Due to recent advances in RF technology, RFA also has been used to treat patients with intermediate-stage tumors. Preliminary reports have shown that RFA performed after balloon catheter occlusion of the hepatic artery, transarterial embolization, or chemoembolization results in increased volumes of coagulation necrosis, thus enabling successful destruction of large HCC lesions (Yamasaki et al. 2005; de Baere et al. 2002; Akamatsu et al. 2004; Qian et al. 2003; Kurokohchi et al. 2004).

This chapter reviews the current status of percutaneous, image-guided RFA in the management of HCC by discussing technical issues and clinical results in the treatment of early- and intermediate-stage HCC.

3.3.2 Indications and Contraindications

Patients with HCC not suitable for surgical resection are considered to be eligible for RFA when they have an asymptomatic single tumor smaller than 5 cm or as many as three lesions, each smaller than 3 cm with neither evidence of vascular invasion nor significant extrahepatic spread (Llovet et al. 1999a). Patients with Child-Pugh class A or B cirrhosis can be treated with an acceptable complication rate; controversy, however, exists as to whether Child-Pugh class C patients should be treated with RFA as complications are more common (Curley et al. 2000). Close proximity to the main bile ducts is discussed as being a contradiction for RFA because damage to the bile ducts represents a major problem (Livraghi et al. 1997). Intraductal cooling to protect bile ducts was successfully performed during RFA in three patients with tumors in close proximity to major bile ducts (Elias et al. 2004). Especially in cases where the tumor is located in close proximity to thermosensitive organs such as the kidney, small / large bowel or stomach the dissection of these organs at risk using air or glucose might allow for performing the procedure without harming these structures. Therefore the close proximity is a relative contraindication only. Indications and contraindications are summarized in Table 3.3.1.

3.3.3 Technique and Practical Aspects

At our institution RFA is performed percutaneously as previously described in this book by predominantly using either a radiofrequency system with a

Table 3.3.1. According to the Barcelona-Clinic Liver Cancer (*BCLC*) criteria the indications and contraindications for RFA of HCC are listed in this table

Indications	Contraindications
Single tumor ≤5 cm in diameter	Life expectancy <6 months
Max. 3 lesions ≤3 cm in diameter	Current infection
Non-resectable	Treatment refractory coagulopathy
Child-Pugh class A or B cirrhosis	Treatment refractory ascites
Recurrence after surgical resection	Portal hypertension
Patient declined surgery	Tumor size > 5cm[a]
	>4 lesions
	advanced or terminal-stage HCC
	Tumor adjacent to structures at risk (main bile ducts, pericardium, stomach or bowel)[b]
	Extrahepatic spread[c]

[a] In individual cases depending on the location within the liver parenchyma the ablation of HCC nodules exceeding a diameter of 5 cm is feasible

[b] This applies only if the dissection of structures at risk is not possible using air or glucose

[c] In selected patients RFA is possible even if extrahepatic tumor is present. Note that in carefully selected patients extrahepatic tumors (e.g. bone, lung, pleura or soft tissue) can also be addressed by RFA

460 kHz generator (RITA Medical Systems, Mountain View, Calif., USA) or with the RF3000 generator system (Boston Scientific, Natick, Mass., USA). These systems consist of a generator supplying up to 200 W of power and expandable electrode needles. These designs decrease the distance between the tissue and the individual electrodes, thereby ensuring uniform heating that relies less on heat conduction over a large distance.

Using the Boston system, a LeVeen monopolar array needle electrode (2.0–5.0 cm maximum array diameter) and four indifferent dispersive grounding electrode pads applied to the patient's skin are used. The LeVeen electrode is a 15-gauge, 15- to 25-cm-long insulated cannula containing 10 parachute-like shaped electrodes to be deployed within the tumor. Due to the expected ablation zone the hooks are usually deployed at the posterior interface between the tumor and the surrounding normal liver parenchyma (Fig. 3.3.2).

In larger lesions, the array is withdrawn and redeployed anteriorly at 1.5- to 2.0-cm intervals into the tumor. After the hooks are fully deployed, the electrode is connected to the RF generator. The heating protocol for all the available needles is provided by the manufacturer. In general, the generator is started at a lower power setting and is subsequently increased in 10-W increments at 1-min intervals. The endpoint of RF application is the appearance of a rapid increase in tissue impedance (Roll-off) around the electrode. When this occurs, the RF application is automatically terminated. This process is repeated starting at 70% of the roll-off power until a second increase of the impedance occurs. Since the time point of the rapid increase in tissue impedance cannot be predicted, the ablation time needed varies dramatically between different tumor sizes and nodules. At the end of the procedure the needle track is ablated to prevent any tumor dissemination. Therefore, the tip has to be unisolated prior to the insertion of the needle.

Using the RITA system a 14-gauge expandable electrode needle is available. The needle electrode consists of an insulated outer cannula containing nine curved electrodes that are deployed directly into the tumor (Fig. 3.3.3). Five of the electrodes contain temperature sensors in their tips that are used to measure the temperature of the treated tissue. Two indifferent dispersive grounding pads are placed on the patient's thighs. Probe tip temperatures, tissue impedance and wattage are visualized on the RF generator display. The maximum power output, the extent of electrode deployment and the duration of the ablation time at the target temperature (usually between 95°C and 105°C) depend on the tumor size and therefore on the desired volume of ablation.. Different to the Boston system, the tip of the needle is positioned close to the proximal edge of the lesion, and the electrodes are initially deployed to 2 cm, pronging into the tumor. Energy is applied and the temperature at the tips of the electrodes is controlled, and the power is increased until the target temperature is reached. At this point, the electrodes are deployed stepwise to 3, 4 or 5 cm depending on the tumor size. The time at target temperature for each step depends on the planned maximum deployment. At the end of the procedure the needle track is ablated to prevent tumor dissemination.

We select the type of radiofrequency devices on a case-by-case basis, depending on the size and location of the tumors. Ideally, optimal positioning of the electrodes, regardless of the system used, allows for complete destruction of the tumor and a 1-cm safety zone of surrounding liver parenchyma.

RFA procedures are typically done while the patient is under conscious sedation. The procedure is performed under standard cardiac, pressure, and oxygen monitoring with oxygen administration, if necessary.

A careful post-treatment protocol is mandatory after RFA. We usually perform a contrast-enhanced CT scan of the upper abdomen immediately after the procedure is completed. This is to rule out residual tumor tissue and reassure that complete coverage of the tumor is given by the ablation zone and of course to look for complications such as bleeding. The

Fig. 3.3.2a–h. RFA of HCC as assessed by multi-detector CT. Pre-treatment CT reveals two HCC lesions after TACE performed the day before (**a**, **b**). The RF needle (LeVeen, Boston, Mass.) is placed using CT fluoroscopy and the hooks are deployed at the posterior interface between the tumor and the surrounding normal liver parenchyma (**c**). Immediately after the procedure a peripheral enhancing rim, which is most likely the inflammatory reaction surrounding the coagulation necrosis, can be appreciated in the arterial phase of the CT scan (**d**). The post-treatment scan the day after the RF procedure shows complete coverage of the HCC by the ablation zone (**e**, **f**). Six-months follow-up detects a well-circumscribed ablation zone, shrinking over time, with no evidence for either local tumor recurrence or new HCC lesions. The second HCC nodule is treated adequately as well (**g**, **h**)

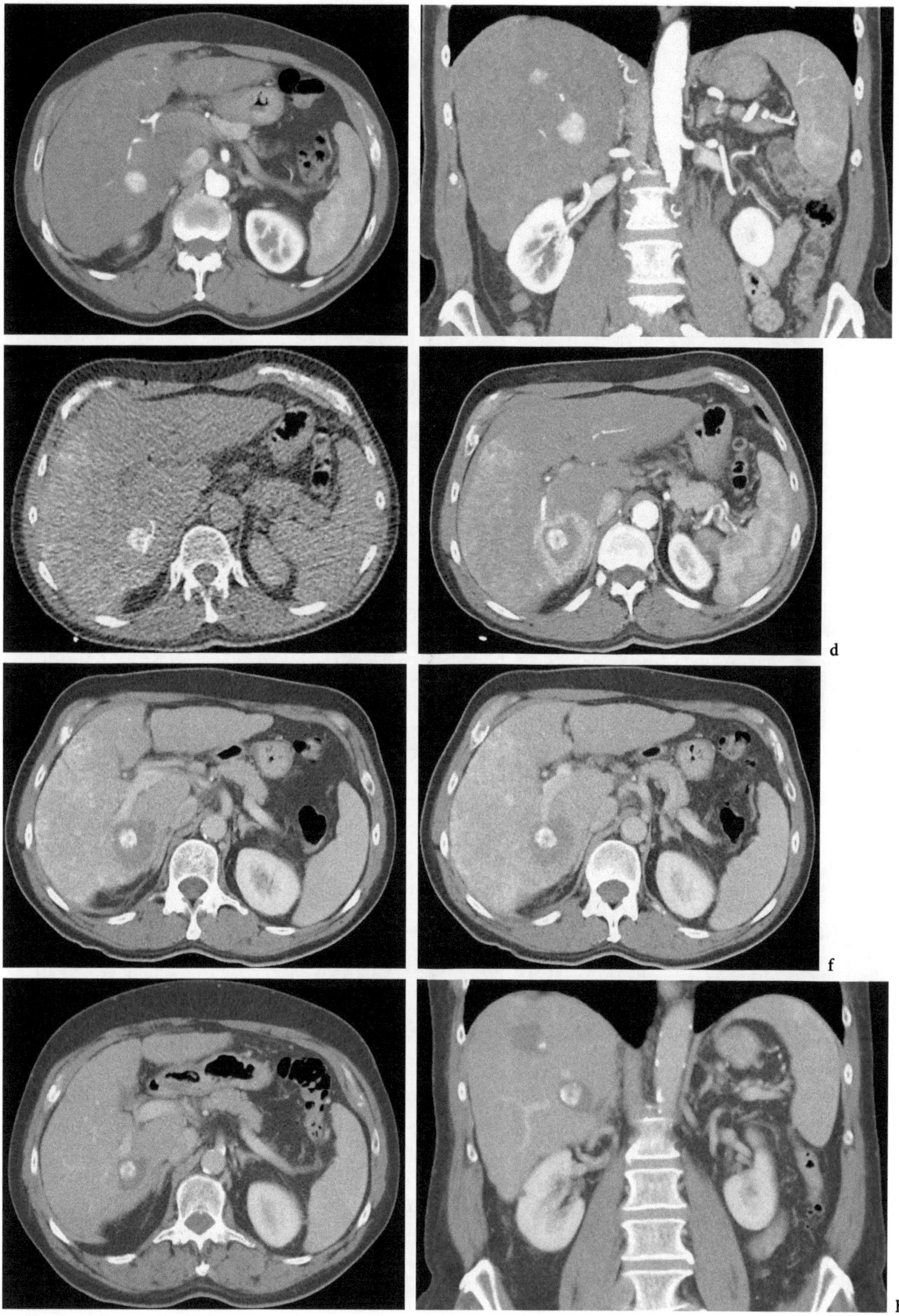

a b c d e f g h

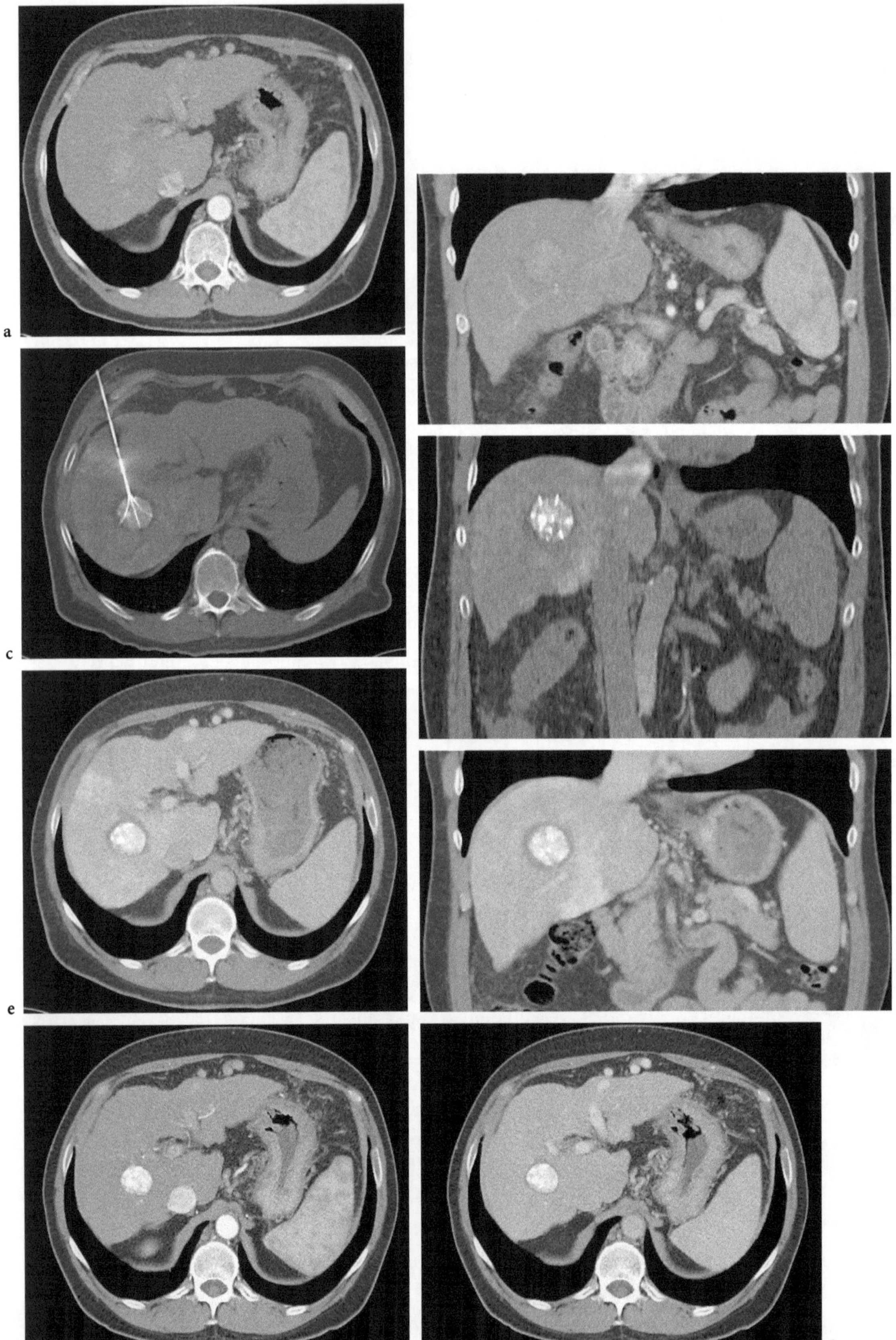

patient is usually kept under close medical observation for 24 h and rescanned with contrast-enhanced CT prior to discharge to provide a baseline study for further follow-up.

Subsequent follow-up monitoring of patients includes physical examination, serum alpha fetoprotein (AFP) level measurements (if applicable) and multiphase CT scans performed at 6 weeks after the initial procedure and then every 3 months during the first 2 years and every 6 months thereafter.

3.3.4 Combination of TACE and RFA

According to our own experience and the literature, the combination of TACE and RFA results in a higher percentage of complete tumor necrosis (Dupuy and Goldberg 2001; Yamakado et al. 2002; Bloomston et al. 2002). Hence, the hypoxic injury due to arterial embolization associated with damage caused by chemotherapeutic agents is synergic to the thermal ablation effect; moreover, ischemia causes reduction of heat dispersion thus increasing the range of therapeutic isotherms. Furthermore, the deposition of lipiodol as part of the embolic material helps to detect the HCC nodule using non-enhanced CT fluoroscopy and therefore increases the confidence of the interventional radiologist to deploy the hooks of the RF needle as appropriate.

3.3.5 Results

Treatment success, in terms of initial technical performance as well as long-term survival, varies with the size of the ablated lesion and the surrounding environment. The reported experience of Buscarini (Buscarini and Buscarini 2001; Buscarini et al. 2001) in 88 patients shows that complete tumor necrosis is achievable in tumors smaller than 3.5 cm in maximum diameter. However, this group stated that in some patients multiple sessions were required to achieve complete destruction of the tumor. Poon et al. (2002) reviewed several papers addressing local-regional therapies for HCC and reported on studies in which a complete tumor necrosis was achieved with a single treatment session in 80%–90% of tumors smaller than 3–5 cm in size. Limited success concerning RFA of larger HCC tumors (mean diameter 5.4 cm; range 3.1–9.5 cm) is reported by Livraghi et al. (2000) in a study including 126 patients. Here, the success rate for achieving complete necrosis was 48% only. However in a study published by Poon et al. (2002) the complete ablation rate after a single session of RFA assessed by means of computed tomography 1 month after treatment was 91% in 35 patients with HCC nodules ranging from 3.1 to 8.0 cm. This result did not differ significantly from the group containing 51 HCC patients with tumors smaller than 3 cm and a complete ablation rate of 94%.

A recently published prospective clinical trail performed on 187 patients showed promising results concerning long-term survival in HCC patients after RFA (Lencioni et al. 2005a). In this study patients were treated according to the BCLC criteria described before. Overall survival rates were 97% at 1 year, 89% at 2 years, 71% at 3 years, 57% at 4 years and 48% at 5 years of follow-up. The survival rates of patients with a Child-Pugh class A cirrhosis ($n=144$; 76% at 3 years and 51% at 5 years) were significantly higher than those of patients with a Child-Pugh class B cirrhosis ($n=43$; 46% at 3 years and 31% at 5 years). Interestingly, in a subgroup of 116 patients with a Child-Pugh class A cirrhosis and a solitary HCC only, the 3- and 5-year survival rates are reported to be 89% and 61%, respectively.

Tateishi et al. (2005) published interesting data concerning percutaneous RFA for HCC in 664 patients. The authors assessed the cumulative survival in patients who received RFA as the primary treatment ($n=319$, naive patients) as well as in patients who received RFA for recurrent tumor ($n=345$, non-

Fig. 3.3.3a–h. RFA of a single HCC as assessed by multi-detector CT. Pre-treatment CT acquired in the arterial phase demonstrates a native tumor as a faint enhancing lesion in the axial and coronal view (**a**, **b**). Para-axial and coronal reformats of the CT scan (after TACE the day before) with the RF needle (RITA Starburst XL) in place demonstrate complete coverage of the lesion with the fully deployed hooks (**c**, **d**). The post-treatment scan the day after the RF procedure shows complete coverage of the HCC by the ablation zone (**e**, **f**). CT scan at 6 months follow-up displays in the arterial (**g**) as well as in the porto-venous phase (**h**) a well-circumscribed ablation zone, stable in size, with no evidence for local tumor recurrence naive patients) after previous treatment including surgical resection, microwave coagulation therapy, PEI and TACE. The cumulative survival rates at 1, 2, 3, 4, and 5 years were 94.7%, 86.1%, 77.7%, 67.4%, and 54.3% for naive patients, whereas the cumulative survival rates were 91.8%, 75.6%, 62.4%, 53.7%, and 38.2% for non-naive patients, respectively. If the cumulative survival rates are divided by Child-Pugh classes, the authors report on survival rates of 96.4%, 90.4%, 83.4%, 72.9% and 63.1% for Child-Pugh class A patients at 1, 2, 3, 4 and 5 years and 90.7%, 79.0%, 65.0%, 53.9% and 31.4% for Child-Pugh class B/C patients, respectively. Regarding the tumor size, the cumulative survival rates at 1, 2, 3, 4 and 5 years were 100%, 93.2%, 90.8%, 90.8%, and 83.8% for patients with tumors ≤2 cm, 93.0%, 85.4%, 74.3%, 63.0% and 45.2% for patients with tumors between 2.1 and 5.0 cm, and 87.5%, 73.4%, 58.7%, 33.6% and 33.6% for patients with HCCs > 5.0 cm, respectively.

3.3.6 Morbidity and Mortality

Mulier et al. (2002) published an exhaustive review of the world literature concerning morbidity and mortality in patients who received RFA of the liver. The authors identified 3670 patients as being eligible for this evaluation. In these patients, the complication rate was 8.9% and the mortality rate was 0.5%. Depending on the technique, the complication rate was 7.2%, 9.5%, 9.9%, and 31.8% for a percutaneous, laparoscopic, simple open, and combined open approach, respectively. The mortality rate was 0.5%, 0% and 4.5% respectively.

Livraghi et al. (2003) recently reported in a multi-center study on complications encountered in patients treated with RFA of liver tumors; 2320 patients with 3554 lesions treated were analyzed. Of these patients 1610 patients were suffering from HCC. The depicted mortality rate and major complications rate was 0.3% ($n=3$) and 2.2% ($n=50$), respectively. The most frequent complications were peritoneal hemorrhage, neoplastic seeding, intrahepatic abscesses, and intestinal perforation. The incidence of complications was related to the number of RF sessions performed in the individual patient. Minor complications (no further action required, no prolonged hospital stay) were observed in less than 5% of the patients.

Tumor seeding after RFA of HCCs is a very important issue. In a study containing 241 patients with HCC and a median follow-up of 37 months, neoplastic seeding was identified in 12 patients (0.9%) (Livraghi et al. 2005). However, previous biopsy was significantly associated with the occurrence of tumor seeding. Therefore, the authors conclude that RFA is associated with a low risk of neoplastic seeding, but biopsy before RFA is to be discouraged, particularly when liver transplantation might be a possibility at a later date.

3.3.7 Bridging for Transplantation

HCC is the only solid neoplasm in which transplantation plays an important role. Cadaveric liver transplantation has been a major breakthrough, especially since transplantation might simultaneously cure the tumor and the underlying chronic liver disease. The patients eligible for cadaveric liver transplantation have one HCC smaller than 5 cm or up to three tumor nodules smaller than 3 cm, who, according to the literature, achieve 70% survival at 5 years, with a recurrence rate lower than 15% (Llovet et al. 1999c; Mazzaferro et al. 1996). However, the shortage of donor livers results in a prolonged waiting time for transplantation. This may worsen post-transplantation prognosis as a result of interval tumor progression. Since, especially in some Western countries, the waiting time can easily exceed 12 months, there is a drop-out rate of 20%–50% of cases. Living donor liver transplantation is emerging as the most feasible alternative to cadaveric liver transplantation, but discussed controversially. Therefore, adjuvant multi-modality ablative treatments (including RFA) are applied to prevent tumor progression while patients are on the waiting list.

Several recently published papers support the theory that RFA is a safe and effective treatment for HCCs <3 cm in patients with cirrhosis awaiting liver transplantation. Mazzaferro et al. (2004) determined the histopathological response rate of 60 HCCs in 50 patients who underwent liver transplantation after single-session RFA. The authors reported a complete response rate of 63% in tumor nodules <3 cm in the histopathological work-up, corresponding to a 70% response rate provided by adequate imaging. The tumor persistence after RFA increased over time (59% at 12 months; 70% at 18 months). Therefore, they concluded that tumor size exceeding 3 cm and a time interval longer than 1 year after ablation predicts an increased likelihood of the targeted tumor. That aggressive ablation therapy with a short period of time on the waiting list optimizes the results of liver transplantation in carefully selected cirrhotic HCC patients is supported by various authors (Fisher et al. 2004; Fontana et al. 2002; Lu et al. 2005).

3.3.8 Conclusion

RFA performed with currently available technology and an experienced hand is a valuable option in the armamentarium of interventional radiologists in the treatment of patients with HCC. Considering that only a limited number of patients are eligible for either surgical resection or liver transplantation, local ablative techniques such as RFA will play a central role in the therapeutic management of patients suffering from early-stage HCC. In patients meeting the BCLC criteria (single tumor <5 cm, 3 nodules <3 cm, Child-Pugh class A/B cirrhosis, good performance status) it is a reasonable expectation to have success in terms of local tumor control using RFA. The 5-year survival rates appear to be superior to the other local ablative treatment options such as PEI. For sure, the survival rates are obviously better than the natural course of the disease. Percutaneous RFA is an effective bridge to liver transplantation for patients with compensated liver function, and in addition it decreases the tumor-related dropout rate and optimizes the post-transplantation outcome. Appropriate use of this technique, careful patient selection and tailored tumor therapy are mandatory for the benefit of the individual patient.

References

Akamatsu M, Yoshida H, Obi S et al (2004) Evaluation of transcatheter arterial embolization prior to percutaneous tumor ablation in patients with hepatocellular carcinoma: a randomized controlled trial. Liver Int 24:625–629

de Baere T, Bessoud B, Dromain C et al (2002) Percutaneous radiofrequency ablation of hepatic tumors during temporary venous occlusion. AJR Am J Roentgenol 178:53–59

Bloomston M, Binitie O, Fraiji E et al (2002) Transcatheter arterial chemoembolization with or without radiofrequency ablation in the management of patients with advanced hepatic malignancy. Am Surg 68:827–831

Bruix J, Llovet JM (2002) Prognostic prediction and treatment strategy in hepatocellular carcinoma. Hepatology 35:519–524

Bruix J, Llovet JM, Castells A et al (1998) Transarterial embolization versus symptomatic treatment in patients with advanced hepatocellular carcinoma: results of a randomized, controlled trial in a single institution. Hepatology 27:1578–1583

Bruix J, Sherman M, Llovet JM et al (2001) Clinical management of hepatocellular carcinoma. Conclusions of the Barcelona-2000 EASL conference. European Association for the Study of the Liver. J Hepatol 35:421–430

Buscarini L, Buscarini E (2001) Therapy of HCC-radiofrequency ablation. Hepatogastroenterology 48:15–19

Buscarini L, Buscarini E, Di Stasi M, Vallisa D, Quaretti P, Rocca A (2001) Percutaneous radiofrequency ablation of small hepatocellular carcinoma: long-term results. Eur Radiol 11:914–921

Chen MH, Yan K, Yang W et al (2005) [Efficacy of radiofrequency ablation of 343 patients with hepatic tumor and the relevant complications]. Beijing Da Xue Xue Bao 37:292–296

Curley SA, Izzo F, Ellis LM, Nicolas Vauthey J, Vallone P (2000) Radiofrequency ablation of hepatocellular cancer in 110 patients with cirrhosis. Ann Surg 232:381–391

Dupuy DE, Goldberg SN (2001) Image-guided radiofrequency tumor ablation: challenges and opportunities-part II. J Vasc Interv Radiol 12:1135–1148

Elias D, Sideris L, Pocard M, Dromain C, De Baere T (2004) Intraductal cooling of the main bile ducts during radiofrequency ablation prevents biliary stenosis. J Am Coll Surg 198:717–721

Fan ST, Lai EC, Lo CM, Ng IO, Wong J (1995) Hospital mortality of major hepatectomy for hepatocellular carcinoma associated with cirrhosis. Arch Surg 130:198–203

Fisher RA, Maluf D, Cotterell AH et al (2004) Non-resective ablation therapy for hepatocellular carcinoma: effectiveness measured by intention-to-treat and dropout from liver transplant waiting list. Clin Transplant 18:502–512

Fontana RJ, Hamidullah H, Nghiem H et al (2002) Percutaneous radiofrequency thermal ablation of hepatocellular carcinoma: a safe and effective bridge to liver transplantation. Liver Transpl 8:1165–1174

Gadaleta C, Mattioli V, Colucci G et al (2004) Radiofrequency ablation of 40 lung neoplasms: preliminary results. AJR Am J Roentgenol 183:361–368

Gillams AR (2003) Radiofrequency ablation in the management of liver tumours. Eur J Surg Oncol 29:9–16

Gillams AR (2005) The use of radiofrequency in cancer. Br J Cancer 92:1825–1829

Goldberg SN, Ahmed M (2002) Minimally invasive image-guided therapies for hepatocellular carcinoma. J Clin Gastroenterol 35:S115–S129

Goldberg SN, Gazelle GS, Halpern EF, Rittman WJ, Mueller PR, Rosenthal DI (1996) Radiofrequency tissue ablation: importance of local temperature along the electrode tip

exposure in determining lesion shape and size. Acad Radiol 3:212–218
Koda M, Murawaki Y, Mitsuda A et al (2000) Predictive factors for intrahepatic recurrence after percutaneous ethanol injection therapy for small hepatocellular carcinoma. Cancer 88:529–537
Kurokohchi K, Masaki T, Miyauchi Y et al (2004) Efficacy of combination therapies of percutaneous or laparoscopic ethanol-lipiodol injection and radiofrequency ablation. Int J Oncol 25:1737–1743
Lai EC, Fan ST, Lo CM, Chu KM, Liu CL, Wong J (1995) Hepatic resection for hepatocellular carcinoma. An audit of 343 patients. Ann Surg 221:291–298
Lencioni R, Bartolozzi C, Caramella D et al (1995) Treatment of small hepatocellular carcinoma with percutaneous ethanol injection. Analysis of prognostic factors in 105 Western patients. Cancer 76:1737–1746
Lencioni R, Cioni D, Crocetti L, Bartolozzi C (2004) Percutaneous ablation of hepatocellular carcinoma: state-of-the-art. Liver Transpl 10:S91–S97
Lencioni R, Cioni D, Crocetti L et al (2005a) Early-stage hepatocellular carcinoma in patients with cirrhosis: long-term results of percutaneous image-guided radiofrequency ablation. Radiology 234:961–967
Lencioni R, Della Pina C, Bartolozzi C (2005b) Percutaneous image-guided radiofrequency ablation in the therapeutic management of hepatocellular carcinoma. Abdom Imaging 30:401–408
Liver Cancer Study Group of Japan (1990) Primary liver cancer in Japan Clinicopathologic features and results of surgical treatment. Ann Surg 211:277–287
Livraghi T, Giorgio A, Marin G et al (1995) Hepatocellular carcinoma and cirrhosis in 746 patients: long-term results of percutaneous ethanol injection. Radiology 197:101–108
Livraghi T, Goldberg SN, Monti F et al (1997) Saline-enhanced radio-frequency tissue ablation in the treatment of liver metastases. Radiology 202:205–210
Livraghi T, Goldberg SN, Lazzaroni S et al (2000) Hepatocellular carcinoma: radio-frequency ablation of medium and large lesions. Radiology 214:761–768
Livraghi T, Solbiati L, Meloni MF, Gazelle GS, Halpern EF, Goldberg SN (2003) Treatment of focal liver tumors with percutaneous radio-frequency ablation: complications encountered in a multicenter study. Radiology 226:441–451
Livraghi T, Lazzaroni S, Meloni F, Solbiati L (2005) Risk of tumour seeding after percutaneous radiofrequency ablation for hepatocellular carcinoma. Br J Surg 92:856–858
Llovet JM, Bru C, Bruix J (1999a) Prognosis of hepatocellular carcinoma: the BCLC staging classification. Semin Liver Dis 19:329–338
Llovet JM, Bustamante J, Castells A et al (1999b) Natural history of untreated nonsurgical hepatocellular carcinoma: rationale for the design and evaluation of therapeutic trials. Hepatology 29:62–67
Llovet JM, Fuster J, Bruix J (1999c) Intention-to-treat analysis of surgical treatment for early hepatocellular carcinoma: resection versus transplantation. Hepatology 30:1434–1440
Llovet JM, Real MI, Montana X et al (2002) Arterial embolisation or chemoembolisation versus symptomatic treatment in patients with unresectable hepatocellular carcinoma: a randomised controlled trial. Lancet 359:1734–1739
Llovet JM, Burroughs A, Bruix J (2003) Hepatocellular carcinoma. Lancet 362:1907–1917
Lu DS, Yu NC, Raman SS et al (2005) Percutaneous radiofrequency ablation of hepatocellular carcinoma as a bridge to liver transplantation. Hepatology 41:1130–1137
Mazzaferro V, Regalia E, Doci R et al (1996) Liver transplantation for the treatment of small hepatocellular carcinomas in patients with cirrhosis. N Engl J Med 334:693–699
Mazzaferro V, Battiston C, Perrone S et al (2004) Radiofrequency ablation of small hepatocellular carcinoma in cirrhotic patients awaiting liver transplantation: a prospective study. Ann Surg 240:900–909
Moreno Planas JM, Lopez Monclus J, Gomez Cruz A et al (2005) Efficacy of hepatocellular carcinoma locoregional therapies on patients waiting for liver transplantation. Transplant Proc 37:1484–1485
Mulier S, Mulier P, Ni Y et al (2002) Complications of radiofrequency coagulation of liver tumours. Br J Surg 89:1206–1222
Poon RT, Fan ST, Tsang FH, Wong J (2002) Locoregional therapies for hepatocellular carcinoma: a critical review from the surgeon's perspective. Ann Surg 235:466–486
Qian J, Feng GS, Vogl T (2003) Combined interventional therapies of hepatocellular carcinoma. World J Gastroenterol 9:1885–1891
Raut CP, Izzo F, Marra P et al (2005) Significant long-term survival after radiofrequency ablation of unresectable hepatocellular carcinoma in patients with cirrhosis. Ann Surg Oncol 12:616–628
Sarasin FP, Giostra E, Mentha G, Hadengue A (1998) Partial hepatectomy or orthotopic liver transplantation for the treatment of resectable hepatocellular carcinoma? A cost-effectiveness perspective. Hepatology 28:436–442
Tateishi R, Shiina S, Teratani T et al (2005) Percutaneous radiofrequency ablation for hepatocellular carcinoma. An analysis of 1000 cases. Cancer 103:1201–1209
Ulmer SC (2000) Hepatocellular carcinoma. A concise guide to its status and management. Postgrad Med 107:117–124
Yamakado K, Nakatsuka A, Ohmori S et al (2002) Radiofrequency ablation combined with chemoembolization in hepatocellular carcinoma: treatment response based on tumor size and morphology. J Vasc Interv Radiol 13:1225–1232
Yamasaki T, Kimura T, Kurokawa F et al (2005) Percutaneous radiofrequency ablation with cooled electrodes combined with hepatic arterial balloon occlusion in hepatocellular carcinoma. J Gastroenterol 40:171–178

Liver

Primary Tumors

3

3.4 LITT-HCC

Katrin Eichler, Martin G. Mack, and Thomas J. Vogl

CONTENTS

Hepatocellular carcinoma (HCC) is one of the most common cancers worldwide, due to its high rate of incidence in Africa (south of the Sahara), and a high association with hepatitis viruses (HBV and HCV), consumption of alcohol, aflatoxin B1, and hepatic cirrhosis (Bruix et al. 1991). The incidence of HCC has increased both because of a real increase in the occurrence of the disease, and because modern imaging techniques allow diagnosis at an earlier stage of disease. Surgical resection and liver transplantation remain the most effective treatment strategies for small and oligonodular (five or fewer intrahepatic lesions) HCCs. Some studies yield excellent survival rates using percutaneous ethanol injection (PEI) (Bruix et al. 1991; Sironi et al. 1991, 1993; Amin et al. 1993; Livraghi et al. 1995; Kawai et al. 1997).

Transcatheter arterial embolization is also an established treatment modality for patients with HCC, and in some studies it has proven to be effective in reducing tumor volume and increasing survival (Kanematsu et al. 1993; Kawai et al. 1997). Radiofrequency ablation (RF) has recently been introduced in the clinical setting by a number of groups (Rossi et al. 1993, 1996; Solbiati et al. 1997; Livraghi et al. 1999). MR-guided laser-induced thermotherapy (LITT) is a minimally invasive technique for local tumor destruction within solid organs (Jolesz et al. 1988; Anzai et al. 1991; Matsumoto et al. 1992; Amin et al. 1993a, 1993b; Rossi et al. 1993, 1996; Solbiati et al. 1997; Vogl et al. 1997, 1998; Livraghi et al. 1999). Experimental work has shown that a well-defined area of coagulative necrosis is obtained around the fiber tip of a laser applicator that disperses light energy delivered through optical fibers (Dickinson et al. 1986). This causes destruction of the tumor by directly applied thermal energy, substantially limiting damage to surrounding structures, such as nerves or vessels. The possibility of performing online MR thermometry allows exact timing and dosing of the applied energy to the tumorous tissue and surrounding normal parenchyma.

The purpose of the present study was to evaluate the therapeutic potential of MR-guided LITT in oligonodular and small HCC. The success of LITT in the treatment of HCC depends on optimal positioning of the specially designed laser-emitting tip of the optical fibers in the target area. MRI has proven to be an ideal instrument for real-time monitoring of the progress of the hyperthermic effects of LITT and the subsequent evaluation of the extent of induced coagulative necrosis. In this prospective study we analyzed the local tumor control and survival data of MR-guided LITT in patients with oligonodular HCC.

Recently there has been great interest in the further developments of interstitial procedures such as laser-induced interstitial thermotherapy (LITT), RF ablation, and microwave ablation and cryotherapy.

The purpose of this chapter is to present the technical data, the practical performance, and the application data of MR-guided LITT for primary liver tumors.

K. Eichler, MD; M. G. Mack, MD, PD
T. J. Vogl, MD, Professor
Institute for Diagnostic and Interventional Radiology, University Hospital, Johann Wolfgang Goethe University, Theodor-Stern-Kai 7, 60590 Frankfurt am Main, Germany

Between June 1993 and April 2007, 84 patients with 115 intrahepatic lesions were treated with MR-guided LITT. The male:female ratio was 63:21 and 56 patients had percutaneous transarterial chemoembolization as their initial treatment. We also included patients with recurrent liver metastases after partial liver resection, patients with metastases in both liver lobes, patients with locally non-resectable lesions, and patients who had general contraindications for surgery or refused surgical resection.

The Nd-YAG laser fiber was introduced with a percutaneously positioned irrigated laser application system. Qualitative and quantitative MR parameters and clinical data were evaluated. Survival data were calculated using the Kaplan–Meier method.

See Chapter 2.3 for technical data.

3.4.1 During Therapy

The HCC nodules were localized on computed tomographic (CT) scans and the injection site was infiltrated with 20 ml of 1% lidocaine. Under CT guidance, up to four sheaths were inserted using the Seldinger technique. A special heat-resistant protective fiber was then introduced. For the positioning of the applicators we routinely used the CT guidance in all patients; this is because of later procedures and because it allows immediate reaction in cases of bleeding or pneumothorax. After the patient was positioned on the MRI table, the laser fiber was inserted into the protective catheter. MR sequences

a

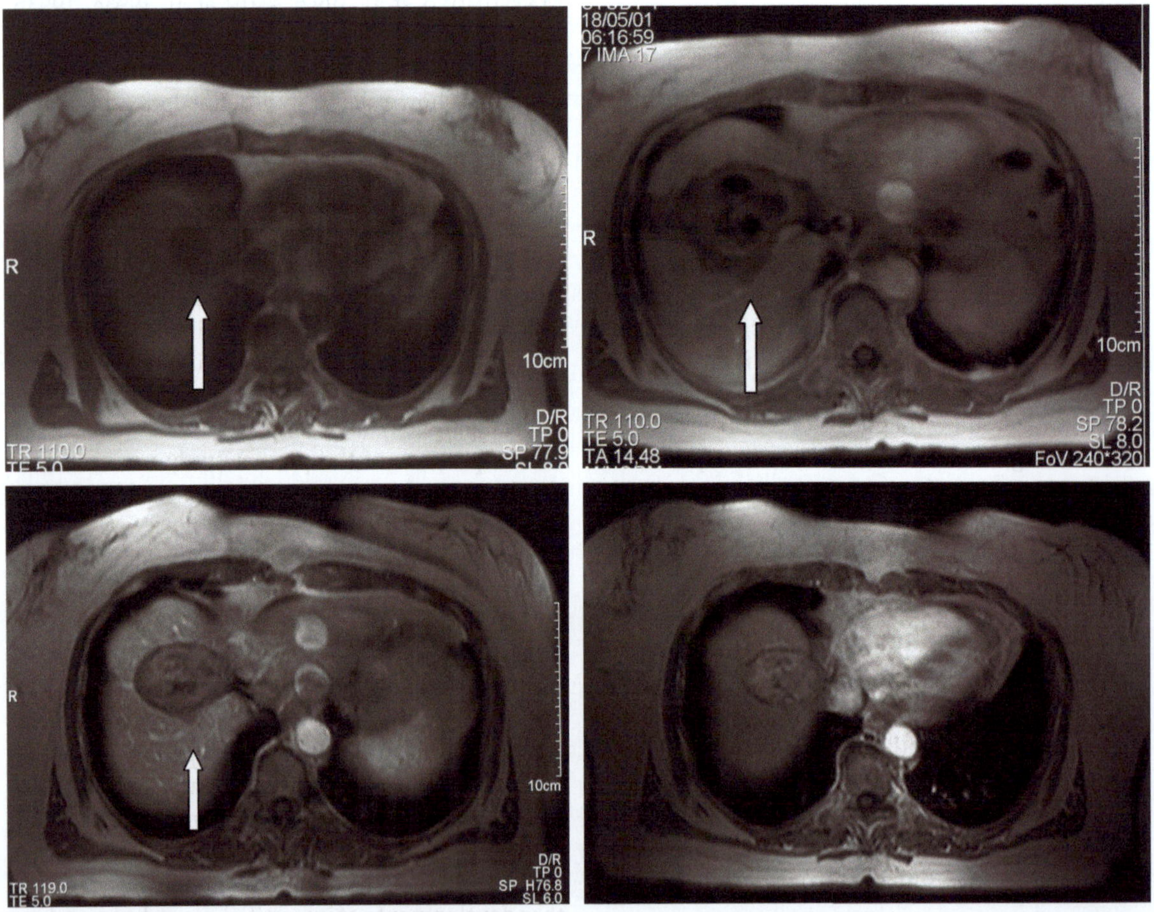

b c d

Fig. 3.4.1a–d. An axial contrast-enhanced FLASH-2D image (**a**) reveals the size and location of the hepatocellular carcinoma (*HCC*) in liver segment 8 (*arrow*) of a 62-year-old patient with recurrence of HCC in the right liver lobe. **b** An axial contrast-enhanced FLASH-2D image 2 days after laser-induced thermotherapy (*LITT*; 25 min with four power lasers 25 W) demonstrates induced coagulative necrosis (*arrow*), presumably a sign of total destruction of the tumor with a 5-mm safety margin around the primary lesion. **c** Contrast-enhanced T1-weighted image 18 months after laser intervention demonstrates reduction in the volume of necrosis. There are no primary or secondary signs hinting that the tumor is still active (*arrow*). **d** The axial T1-weighted image reveals no viable tumor 60 months after LITT were performed in axial, coronal, and sagittal orientations before and during LITT. Magnetic resonance (MR) thermometry was carried out using a specially designed FLASH-2D (TR 102/TE 8/flip angle 15°) sequence, which is more sensitive at detecting thermal changes in the signal (Fig. 3.4.1).

Depending on the geometry and intensity of the signal loss, the position of the laser fibers was readjusted within the thermostable catheter. Using a pull-back technique, the laser energy was applied in order to adapt thermally induced changes individually to the geometry of the given lesion.

After switching off the laser, FLASH-2D (TR 154/TE 6/flip angle 70°) contrast-enhanced [GD-DTPA, 0.1 mmol/kg body weight (b.w.) in a bolus administration] images were obtained to determine the degree of necrosis induced (Fig. 3.4.2). After the procedure the cannulation channel was closed with

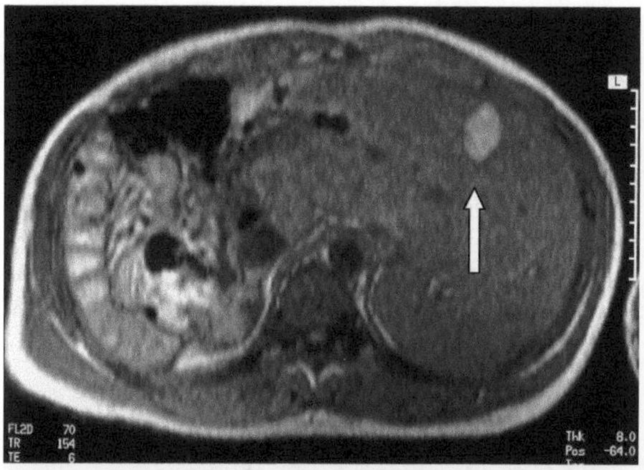
a

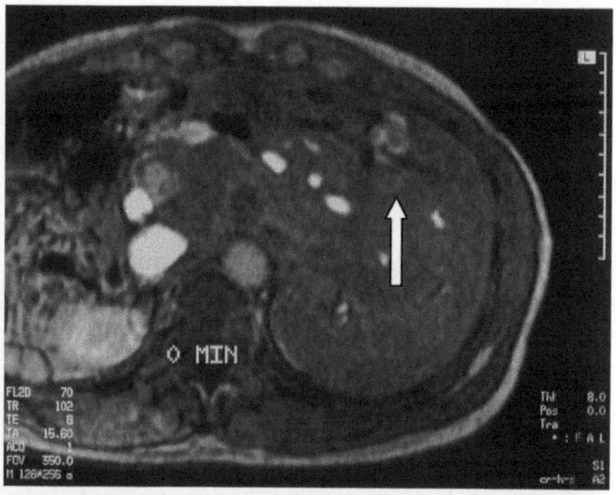

b

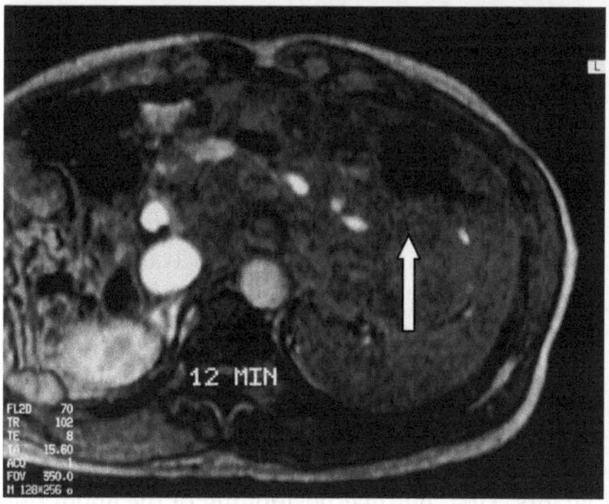

c

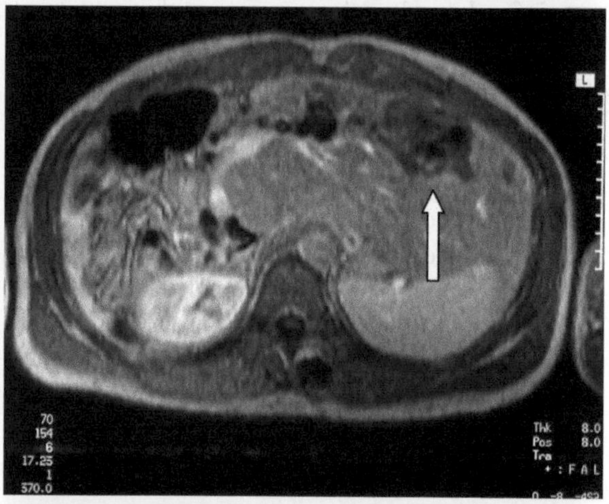
d

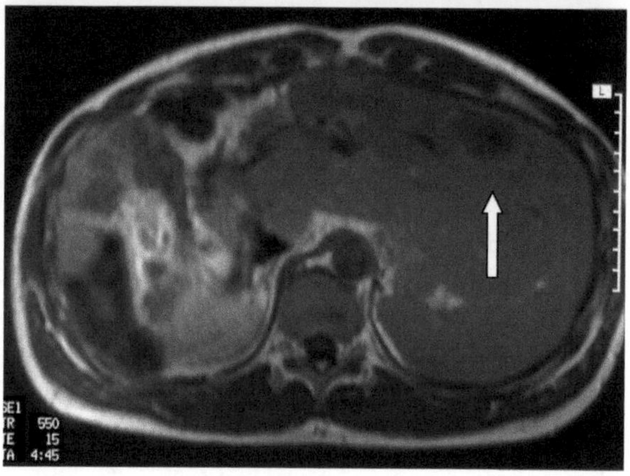
e

Fig. 3.4.2a–e. The axial plain FLASH-2D image (**a**) (TR 154/TE 6/flip angle 70°) shows untreated HCC as a hypointense lesion in a 38-year-old patient (*arrow*). **b** MR thermosensitive FLASH-2D images (TR 102/TE 8/flip angle 15°) before commencing laser intervention (*arrow*). **c** Axial MR thermosensitive FLASH-2D images (TR 102/TE 8/flip angle 15°) during laser application: 12 min into application of heat, the hypointense area shows the distribution of thermal energy in the tissue and allows an early assessment of the expected necrosis (*arrow*). **d** The axial T1-weighted MR image 2 days after LITT shows a significant signal change with a thin hypointense border, promising sufficient tumor destruction (*arrow*). **e** HCC nodule 11 months after MR-guided LITT. The axial contrast-enhanced treated T1-weighted image (TR 550/TE 15) shows only residual signal changes in the liver parenchyma (*arrow*) fibrin glue (Tissucol Duo S 2ml, Immuno Baxter, Unterschleissheim, Germany).

3.4.2 Qualitative and Quantitative Evaluation / Survival

The qualitative evaluation of laser-induced effects was based on an analysis of lesions and surrounding liver parenchyma before and after the evaluation periods, and included documentation of the morphology of lesions as seen in T2- and T1-weighted spin-echo (SE) and gradient recalled echo (GRE) sequences. Quantitative data were obtained by volumetric calculation of tumor and necrosis volumes before and after intervention with the formula $(a \times b \times c) \times 0.5$, where a was the maximum anterior–posterior diameter, b was the maximum lateral–medial diameter and c was maximum cranial–caudal diameter.

Spontaneous or therapeutically induced necrosis was defined as a hypointense area with no contrast enhancement after i.v. application of 0.1 mmol/kg b.w. Gd-DTPA in T1-weighted (TR 154/TE 6/flip angle 70°) sequences. Geographical or confluent areas with subtle enhancement in postinterventional sequences were interpreted as residual tumor tissue if the lesions could be topographically identified in the area of the previous tumor. Surrounding rim structures with a high degree of contrast enhancement and a width of up to 3 mm were defined as reactive hypervascular changes, induced by the therapy itself.

3.4.3 Clinical Data of MR-Guided LITT of HCC

All patients tolerated the procedure well under local anesthesia. The total procedure time was on average 90 min and all patients were treated on an outpatient basis. All complications observed were minor and no further treatment was necessary. Online MR thermometry allowed exact visualization of the extension of laser-induced changes and their relationship to the neighboring anatomy. Lesions up to 2 cm in diameter could be efficiently treated with a single laser application; larger lesions were treated with a dual, triple, and quadruple simultaneous application.

It was found that 22.4% of the lesions were 2 cm or less in diameter (mean applied energy 41.1 kJ), 30.4% were between 2 and 3 cm (mean applied energy 73.4 kJ), 20% were between 3 and 4 cm (mean applied energy 117.9 kJ), and 27.2% were larger than 4 cm in maximum diameter (mean applied energy 146.1 kJ). In 98.5 % we achieved complete necrosis of the tumor and a 5-mm safety margin, resulting in complete destruction of the tumor without local recurrences. The mean survival rate, starting the calculation at the date of diagnosis of the HCC nodule, was 4.7 years [95% confidence interval (CI) 3.9–5.5 years, 1-year survival 93%, 2-year survival 76%, 3-year survival 59%, 5-year survival 41%]. Mean survival after the first laser treatment was 4.1 years (95% CI 3.1–5.0 years, 1-year survival 81%, 2-year survival 63%, 3-year survival 47%, 5-year survival 32%).

At present, HCC accounts for 4% of all malignant tumors worldwide and represents the seventh most common tumor in males and the ninth most common in females (Bruix et al. 1991). At this time, liver resection and transplantation are considered to represent the only curative strategies in the treatment of HCC (Bismuth et al. 1993). Clinical conditions, the presence of larger lesions, lesions in both hepatic lobes, or poor clinical status preclude surgical treatment. Liver resection and transplantation can therefore be offered to only a small number of patients with a good chance of success: there is a need for adjunct treatments to improve the success of resection and to diminish the incidence of recurrence after surgery (Bismuth et al. 1993). The clinical success of MR-guided LITT depends on many factors. First, optimal positioning of the applicator in the center of the lesion must be ensured, as determined in three dimensions. The real advantage of MR over CT and ultrasound lies in the thermosensitivity of the MR sequence. It allows for rapid acquisition temperature maps, allowing near real-time documentation of LITT effects. Monitoring of these effects during ongoing therapy is advantageous for a number of reasons. The technique can be used to ensure that the entire lesion has been treated, and, if there is residual tissue within the lesion that has not been treated, the applicator can be re-positioned under MR guidance during the same session.

Monitoring also minimizes destruction of healthy tissue, thus enhancing the safety of the procedure, particularly in the vicinity of vital structures such as large vessels or the central bile ducts in the liver. MR provides unparalleled topographical accuracy due to its excellent soft-tissue contrast and high spatial resolution. This allows early detection of complications. In the group with HCC only two pleural effusions were observed. However, potential further complications of this method can be subcapsular hematoma, injuries to bile ducts and bowel, infections, liver failure, bleeding, and damage to vessels or other structures.

Several factors may influence the size and morphology of the areas of induced necrosis, including tumor geometry and adjacent structures such as arteries, portal and hepatic veins, and the biliary tree. The relationship of the tumor to the liver capsule is an essential factor in planning treatment of the lesion. Analgesia must be significantly increased if a lesion lies close to the liver capsule. Conventional MR applicator systems should only be used for HCC nodules < 10 mm. The multiapplicator technique using conventional applicators should be rejected due to the need for multiple accesses to the tumor and the promising results of the power LITT system. Liquid-cooled application systems have also been investigated, and, compared to the conventional system, they yield larger coagulation volumes, better visualization of the hyperthermic changes, and homogeneity of the induced changes but with fewer punctures necessary (Vogl et al. 1998). For a 5-cm lesion three to four laser applicators are necessary. The number of inserted laser applicators depends on the size of the lesion, the relationship to vessels, and the geometrical configuration.

The results presented here must still be compared with a variety of other minimally invasive techniques. Transarterial chemoembolization is a procedure involving the injection of lipiodol and a chemotherapeutic agent into the hepatic artery. The intention is to produce selective ischemic injury to the tumor, which relies mainly on the arterial circulation. Kanematsu et al. (1993) did the first comparative study between hepatic resection in 67 patients and transcatheter arterial embolization (TAE) in 20 patients with resectable disease. The 1-year, 3-year, and 5-year cumulative survival rates for 67 patients undergoing surgery were 89.1%, 74.6%, and 54.6% respectively; and for the 20 patients treated with TAE, 90%, 50%, and 17.50% respectively. Surgery therefore provided more favorable results (Kanematsu et al. 1993).

Percutaneous ethanol injection (PEI) is a technique for the treatment of HCC which is now considered to represent a reliable alternative to surgical resection. Ethanol shows selective diffusion in HCC, due to the softer consistency and hypervascularity of these lesions; it carries little or no risk to the remaining parenchyma. Livraghi et al. (1999), in a multicentric trial involving nine centers, observed in patients with solitary lesions of less than 5 cm diameter a 3-year survival rate of 79%, and a 5-year survival rate of 47%. The results obtained with PEI certainly compete with the results of surgery and are influenced by the size of the lesions and the severity of cirrhosis (Livraghi et al. 1995).

RF lesion ablation is another method for thermocoagulating tissue. RF energy is emitted from the exposed portion of an electrode. This energy translates into ion agitation that is converted into heat, which induces cellular death as a result of coagulation necrosis. Rossi et al. (1993, 1996) reported on experiences by an expandable RF needle electrode in 21 patients with small HCC (mean diameter of the tumor nodules was 2.5 cm): 6 patients showed recurrences and 15 remained disease-free (follow up 6–19 months). Pacella et al. (1997) reported on 3 years of experience with percutaneous US-guided interstitial laser photocoagulation (ILP) in the treatment of HCC; here, 47 small HCCs (diameter 13–30 mm), histologically confirmed, were treated in 29 patients. This group describes local recurrences in four patients and metachronous lesions in 13 patients. The survival rate is reported to be as high as 100% after 1 year, and 85% after 2 years (Pacella et al. 1997).

Livraghi et al. (1999) compared the effectiveness of RF ablation with that of PEI in the treatment of small HCC in 86 patients. Complete necrosis was achieved in 47 of 52 tumors with RF ablation (90%) and in 48 of 60 tumors with PEI (80%). One hour before RF ablation the patients received an orally administered sedative and an intravenously administered analgesic and were monitored continuously before, during, and after the procedure. Most patients experienced moderate pain, but occasionally the treatment had to be interrupted due to severe pain; an anesthesiologist administered propofol and performed assisted ventilation for the duration of the procedure (Livraghi et al. 1999).

The major advantage of MR-guided LITT is that it is performed under MR and that the procedure can be monitored more carefully than is the case with some other techniques.

The long-term studies revealed a local tumor control rate that depended largely on the technique used and the experience of the interventional group performing the procedure.

The therapy's minimally invasive character, its lack of short- or long-term side-effects, and the good tolerance patients have for it, allowing it to be carried out on an outpatient basis, are the main benefits of our MR-guided LITT protocol (Vogl et al. 1997, 1998).

In summary, MR-guided thermotherapy has been proved to be a safe and effective palliative treatment protocol for oligonodular HCC.

References

Amin Z, Donald JJ, Masters A et al (1993a) Hepatic metastases: interstitial laser photocoagulation with real-time US monitoring and dynamic CT evaluation of treatment. Radiology 187:339–347

Amin Z, Bown SG, Lees WR (1993b) Local treatment of colorectal liver metastases: a comparison of interstitial laser photocoagulation (ILP) and percutaneous alcohol injection (PAI). Clin Radiol 48:166–171

Anzai Y, Lufkin RB, Castro DJ et al (1991) MR imaging-guided interstitial Nd:YAG laser phototherapy: dosimetry study of acute tissue damage in an in vivo model. J Magn Reson Imaging 1:553–559

Bismuth H, Chiche L, Adam R, Castaing D, Diamond T, Dennison A (1993) Liver resection versus transplantation for hepatocellular carcinoma in cirrhotic patients. Ann Surg 218:145–151

Bruix J, Castells A, Bru C (1991) Caracteristicas clinicas y prognostico del carcinoma hepatocelular. Existen difirencias geograficas? Gastroenterol Hepatol 14:520–524

Dickinson RJ, Hall AS, Hind AJ, Young IR (1986) Measurement of changes in tissue temperature using MR imaging. J Comput Assist Tomogr 10:468–472

Jolesz FA, Bleier AR, Jakab P, Ruenzel PW, Huttl K, Jako GJ (1988) MR imaging of laser-tissue interactions. Radiology 168:249–253

Kanematsu T, Matsumata T, Shirabe K (1993) A comparative study of hepatic resection and transcatheter arterial embolization for the treatment of primary hepatocellular carcinoma. Cancer 71:2181–2186

Kawai S, Tani M, Okumura J, Ogawa M et al (1997) Prospective and randomized clinical trial of lipiodol-transcatheter arterial chemoembolization for treatment of hepatocellular carcinoma: a comparison of epirubicin and doxorubicin (second cooperative study). Semin Oncol 24:38–45

Livraghi T, Giorgio A, Marin G et al (1995) Hepatocellular carcinoma and cirrhosis in 746 patients: long-term results of percutaneous ethanol injection. Radiology 197:101–108

Livraghi T, Goldberg SN, Lazzaroni S, Meloni F, Solbiati L, Gazelle GS (1999) Small hepatocellular carcinoma: treatment with radio-frequency ablation versus ethanol injection. Radiology 210:655–661

Matsumoto R, Oshio K, Jolesz FA (1992) Monitoring of laser and freezing-induced ablation in the liver with T1-weighted MR imaging. J Magn Reson Imaging 2:555–562

Pacella CM, Bizarri G, Anelli V (1997) Treatment of small hepatocellular carcinoma: value of percutaneous laser interstitial photocoagulation. Radiology 205(P):200

Rossi S, Fornari F, Buscarini L (1993) Percutaneous ultrasound-guided radiofrequency electrocautery for the treatment of small hepatocellular carcinoma. J Interv Radiol 8:97–103

Rossi S, Di Stasi M, Buscarini E et al (1996) Percutaneous RF interstitial thermal ablation in the treatment of hepatic cancer. AJR Am J Roentgenol 167:759–768

Sironi S, Livraghi T, DelMaschio A (1991) Small hepatocellular carcinoma treated with percutaneous ethanol injection: MR imaging findings. Radiology 180:333–336

Sironi S, Livraghi T, Angeli E et al (1993) Small hepatocellular carcinoma: MR follow-up of treatment with percutaneous ethanol injection. Radiology 187:119–123

Solbiati L, Goldberg SN, Ierace T et al (1997) Hepatic metastases: percutaneous radio-frequency ablation with cooled-tip electrodes. Radiology 205:367–373

Vogl TJ, Mack MG, Straub R, Roggan A, Felix R (1997) Percutaneous MRI-guided laser-induced thermotherapy for hepatic metastases for colorectal cancer. Lancet 350:29

Vogl TJ, Mack MG, Roggan A et al (1998) Internally cooled power laser for MR-guided interstitial laser-induced thermotherapy of liver lesions: initial clinical results. Radiology 209:381–385

Liver

Secondary Tumors

3.5 Radiofrequency Ablation (RFA)

Ralf-Thorsten Hoffmann, Tobias F. Jakobs, Thomas K. Helmberger, and Maximilian F. Reiser

CONTENTS

3.5.1 Introduction

In most patients suffering from cancer, the primary tumor can be resected in a curative intention. However, during patient's history, liver metastases occur – depending on the tumor – in up to 70%. There are data from large autopsy studies showing that liver metastases are detectable in more than 40% of all malignancies (Tranberg 2004). Liver metastases therefore have the highest impact on patient's long-term survival and are responsible for the largest part of cancer-related deaths worldwide (Tranberg 2004). In the western world metastases of colorectal cancer are the most common indication for resection, followed by metastases of breast cancer. It has been shown that the 3-, 5-, and 10-year survival rates after a successful resection of liver metastases are as high as 45%, 30%, and 20% respectively (Ohlsson et al. 1998; Scheele et al. 1995). For this reason, in recent years surgical resection was considered to be the only curative option in liver metastases, while chemotherapy and radiation therapy were viewed as only palliative treatment options. However, the restricted inclusion criteria for surgical resection – only 10%–25% of all patients suffering from liver metastases are suitable candidates to undergo surgery – have stipulated an increasing demand for minimally invasive treatments achieving effective and reproducible percutaneous tumor ablation while simultaneously lowering both morbidity and costs. Recently, several interstitial ablative techniques, including freezing, heating or chemical ablation, have demonstrated promising results. The first experiments in thermal ablation of living tissue were described by d'Arsonval as early as 1868 (Erce and Parks 2003), while the use of thermal ablation for treatment of malignant hepatic lesions was first suggested by McGahan et al. and Rossi et al. in 1990 (McGahan et al. 1990; Rossi et al. 1990). Since then, the use of thermal ablation to treat both primary and secondary hepatic tumors has dramatically increased and has generated international interest with a multitude of clinical investigations. Although it is a relatively new procedure with rapidly changing patterns of clinical practice, thermal ablation is already challenging surgical resection as the treatment of choice for patients with circumscript hepatic tumors.

R.-T. Hoffmann, MD; T. F. Jakobs, MD;
M. F. Reiser, MD, Professor
Department of Cinical Radiology, University Hospitals – Grosshadern, Ludwig-Maximilians-University of Munich, Marchioninistrasse 15, 81377 Munich, Germany
T. K. Helmberger, MD
Professor, Department of Diagnostic and Interventional Radiology and Nuclear Medicine, Klinikum Bogenhausen, Engelschalkinger Strasse 77, 81925 Munich, Germany

3.5.2 Indications and Contraindications

The ultimate goal for radiofrequency ablation (RFA) is to prolong survival of the patients. Therefore, the indications for local ablative treatment are similar to those established for resection – however with some modifications (Table 3.5.1). There is general

Table. 3.5.1. Indications and contraindications for local ablative treatment

Indications	Contraindications
Single tumor ≤5 cm in diameter	Life expectancy <6 months
Max. 3 lesions ≤3 cm in diameter	Current infection
Nonresectable	Treatment refractory coagulopathy
Recurrence after surgical resection	Treatment refractory ascites
Patient declined surgery	Portal hypertension
Combination with resection	Tumor size >5 cm[a]
	>4 lesions
	Extrahepatic spread[b]
	Tumor adjacent to structures at risk (main bile ducts, pericardium, stomach or bowel)[c]

[a] In individual cases depending on the location within the liver parenchyma an ablation might be possible.
[b] In selected patients RFA is possible even if extrahepatic tumor (e.g. stable bone metastases, slow growing lymph nodes) is present
[c] Only if a dissection of structures at risk by injection of air or glucose is not possible.

consent that RFA is indicated for patients suffering from unresectable metastases due to a multilocular tumor or due to contraindications to surgical treatment, e.g. cardiovascular risk factors. It may also be used in combination with surgical resection as an adjuvant therapy or as a neoadjuvant therapy for bilobar tumors. Most investigators have limited ablative treatment to patients with four or fewer hepatic tumors with a diameter of 5 cm or smaller, due to a significantly higher local recurrence rate in tumors larger than 3 cm (Curley et al. 1999, 2000). Contraindications include the presence of extrahepatic metastatic disease, a tumor volume of more than 30% of the total liver volume, sepsis, severe debilitation, and uncorrectable coagulopathies. However, patients with renal or breast cancer – usually associated with disseminated disease – can be considered suitable if they had effective systemic therapy and have only liver metastases left (Curley 2003). Additionally, tumor location next to the large portal triads is a relative contraindication due to the risk of harming the bile duct. Ideally, tumors are smaller than 3.5 cm in diameter and completely surrounded by hepatic parenchyma, with a distance of at least 1 cm to the liver capsule and of more than 2 cm to the large hepatic or portal veins (Gazelle et al. 2000). Even though subcapsular liver tumors can be treated with RFA, the treatment is usually associated with greater procedural and post-procedural pain and often associated with a higher complication rate (Lencioni et al. 2001). Furthermore, tumors larger than 3–4 cm can now be treated, using newer RF generators, multiple needle positions or angiographically assisted RFA (Gazelle et al. 2000; Lencioni et al. 2001). Tumors adjacent to large blood vessels are more difficult to treat because perfusion-mediated tissue cooling reduces the extent of coagulation necrosis produced by thermal ablation (Gazelle et al. 2000). However the blood flow-mediated so-called heat sink effect also protects the vascular endothelium from thermal injury, allowing us to place the electrodes as close as necessary to the vessels.

3.5.3 Results

Assessing outcome after ablation is difficult because few studies with good long-term follow-up have evaluated local recurrence, disease-free survival, and overall survival after ablation. The best way to evaluate the benefit of any local ablative therapy is to examine the rate of local tumor control and the local recurrence rate respectively. Many studies have shown that completeness of tumor ablation is directly related to survival (Bilchik et al. 2001), comparable to a free resection margin after surgery (Ohlsson et al. 1998; Scheele et al. 1995). The major objective – the local recurrence rate – strongly depends on the size of the treated metastases (Curley 2003; Solbiati et al. 2001; Wood et al.

2000). In the study by Curley (Curley 2003) a local relapse in only about 7% of the patients was shown after RFA of colorectal metastases, however, 80% of the local recurrences developed in the periphery of tumors larger than 5 cm in diameter.

A report of RFA of hepatic tumor showing the results from 109 patients with 172 metastatic lesions who underwent RFA was published by Solbiati and colleagues (Solbiati et al. 2001). The median follow-up in this study was 3 years (with a range between 5 and 52 months). Local tumor control was achieved in 70% of the lesions, but local recurrence developed in 30%. As described above, the tumor control depends mainly on tumor diameter. The authors of this study were also able to show a significant difference in local recurrence comparing lesions smaller than 3 cm and larger than 3 cm in diameter with a local relapse of 16.5% versus 56.1%, respectively. The overall 2- and 3-year survival rates were 67% and 33%, respectively, with a median survival of 30 months (Solbiati et al. 2001). The patients in this study were treated with percutaneous, ultrasound-guided RFA, leading to a quite high incomplete treatment rate, associated with a higher local recurrence rate due to a limited resolution with transabdominal ultrasonography, making correct needle electrode placement much more difficult. A study from France (de Baere et al. 2000) analyzed 68 patients with 121 hepatic metastases who underwent 76 sessions of RFA with or without additional surgery. Forty-seven patients with 88 metastases ranging from 1 to 4.2 cm in diameter were treated with RFA alone while the remaining 21 patients underwent a combination of surgery and intraoperative RFA for remaining small tumors. In 33 patients with 67 metastases who underwent percutaneous RFA a follow-up of at least 4 months was available, showing a local relapse in only 10% of the lesions (21% of the patients). A mean follow-up of 13.7 months was available for all patients showing 79% of the patients treated with percutaneous RFA were alive, 42% had no evidence of new or recurrent malignant hepatic disease, but only 27% were completely tumor free. A very interesting finding was that the 21 patients with otherwise unresectable metastatic lesions which underwent a combination of intraoperative RFA (33 lesions) and surgical resection had 2-year overall and disease-free survival rates of 94.7% and 22%, respectively (de Baere et al. 2000). This finding suggests that RFA can be used safely in combination with resection to increase the number of patients who are surgical candidates in an attempt to improve overall survival rates. A study recently published by Gillams (Gillams and Lees 2004) referred to a cohort of 167 patients with colorectal liver metastases treated with percutaneous RFA. The authors were able to show a median survival period of 38 months, with a 5-year survival rate of 30% after the diagnosis of liver metastases. Furthermore, a survival period of 31 months, with a 5-year survival rate of 25%, after the first ablation was reported. The authors concluded from their results that RFA increases the therapeutic options for patients with colorectal metastases. Furthermore their conclusion was that until controlled trials can better define the role of RFA, there are several groups of patients who are not surgical candidates and can be considered for RFA.

Neuroendocrine tumors are metastatic and treatable with RFA. Liver metastases from neuroendocrine tumors often produce severe clinical symptoms caused by excessive hormone production and release. Only a minority of these patients with neuroendocrine liver metastases are curable by surgical resection. However, a significant relief of symptoms can be obtained by "debulking," which includes resection, resection combined with RFA or RFA alone. There is one publication reporting on 18 patients with more than 100 neuroendocrine tumors (carcinoid, islet cell, or medullary thyroid cancers) treated with RFA (Siperstein and Berber 2001). Unfortunately, the exact number of patients was not indicated. However, the authors reported that most patients had significant improvement in symptoms related to reduced hormone release after RFA (Siperstein and Berber 2001). However, the major drawback is that there are no prospective randomized trials so far, comparing local ablation with hepatic resection or with chemotherapy alone and there are no randomized studies comparing the outcome of patients after different ablative methods.

3.5.4 Complication Rates

A recently published multicenter study by Livraghi et al. (Livraghi et al. 2003) reported the complication rates after treating 2320 patients with a total number of 3554 lesions. Six deaths (0.3%) were noted, including two fatalities caused by multiorgan failure following intestinal perforation. One case of septic shock following *Staphylococcus aureus* peritonitis was reported. One patient died due to massive hemorrhage following tumor rupture, another due to liver failure following stenosis of the right bile duct; and one death of unknown cause occurred 3 days after the procedure. Furthermore, 50 patients (2.2%) had major complications. The most frequently observed major complications were peritoneal hemorrhage, intrahepatic abscess formation, and intestinal perforation. Tumor seeding along the needle tract has been a rare complication as track ablation was performed after every thermal ablation (Livraghi and Meloni 2001). Peritoneal hemorrhage mostly occurred in patients with superficial metastases, whereas intrahepatic abscesses were mostly observed in diabetic patients without peri-procedural antibiotics. Furthermore, thermal damage to adjacent organs (colon, stomach) has rarely been described in patients with minimal hepatic reserve (Livraghi et al. 2003). Minor complications, including post- or peri-procedural pain, fever and asymptomatic pleural effusion, were observed in less than 5% of patients. Fever with a temperature of up to 39°C has been reported as part of the comparatively common postablation syndrome, the occurrence of which seems to be dependent on the volume of ablated tumor tissue. Pleural effusion is a relatively common feature, especially when using an intercostal approach or when the lesion is located in the dome of the liver. Furthermore, Livraghi et al. (2003) reported the rate of complications to be directly related to the number of required RF sessions. However, the tumor size itself or the type of electrode used appears to have no significant influence on the number and extent of reported complications. The results of the study by Livraghi (Livraghi et al. 2003) confirmed – in accordance with the experience of other authors – RFA to be a relatively low-risk procedure for the treatment of focal liver tumors (Curley et al. 2004; Liu et al. 2002; Mulier et al. 2002; Pereira et al. 2003).

3.5.5 Control of Effectiveness

The main problem with local ablative therapies (including RFA) is the lack of an immediate direct control to determine the extent of tissue necrosis and therefore the success of the therapy. As an indirect control of the effectiveness of the RFA, unenhanced CT scans can be obtained immediately after ablation. These native CT examinations commonly reveal an increased density at the center of the treatment zone, which is most often surrounded by a region of hypoattenuation. Furthermore, contrast-enhanced CT immediately after thermal ablation may aid in discriminating between ablated tissue and residual viable tumor. Post-therapeutic CT scans usually demonstrate regions of hypoattenuation in the treated portions of the tumor devoid of characteristic tumorous or parenchymal enhancement. Ideally, the lesion created by RFA of a hepatic tumor should be larger (at least 1 cm in each diameter) on post-treatment images when compared to pretreatment images to assure a complete ablation including a safety margin (Fig. 3.5.1). Furthermore, imaging during the arterial phase may show a thin rim of contrast enhancement corresponding to an early inflammatory reaction in the periphery of the ablated area due to the thermal damage.

Long-term follow-up examinations are indispensable for detecting untreated or insufficiently treated neoplastic areas or for documenting complete treatment. In our opinion, contrast-enhanced CT has established itself as the state of the art imaging method in long-term follow-up. However, some authors use MRI or contrast-enhanced ultrasound (Cioni et al. 2001; Lencioni et al. 2002) for the follow-up. Coagulated non-enhancing regions are more clearly delineated 24 h after ablation. Imaging 6–12 months after RFA normally demonstrates – depending on the regeneration capacity of the liver – a marked regression of the volume of both the lesion and the region of induced coagulation necrosis (Fig. 3.5.2). A densely enhancing peripheral rim on delayed images often surrounds the region of coagulation. This rim normally represents an inflammatory reaction to the thermally induced damage, whereas a bulky irregularity at the edge of a treatment site is the most common appearance of an incompletely treated lesion. If residual viable tumor tissue is detected, a second treatment cycle needs to be considered to reach complete necrosis. Another possibility for controlling the effectiveness of the locally ablative therapy is to monitor the tumor markers (CEA, CA 15-3 and others). Tumor markers have been reported to normalize or decrease in the first month after RFA in 81%–100% of patients that had raised levels before therapy (Erce and Parks 2003). PET scan or a combination of PET and helical CT (PET-CT) can make a valuable contribution

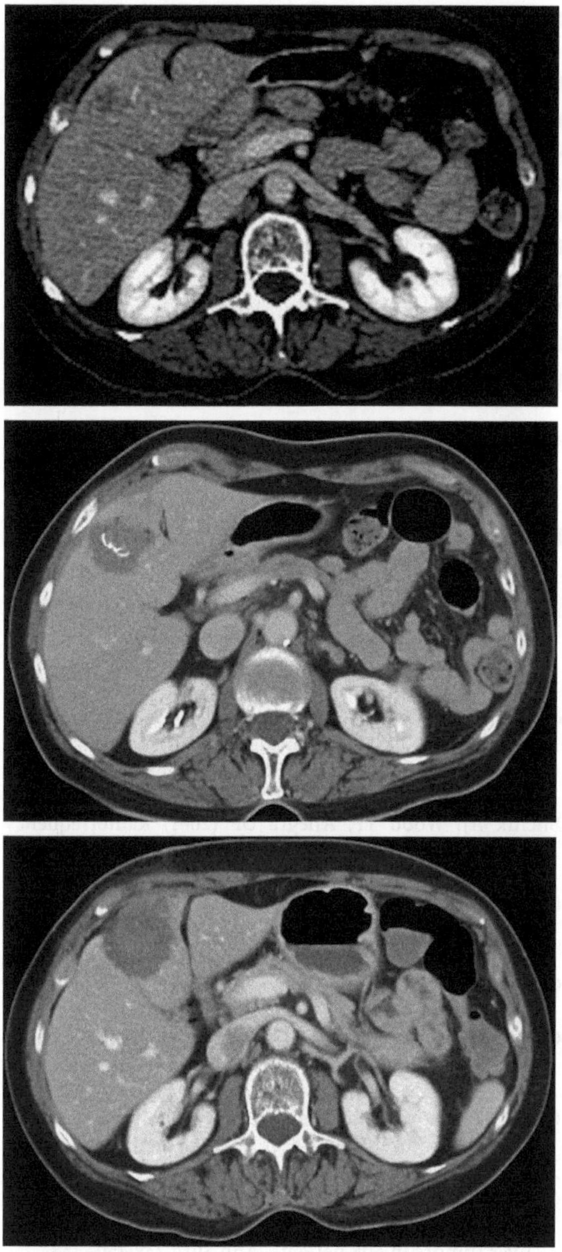

a

b

c

Fig. 3.5.1a–c. Patient suffering from metastasis of a colorectal carcinoma; not a suitable candidate for surgery. **a** Pretherapy CT scan showed a 2-cm lesion within segment 5. **b** RF ablation was performed under CT-fluoroscopic guidance using a 3.0-cm umbrella-shaped needle. CT scan immediately after treatment with a reduced amount of contrast agent showed the lesion completely covered by the ablation. **c** Twenty-four hours after ablation the thermal lesion has grown, covering the metastasis with a margin of at least 1 cm

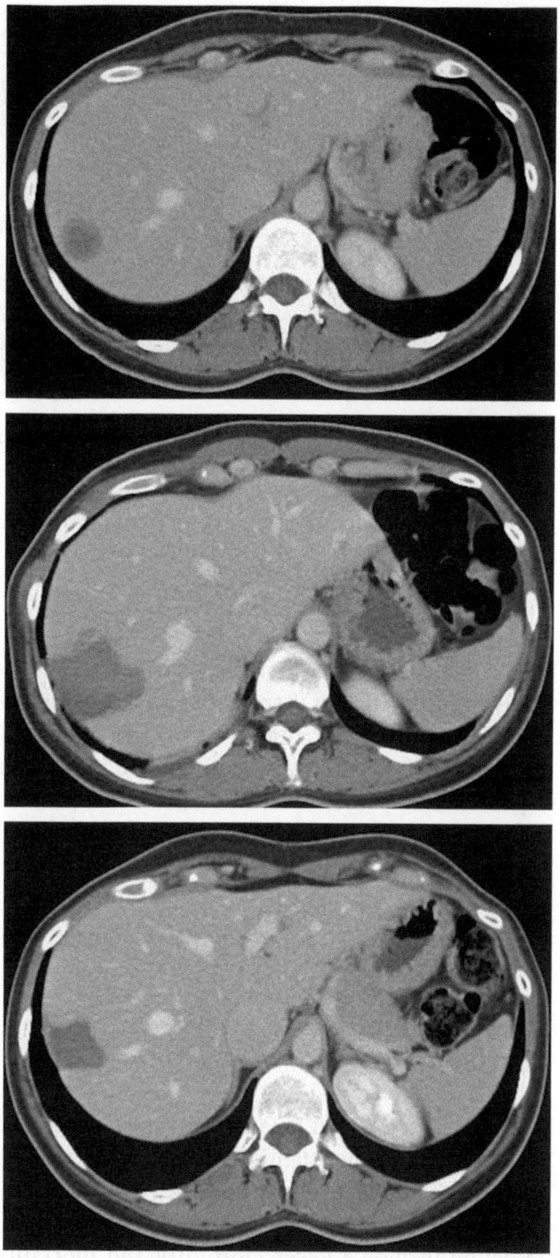

a

b

c

Fig. 3.5.2a–c. Patient refused to undergo surgery. **a** Contrast-enhanced CT images show a solitary metastasis in liver segment 7 with a diameter of about 3 cm. **b** Twenty-four hours after treatment – using a 4-cm umbrella-shaped electrode in composite ablation technique to create sufficient thermal necrosis – CT scan showed a huge ablation area with a sufficient safety margin. **c** A control scan 6 months after RF ablation shows scarring and shrinkage of the formerly treated area indicating a sufficient ablation procedure with no local recurrence detectable

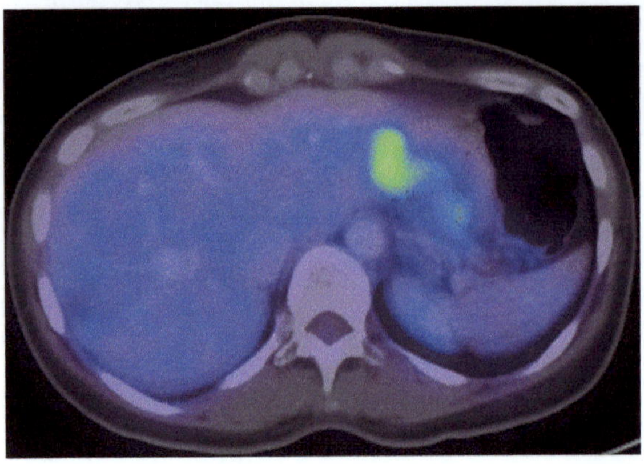

Fig. 3.5.3. PET-CT image taken from a follow-up study from the patient shown in Fig. 3.5.2 12 months after treatment. There is no elevated fluorodeoxyglucose uptake in the formerly treated area; however, a new metastasis can be detected in segment 2, not visible in the contrast-enhanced CT scan

in the detection of residual tumor after RFA. Especially in inconclusive CT scans the additional information regarding the vitality of tumors shown by an elevated fluorodeoxyglucose uptake can prove a possible relapse of the tumor (Anderson et al. 2003; Donckier et al. 2003; Joosten et al. 2005) (Fig. 3.5.3).

3.5.6 Conclusion

Percutaneous thermal ablative therapies have been receiving increasing attention as a potential curative treatment for focal liver metastases. Possible advantages of ablative therapies as compared to surgical resection include a lower morbidity and mortality rate, lower costs, a suitability for real-time imaging guidance, the option of performing ablative procedures on outpatients and the potential application to a wider spectrum of patients, including those who are unsuitable as surgical candidates (Goldberg and Ahmed 2002). Other advantages are the possibility of causing selective damage with less immunosuppression and a smaller release of growth factors and the possibility of starting chemotherapy before or at the time of local therapy (Tranberg 2004).

In our opinion, the major advantage of RFA is its ability to create a well-controlled focal thermal injury in the liver resulting in high success rates in treating metastases smaller than 3 cm in diameter with long-term results comparable to surgery. Furthermore RFA – together with a multimodal therapeutic concept – appears to significantly improve the outcome of the patients. However, surgery or a combination of surgery and RFA seems to currently remain the treatment of choice for tumors larger than 3 cm and for multinodular metastases due to the unsatisfactory results of RFA in this tumor type. Nonetheless, more randomized trials are required to establish a definite treatment protocol for RFA for patients with malignant hepatic tumors.

References

Anderson GS, Brinkmann F, Soulen MC et al (2003) FDG positron emission tomography in the surveillance of hepatic tumors treated with radiofrequency ablation. Clin Nucl Med 28:192–197

de Baere T, Elias D, Dromain C et al (2000) Radiofrequency ablation of 100 hepatic metastases with a mean follow-up of more than 1 year. AJR Am J Roentgenol 175:1619–1625

Bilchik AJ, Wood TF, Allegra DP (2001) Radiofrequency ablation of unresectable hepatic malignancies: lessons learned. Oncologist 6:24–33

Cioni D, Lencioni R, Bartolozzi C (2001) Percutaneous ablation of liver malignancies: imaging evaluation of treatment response. Eur J Ultrasound 13:73–93

Curley SA (2003) Radiofrequency ablation of malignant liver tumors. Ann Surg Oncol 10:338–347

Curley SA, Izzo F, Delrio P et al (1999) Radiofrequency ablation of unresectable primary and metastatic hepatic malignancies: results in 123 patients. Ann Surg 230:1–8

Curley SA, Izzo F, Ellis LM et al (2000) Radiofrequency ablation of hepatocellular cancer in 110 patients with cirrhosis. Ann Surg 232:381–391

Curley SA, Marra P, Beaty K et al (2004) Early and late complications after radiofrequency ablation of malignant liver tumors in 608 patients. Ann Surg 239:450–458

Donckier V, Van Laethem JL, Goldman S et al (2003) [F-18] fluorodeoxyglucose positron emission tomography as a tool for early recognition of incomplete tumor destruction after radiofrequency ablation for liver metastases. J Surg Oncol 84:215–223

Erce C, Parks RW (2003) Interstitial ablative techniques for hepatic tumours. Br J Surg 90:272–289

Gazelle GS, Goldberg SN, Solbiati L et al (2000) Tumor ablation with radio-frequency energy. Radiology 217:633–646

Gillams AR, Lees WR (2004) Radio-frequency ablation of colorectal liver metastases in 167 patients. Eur Radiol 14:2261–2267

Goldberg SN, Ahmed M (2002) Minimally invasive image-guided therapies for hepatocellular carcinoma. J Clin Gastroenterol 35:S115–S129

Joosten J, Jager G, Oyen W, Wobbes T, Ruers T (2005) Cryosurgery and radiofrequency ablation for unresectable colorectal liver metastases. Eur J Surg Oncol 31:1152–1159

Lencioni R, Cioni D, Bartolozzi C (2001) Percutaneous radiofrequency thermal ablation of liver malignancies: techniques, indications, imaging findings, and clinical results. Abdom Imaging 26:345–360

Lencioni R, Cioni D, Crocetti L et al (2002) Ultrasound imaging of focal liver lesions with a second-generation contrast agent. Acad Radiol 9 [Suppl 2]:S371–374

Liu LX, Jiang HC, Piao DX (2002) Radiofrequency ablation of liver cancers. World J Gastroenterol 8:393–399

Livraghi T, Meloni F (2001) Removal of liver tumours using radiofrequency waves. Ann Chir Gynaecol 90:239–245

Livraghi T, Solbiati L, Meloni MF et al (2003) Treatment of focal liver tumors with percutaneous radio-frequency ablation: complications encountered in a multicenter study. Radiology 226:441–451

McGahan JP, Browning PD, Brock JM et al (1990) Hepatic ablation using radiofrequency electrocautery. Invest Radiol 25:267–270

Mulier S, Mulier P, Ni Y et al (2002) Complications of radiofrequency coagulation of liver tumours. Br J Surg 89:1206–1222

Ohlsson B, Stenram U, Tranberg KG (1998) Resection of colorectal liver metastases: 25-year experience. World J Surg 22:268–276; discussion 276–267

Pereira PL, Trubenbach J, Schmidt D (2003) Radiofrequency ablation: basic principles, techniques and challenges. Rofo Fortschr Geb Rontgenstr Neuen Bildgeb Verfahr 175:20–27

Rossi S, Fornari F, Pathies C et al (1990) Thermal lesions induced by 480 kHz localized current field in guinea pig and pig liver. Tumori 76:54–57

Scheele J, Stang R, Altendorf-Hofmann A et al (1995) Resection of colorectal liver metastases. World J Surg 19:59–71

Siperstein AE, Berber E (2001) Cryoablation, percutaneous alcohol injection, and radiofrequency ablation for treatment of neuroendocrine liver metastases. World J Surg 25:693–696

Solbiati L, Ierace T, Tonolini M et al (2001) Radiofrequency thermal ablation of hepatic metastases. Eur J Ultrasound 13:149–158

Tranberg KG (2004) Percutaneous ablation of liver tumours. Best Pract Res Clin Gastroenterol 18:125–145

Wood TF, Rose DM, Chung M et al (2000) Radiofrequency ablation of 231 unresectable hepatic tumors: indications, limitations, and complications. Ann Surg Oncol 7:593–600

Liver

Secondary Tumors

3.6 LITT

Thomas J. Vogl and Martin G. Mack

CONTENTS

3.6.1 Introduction

Although percutaneous tumor ablation has been used in the treatment of various organs, the liver has proven to be an ideal target for this interventional treatment technique. Simultaneously, three different techniques were developed worldwide, namely cryotherapy, laser-induced thermotherapy (LITT), and radiofrequency ablation (RF). The liver plays a central role in human metabolism and so represents one of the organ systems most often affected, especially by tumorous diseases. In principle the liver can be affected by both primary malignant tumors such as hepatocellular carcinoma and, more frequently, by secondary manifestations such as liver metastases. A large number of primary tumors often cause liver metastases as well as bone, lung, and brain metastases. The group of colorectal carcinomas attack this organ metastatically almost exclusively, which, according to studies by Weiss et al., can be attributed to the venous drainage of the intestines through the portal vein (Weiss 1994; Weiss et al. 1986). After curative treatment of the primary tumor, the liver manifestation has a decisive influence on the survival time of affected patients in many cases. A number of factors, such as the underlying primary tumor, the stage the tumor has reached, the localization, and general factors such as age or any existing concomitant disease, influence the prognosis of the patients. Interstitial procedures such as laser-induced thermotherapy (LITT) or radiofrequency ablation (RFA) show a high rate of controlling the site of the tumor and are currently being clinically evaluated.

Strategies for liver metastases are considerably more complex. Up to now the liver resection of solitary lesions has been the only potential curative treatment (Adson et al. 1984; Fong and Blumgart 1998; Harrison et al. 1997; Hughes et al. 1988; Jenkins et al. 1997; Lorenz and Waldemayer 1997; Maksan et al. 2000; Mariette and Fagniez 1992; Petrelli et al. 1985; Scheele et al. 1996; Yoon and Tanabe 1999). However, the high rate of intrahepatic relapses and possible potentiation of metastatic intrahepatic growth by released growth factors as part of the tumor stimulation process are considered problematic. For this reason, recently there has been great interest in further development of interstitial procedures such as laser-induced interstitial thermotherapy (LITT), RFA, microwave ablation, and cryotherapy.

The purpose of this chapter is to present the technical data, the practical performance, and the application data of MR-guided LITT for secondary liver tumors.

Between June 1993 and May 2005, LITT was performed on 1,750 patients with a total of 4,950 liver

T. J. Vogl, MD, Professor; M. G. Mack, MD, PD
Institute for Diagnostic and Interventional Radiology, University Hospital, Johann Wolfgang Goethe University, Theodor-Stern-Kai 7, 60590 Frankfurt, Germany

metastases and 85 hepatocellular carcinomas. In our institute we include patients with different primary tumors such as colorectal liver metastases, liver metastases from breast cancer, hepatocellular carcinoma, liver metastases from pancreatic cancer and a variety of other tumors (Fig. 3.6.1). We also include patients with recurrent liver metastases after partial liver resection, patients with metastases in both liver lobes, patients with locally non-resectable lesions, and patients who had general contraindications for surgery or refused surgical resection.

In our series a laser application is defined as a laser treatment at one certain position. If the laser applicator is pulled back and another laser treatment is performed to enlarge the coagulative necrosis a second laser application is performed.

3.6.2 Technical Data

3.6.2.1 Laser Equipment and Application Set

Laser coagulation is accomplished using a neodymium-YAG laser light with a wavelength of 1,064 nm (MediLas 5060, MediLas 5100, Dornier Germering, Germany), delivered through optic fibers terminated by a specially developed diffuser. In the beginning a diffuser tip with a glass dome of 0.9 mm in diameter, which was mounted at the end of a 10-m long silica fiber (diameter 400 μm), was used. Since the year 2000 a flexible diffuser tip has been used with a diameter of 1.0 mm, which makes the laser applications much easier due to the fact that the risk of damage to the diffuser tip has dropped to almost zero. The active length of the diffuser tip ranges between 20 and 40 mm in length. The laser power is adjusted to 12 watts per cm active length of the laser applicator.

The laser application kit (SOMATEX, Berlin, Germany) consists of a cannulation needle, a sheath system, and a protective catheter which prevents direct contact of the laser applicator with the treated tissues and allows cooling of the tip of the laser applicator. The closed end of the protective catheter enables complete removal of the applicator even in the unlikely event of damage to the fiber during treatment. This simplifies the procedure and makes it safer for the patient.

The laser itself was installed outside the MR examination room, and the light was transmitted through a 10-m long optical fiber. All patients were examined using an MR imaging protocol including T_1-weighted gradient-echo (GE) plain and contrast-enhanced GD-DTPA 0.1 mmol/kg body weight. T_2- and T_1-weighted images were obtained for localizing the target lesion and planning the interventional procedure. The studies were performed with a conventional 1.5-T system (Siemens, Erlangen, Germany) and a 0.5-T system (Escint).

3.6.3 Imaging During Therapy

After informing patients about potential complications, benefits, and disadvantages of LITT, consent is obtained. The metastasis is localized on computed tomographic scans and the injection site is infiltrated with 20 ml of 1% lidocaine. Under CT guidance the laser application system is inserted using the Seldinger technique. After the patient is positioned on the MR table, the laser catheter is

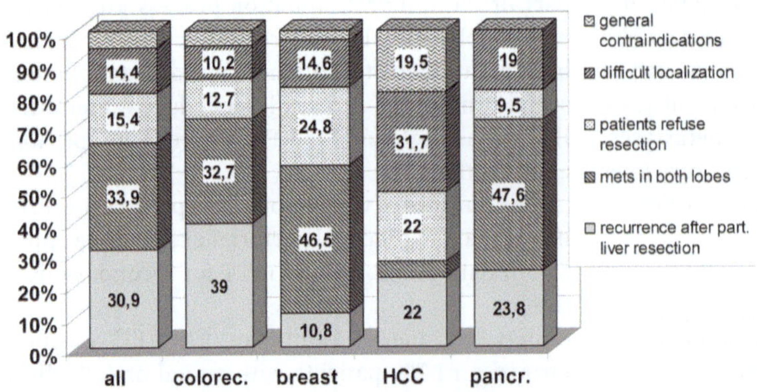

Fig. 3.6.1. Documentation of the distribution of the indications for laser-induced thermotherapy (*LITT*) treatment for all patients (*all*), patients with colorectal liver metastases (*colorec.*), liver metastases from breast cancer (*breast*), hepatocellular carcinoma (*HCC*), and patients with liver metastases from pancreatic cancer (*pancr.*)

inserted into the protective catheter. MR sequences are performed in three perpendicular orientations before and during LITT.

MR sequences are performed every 30 s to assess the progress in heating the lesion and the surrounding tissue. Heating is revealed as signal loss in the T_1-weighted GE images as a result of the heat-induced increase of the T_1 relaxation time. Depending on geometry and intensity of the signal loss and speed of heat distribution, the position of the laser fibers, the laser power and the cooling rate are readjusted. Treatment is stopped after total coagulation of the lesion, and a safety margin from 5 to 15 mm surrounding the lesion is visualized in MR images.

After switching off the laser, T_1-weighted contrast-enhanced FLASH-2D images are obtained for verifying the induced necrosis. After the procedure the puncture channel is sealed with fibrin glue. Follow-up examinations using plain and contrast-enhanced sequences are performed after 24–48 h, and every 3 months following the LITT procedure. Quantitative and qualitative parameters, including size, morphology, signal behavior, and contrast enhancement, are evaluated when deciding whether treatment can be considered successful, or whether subsequent treatment sessions are required.

Laser-induced effects are evaluated by comparing images of lesions and surrounding liver parenchyma with each other before and after laser treatment, and with those obtained at follow-up examinations. Tumor volume and volume of coagulative necrosis are calculated using three-dimensional MR images and measurements of the maximum diameter in three planes (A, B, and C). The volume was calculated using the formula $(A \times B \times C) \times 0.5$. The results are tested for significance using the ANOVA test. Survival rates are calculated using the Kaplan-Meier method.

3.6.4 Clinical Data of MR-Guided LITT of Liver Metastases

All treatments could be performed under local anesthesia and were well tolerated by the patients. All patients treated between June 1993 and September 1998 were hospitalized for 24–48 h after the intervention. All patients treated between October 1998 and May 2005 were strictly treated on an outpatient basis.

Evaluation of the MR thermometry data during MR-guided laser-induced thermotherapy demonstrate that metastatic tissue is very sensitive to heat, showing earlier and more widespread temperature distribution of the delivered thermal energy than does surrounding liver parenchyma. In 90.9% of all cases the area of obviously decreased signal intensity during LITT treatment is identical with the area classified as coagulative necrosis on MR images 24 h after laser treatment. In 8.6% of the cases the size of the coagulative necrosis obtained 24 h after LITT treatment is larger compared to MR thermometry images.

The mean number of treated metastases per patient is 2.8 (median 2). The evaluation of the application details is presented in Table 3.6.1. In 57% of the patients only one or two metastases are treated.

Table 3.6.1. Documentation of the application data for the total patient material including all patients with malignant liver lesions. The number of applicators represents the number of applicators per patient. The number of applications indicates how many LITT treatments were performed per patient

Parameter	Mean	Median	Minimum	Maximum
Age (years)	59.5	60.0	28.4	88.7
Applicators	6.8	5	1	34
Applications	11.4	9	1	56
Metastases	2.8	2	1	21
LITT session	2.4	2	1	13
LITT round	1.5	1	1	9
Applicator per met.	2.5	2	1	9
Session per met.	1.05	1	1	3
Energy per met. (kJ)	104	82.9	5.9	502.4

In 7% more than six metastases are treated in total. The localization of the metastases with respect to the different liver segments showed a quite homogenous distribution of the metastases in the different liver segments taking into account the different volumes of the liver segments.

A total of 49% of the lesions showed a relationship to the liver capsule, 7% presented a relationship to the central portal vein structures and only 29% of the metastases were at a location which was classified as easy.

The mean number of inserted laser applicators for the treatment of one metastasis with a reliable safety margin with regard to the size of the metastases was as follows: in 26.1% of all metastases only one laser applicator was inserted; in 29.8% two laser applicators, in 18.8% three laser applicators, in 18.4% four laser applicators, in 5.3% five laser applicators, and in 1.7% more than five laser applicators were necessary for the treatment of a single metastasis with a reliable safety margin (Fig. 3.6.2).

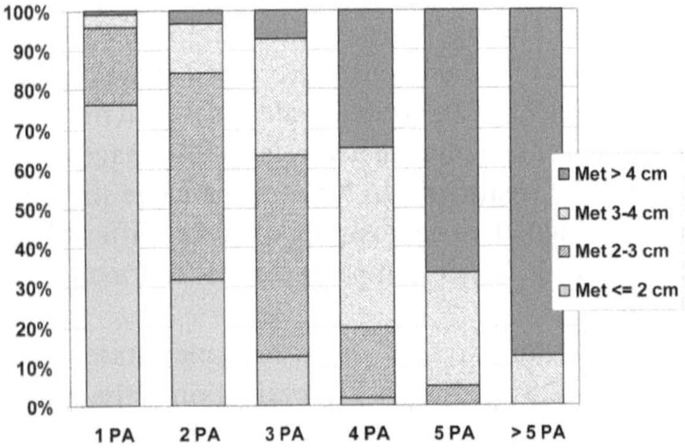

Fig. 3.6.2. The graph shows the number of laser applicators which were inserted for the treatment of one single metastasis with respect to the size of the metastases. (*PA* Power laser applicator)

The mean values of the applied energy were statistically significantly higher in liver metastases of colorectal carcinoma versus liver metastases of breast carcinoma and hepatocellular carcinoma (ANOVA test $p < 0.01$).

The volume of the induced coagulative necrosis 24 h after LITT treatment exceeds the volume of the initial tumor significantly ($p < 0.001$) (Fig. 3.6.5). During follow-up examinations the volume of the induced necrosis gets smaller again due to resorption and shrinking of the lesion. In the 3-month control the volume of the coagulative necrosis is already roughly half of the initial volume of the necrosis, but still larger than the initial tumor volume (Figs. 3.6.3, 3.6.4). The volume of coagulative necrosis 24 h after LITT treatment exceeds the initial tumor volume on average by a factor of 13 (range, 12–17) for lesions with a diameter of 2 cm or less, by a factor of 8 (range, 7.5–8.2) for lesions between 2 and 3 cm in diameter, by a factor of 6 (range, 5.3–6.1) for lesions between 3 and 4 cm in diameter, and by a factor of 2.5 (range, 1.8–2.7) for lesions larger than 4 cm in diameter.

The results achieved to date concerning the survival in patients with liver metastases and primary liver cancer are presented in the following figures (Fig. 3.6.6). So far it can be shown that a survival for more than 5 years is possible in patients with liver metastases, especially of colorectal cancer. The survival was improved in patients with a smaller number of metastases (one or two metastases versus three or more metastases). However, this difference is not statistically significant. Currently all survival data are limited in their scientific value due to the missing randomization of the protocol. However, the presented data show that active local tumor control is possible and a long survival can be achieved.

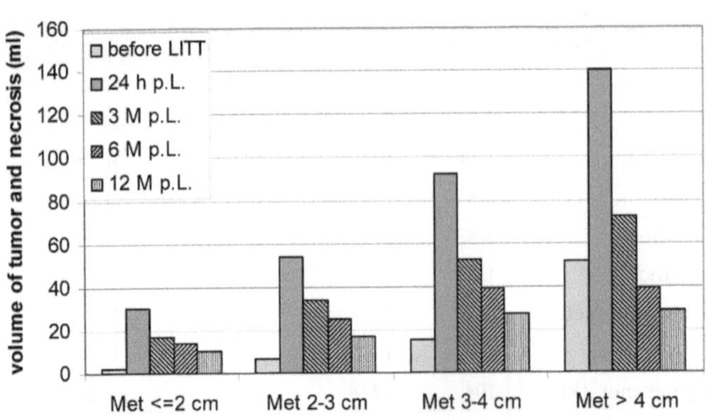

Fig. 3.6.3. The diagram shows the mean values for the initial tumor volume (before LITT) as well as the volumes of the coagulative necrosis obtained 24 h after LITT treatment (*24 h p.L.*), 3 months after LITT (*3 M p.L.*), 6 months (*6 M p.L.*) and 12 months after LITT treatment (*12 M p.L.*). The evaluation included metastases from all primaries

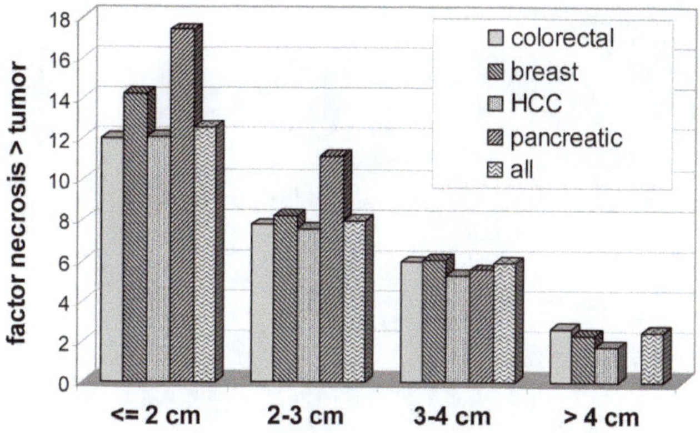

Fig. 3.6.4. The graph shows the factor by which the necrosis measured on contrast-enhanced images 24 h after LITT treatment exceeds the initial tumor volume. The values are separately given for the different primary tumors as well as the different size of the treated metastases

3.6.5 Results and Prognostic Factors of Liver Metastases of Colorectal Carcinoma

MR-guided LITT was performed in 839 patients (mean age 61.6 years) with 2,506 liver metastases of colorectal cancer between 1993 and 2005. The following criteria were analyzed: primary tumor and lymph node staging, localization of the primary tumor (rectum, sigmoid, colon), number of liver metastases at first LITT treatment, synchronous (less than 6 months between diagnosis of tumor and first liver metastases) or metachronous metastases, survival rate, and indication for LITT. The Tarone Ware, Breslow, and Log Rank tests were used for statistical significance.

The following factors had a statistically significant influence on the survival of patients: Lymph node status N0/N1 (mean survival 3.9 years, 95% confidence interval 3.6–4.3) versus N2/N3 (mean survival 3.6 years, 95% CI 3.1–4.0), one to two initial metastases (mean survival 4.3 years, 95% CI 3.9–4.7) versus three to four metastases (mean survival 3.3 years, 95% CI 2.9–3.7) versus five or more metastases (mean survival 2.8 years, 95% confidence interval 2.5–3.1), synchronous metastases (mean survival 3.5 years) versus metachronous (mean survival 4.1 years), patients refused resection (mean survival 5.5 years) versus recurrent liver metastases after resection (mean survival 3.6 years) versus difficult location for surgery (mean survival 3.4 years) versus metastases in both liver lobes (mean survival 3.2 years) versus general contraindications for surgery (mean survival 2.6 years). The primary T staging was not a prognostic factor regarding survival of colorectal liver metastases (T1/T2: mean survival 3.9 years versus T3/T4: mean survival 3.7 years, log rank = 0.45, Breslow = 0.68, Tarone Ware = 0.55). The localization of the primary tumor revealed only statistically significant differences in the Breslow and Tarone Ware tests (rectum: mean survival 3.63 years; sigmoid: mean survival 3.55 years; and colon: mean survival 3.72 years). Survival rates were calculated using the Kaplan–Meier method. Of the lesions, 33.3% were 2 cm or less in diameter (mean applied energy 54.5 kJ; range, 8.2–249.7 kJ), 33.3% were between 2 and 3 cm (mean applied energy 94.9 kJ; range, 11.6–361.4 kJ), 18.1% were between 3 and 4 cm (mean applied energy 133.45 kJ; range, 20.2–452.6 kJ), and 15.6% were larger than 4 cm in maximum diameter (mean applied energy 189.1 kJ, range 10.4–515.0 kJ). Of the patients, 77.6% (n = 651) had five liver metastases or less and no extrahepatic disease at the time of inclusion and were treated with a curative intention; 22.4% (n = 188) were treated with a palliative intention (patients with more than five metastases and/or limited extrahepatic disease). The following number of metastases was treated: one metastasis in 29% of the patients, two metastases in 26.5%, three metastases in 17.8%, four metastases in 10.6%, five metastases in 7.5%, and more than five metastases in 8.6% of the patients.

The mean survival rate for all treated patients, starting the calculation at the date of diagnosis of the metastases which were treated with LITT, was 3.8 years (95% CI 3.5–4.1 years, 1-year survival 93%, 2-year survival 72%, 3-year survival 47%, 5-year survival 24%). The mean survival in the curative group was 4.0 years (95% CI: 3.7–4.4 years). In the palliative group it was 2.8 years (95% CI: 2.4–3.1 years).

The lymph node status, the time interval between primary tumor and liver metastases, and the number of initial liver metastases after MR-guided LITT were prognostic factors regarding the survival of patients. MR-guided LITT yields high local tumor control and survival rates in patients with liver metastases of colorectal carcinoma. In surgical candidates LITT seems to be superior to resection.

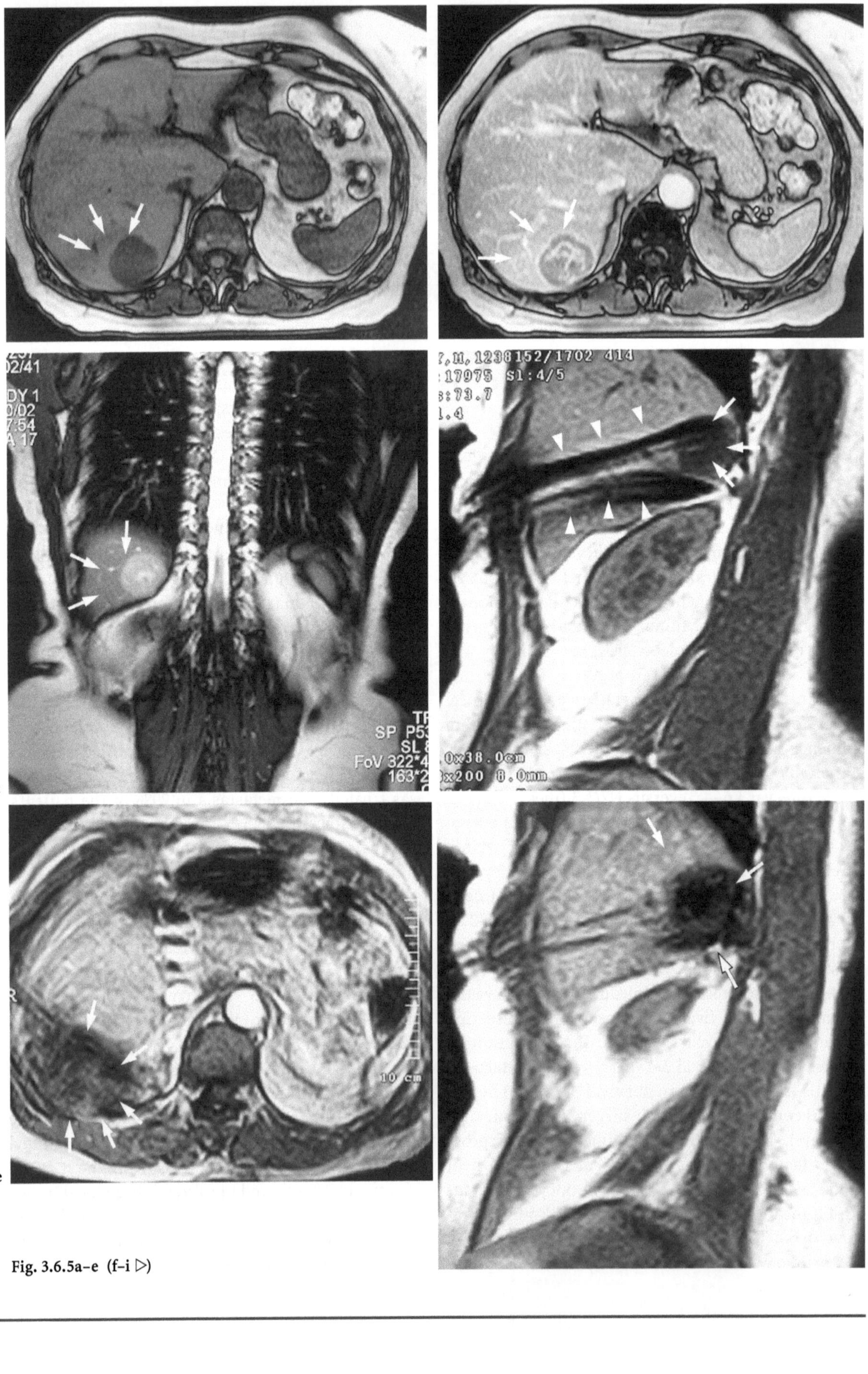

Fig. 3.6.5a–e (f–i ▷)

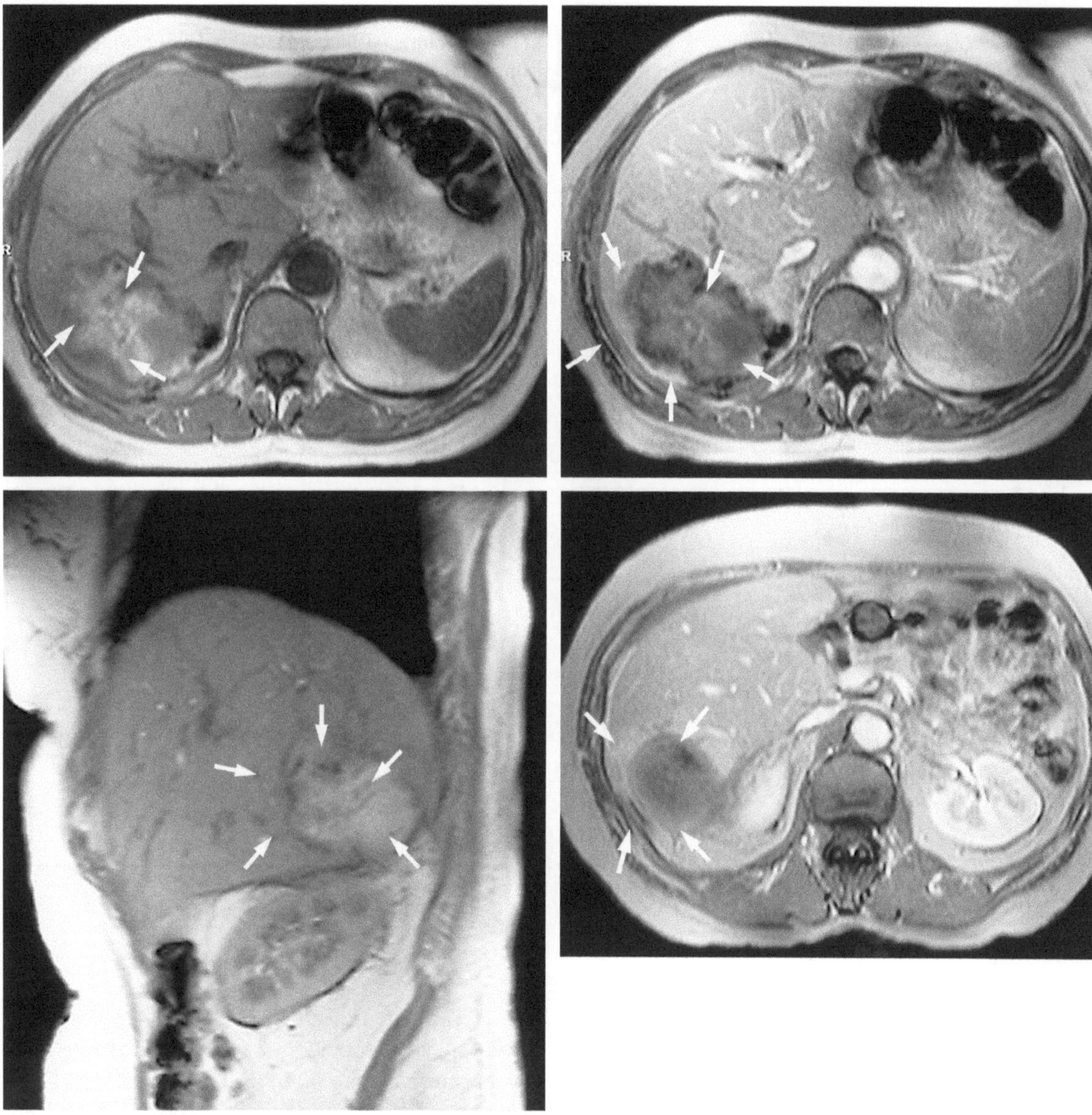

Fig. 3.6.5a–i. A 62-year-old patient with liver metastases from a breast cancer. **a** Transverse unenhanced T_1-weighted GE image (TR/TE = 74/2.6) obtained 2 weeks before laser treatment shows a liver metastasis (*arrows*) in segment 7 with a maximum diameter of 3.8 cm. **b** Transverse contrast-enhanced T_1-weighted GE image (TR/TE = 74/2.6) 2 weeks before LITT treatment shows contrast enhancement in the periphery of the metastases (*arrows*). **c** Coronal unenhanced T_2-weighted GE image (TR/TE = 4.5/2.2) obtained 2 weeks before laser treatment shows a liver metastasies (*arrows*) in segment 7 with a maximum diameter of 3.8 cm. **d** Sagittal unenhanced T_1-weighted FLASH-2D image immediately before starting the LITT treatment shows the metastases (*arrows*) and the positioned laser fibers (*arrow heads*). For better visualization of the application systems a magnetite marker was placed in the protective catheter. **e** Transverse and sagittal unenhanced T_1-weighted images obtained 20 min after starting the laser treatment demonstrate an obvious signal decrease of the lesion and the surrounding tissue (*arrows*) due to the increase of tissue temperature. The temperature in the center of the lesion is around 110°C, in the peripheral zone the temperature is around 60–70°C. **f** Transverse unenhanced T_1-weighted image obtained 24 h after laser treatment shows the induced coagulation area (*arrows*) with some inflammatory changes. **g** Transverse contrast-enhanced T_1-weighted image 24 h after laser treatment shows the induced coagulation area (*arrows*). **h** Sagittal contrast-enhanced T_1-weighted GE obtained 24 h after LITT demonstrates the extension of the necrosis (*arrows*). **i** Transverse contrast-enhanced T_1-weighted image 3 months after laser treatment shows the induced coagulation area (*arrows*)

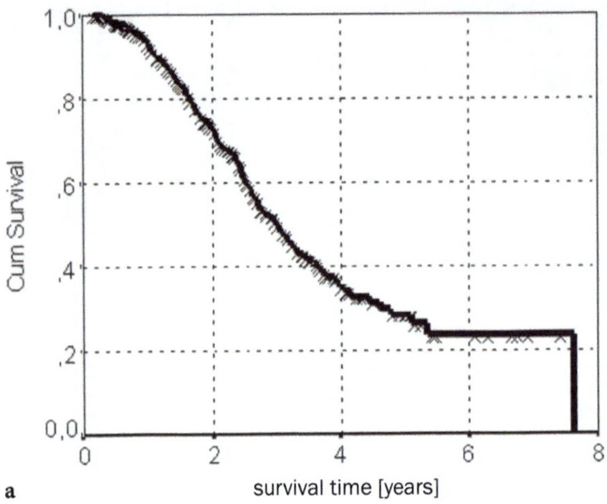

a

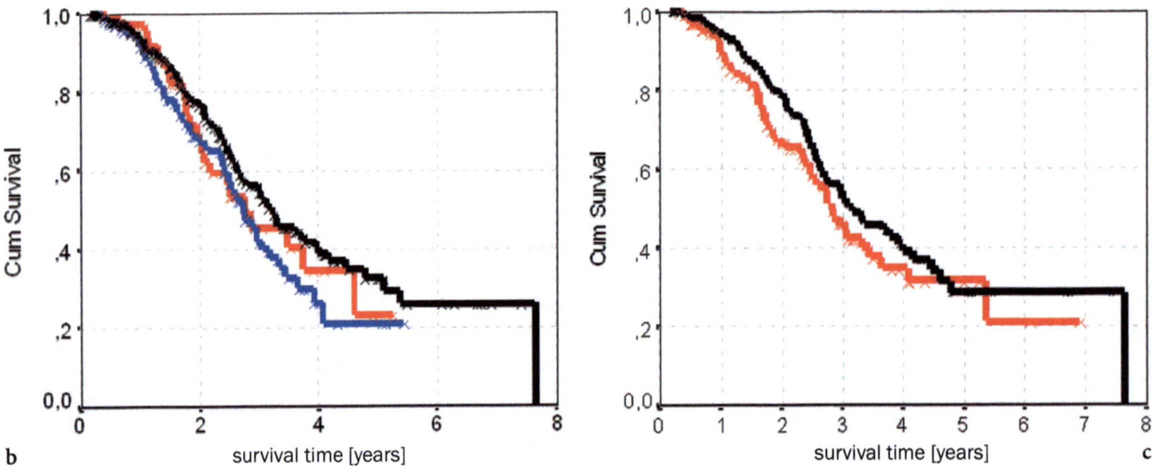

b c

Fig. 3.6.6. a Survival data of all patients ($n=512$) treated with LITT for colorectal liver metastases ($n=1{,}556$). **b** Comparison of survival in patients with respect to the number of initial metastases (*black line*=group 1=1 or 2 metastases, *blue line*=3 or 4 metastases, *red line*=group 2=more than 4 metastases). **c** Comparison of survival in patients with respect to the initial staging of lymph nodes (*black line*=group 1=N0 and N1 stage, *red line*=group 2=N2 or N3 stage)

3.6.6 Liver Metastases of Breast Cancer

Three hundred and thirty-four consecutive patients (average age 54.7 years: range, 23–82 years) were treated. Seven hundred and eighty-one metastases were ablated. Of the patients, 6.6% had recurrent metastases after surgery, 46.4% had metastases in both liver lobes, 28% refused surgical resection, 1.8% had contraindications for surgery, and 17.2% had metastases at a difficult location for surgery. Survival rates were calculated using the Kaplan–Meier method. The influence of prognostic factors such as the number of treated metastases, the presence of bone metastases and the hormone receptor status were evaluated.

The mean survival was 4.3 years (95% CI 3.7–4.8 years; median 3.9 years; 1-year survival rate 85%, 2-year survival rate 66%, 3-year survival rate 50%, and 5-year survival rate 28%) after the first LITT treatment and 4.9 years (95% CI 4.3–5.4 years; 1-year survival rate 95%, 2-year survival rate 78%, 3-year survival rate 60%, and 5-year survival rate 39%) after the diagnosis of metastases, which were treated with LITT. There was a trend that patients with three or more initial metastases had inferior survival compared to patients with one to two initial metastases. However, this was not statistically significant (Tarone Ware $p=0.3$, log rank $p=0.5$, Breslow test $p=0.2$). The presence of bone metastases was not a prognostic factor either. The only proven prognostic factor was the hormone receptor status. Patients with at least one positive hormone receptor status had superior survival versus patients with a negative hormone receptor status (mean survival: 5.5 years; 95% CI 4.8–6.3 versus 3.7 years; 95% CI 2.8–4.6).

MR-guided LITT is a safe and effective treatment option for selected patients with breast cancer liver metastases.

3.6.7 Liver Metastases of Gastric Cancer

A total of 27 patients (22 male, 5 female, average age 61 years, range 36–86 years) were treated. The total number of treated metastases was 58, ablated in 47 treatment sessions. The mean number of treated lesions per patient was 2.1 (range 1–5). Survival rates were calculated using the Kaplan–Meier method. Of the patients 7.4% had recurrent metastases after surgery, 48.1% had metastases in both liver lobes, 25.9% refused surgical resection, 7.4% had general contraindications for surgery, and 11.1% had metastases at a difficult location for surgery; 38.9% of the lesions were 2 cm or less in diameter, 35.2% were between 2 and 3 cm, 14.8% were between 3 and 4 cm, and 11.1% were larger than 4 cm in maximum diameter.

All ablations were performed on an outpatient basis using local anesthesia. The mean survival was 2.3 years (95% CI 1.5–3.1 years, median survival 1.2 years, 1-year survival rate 60%, 2-year survival rate 36%, 5-year survival rate 22%) after the first LITT treatment and 2.7 years after the diagnosis of the metastases, which were treated with LITT (95%CI 1.9–3.5 years; median survival 1.4 years; 1-year survival rate 81%, 2-year survival rate 41%, 5-year survival rate 22%). The mean size of the lesion was 2.4 cm (range, 0.7–7 cm; mean volume 13.9 ml), the mean size of the coagulative necrosis was 4.9 cm (range, 2.0–8.0 cm; mean volume 50 ml). The mean applied energy was 85.1 kJ (median 56.9 kJ; range, 3.1–258.8 kJ).

Local ablation of liver metastases of gastric cancer using MR-guided LITT is a safe, minimally invasive treatment option in well selected cases.

3.6.8 Liver Metastases of Pancreatic Cancer

In total, 26 patients (16 males, 10 females; average age 57 years; range, 40–76 years) were treated. The total number of treated metastases was 69, ablated in 50 treatment sessions. The mean number of treated lesions per patient was 2.7. Survival rates were calculated using the Kaplan–Meier method. We included patients with fewer than five metastases with a maximum diameter of 5 cm. Of the patients 19.2% had recurrent metastases after surgery, 57.7% had metastases in both liver lobes, 7.7% refused surgical resection, and 15.4% had metastases at difficult location for surgery. Six patients had only one metastasis, nine patients had two metastases, seven patients had three metastases, two patients had four metastases and two patients had more than four metastases initially. Sixteen patients had synchronous metastases (within 6 months after the diagnosis of the primary tumor) and ten patients had metachronous metastases.

All ablations were performed on an outpatient basis using local anesthesia. The mean survival was 1.8 years (95% CI 1.1–2.5 years, median survival 0.9 years, 1-year survival rate 46%, 2-year survival rate 38%, 3-year survival rate 14%, 5-year survival rate 9%) after the diagnosis of the metastases, which were treated with LITT. Starting the calculation with the first LITT treatment the mean survival was 1.4 years (95% CI 0.8–2.2 years, median survival 0.8 years, 1-year survival 42%, 2-year survival 21%, 3-year survival 10%). Twenty of twenty-six patients had Whipple's operation before. These patients have a high risk of developing a liver abscess, which was observed in 12.5% of the patients compared to 0.6% in the total LITT patient group.

Local ablation of liver metastases of pancreatic cancer using MR-guided LITT is only indicated in highly selected cases due to the limited survival of the patients and the high risk of developing a liver abscess if the patient had Whipple's operation before.

Liver metastases are the most common tumors in Europe and the United States and are 20 times more common than in Africa, Japan and Eastern countries. The liver is the most common site of metastasis. Colorectal cancer is the third leading cause of death in Western communities, outnumbered only by lung and breast cancer. At the time of death, approximately two-thirds of patients with colorectal cancer have liver metastases. Survival in metastatic liver disease depends on the extent of liver involvement and the presence of metastatic tumors. In several studies, liver metastases of colon carcinoma which were confined to one lobe and involved an area of less than 25% of the liver caused death in 6 months when untreated (Stangl et al. 1994). When 25–75% of the liver was involved, survival was 5.5 months; and when more than 75% of the liver was involved, death occurred in 3.4 months.

Therapeutic alternatives in the treatment of liver metastases include surgery, local ablation such as LITT, RF ablation (Christophi et al. 2004; Gillams 2005; Lubienski 2005; Zhou et al. 2005), cryotherapy (Finlay et al. 2000; Charnley et al. 1989; Seifert et al. 2000; Shapiro et al. 1998; Hewitt et al. 1998), microwave ablation (Wang et al. 2000) and ethanol injection (Bartolozzi and Lencioni 1996; Sato et al. 2000; Shiina et al. 1990; Livraghi et al. 1993) or oncological strategies such as systemic or locoregional chemotherapy (Ardalan et al. 1991; Douillard et al. 2000a, b; Kemeny 1995; Kemeny and Atiq 1999; Kemeny et al. 1999; Lorenz et al. 2000). As a high number of tumors grow in damaged liver parenchyma with reduced hepatic function, it is important for all methods which damage tumor cells to preserve functional reserve capacity, delaying terminal organ failure for as long as possible.

Therefore, many local ablation techniques were developed in order to improve the survival of patients (Dodd et al. 2000). Nowadays, the most common technique is RF ablation. Radiofrequency waves (RF waves) have been used since the 1960s for treating intracerebral tumors, controlled stereotaxically. For some years RF treatment has also been used for treating soft tissue, focusing on the treatment of malignant liver tumors. As in LITT a coagulation necrosis is caused by a local temperature increase. Wavelengths of between 300 and 500 kHz are introduced into the tissue through mono- or bipolar antennae systems resulting in the target area heating up to 90°C, caused by high tissue resistance. In previous studies monopolar systems were almost exclusively used. The necessity for an external second electrode on patients makes an uncontrolled energy flow outside the required target zone possible in theory, as burns cannot be safely ruled out. Bipolar application systems integrate both poles in one applicator. Cooling the tip of the applicator in RF treatment was introduced to increase the size of the induced necrosis up to 5 cm in diameter.

In 1996 Rossi et al. treated 11 patients with 13 metastases using mono- and bipolar systems and the multiapplicator technique. Despite the fact that the tumors were under 3.5 cm in size, 1 year after the operation only one patient was tumor-free and the relapse rate was around 55%. The findings for the 39 patients with HCC were better, as a relapse rate of only 10% and mean survival times of 44 months have been calculated (Rossi et al. 1996).

In 1997 Solbiati et al. (1997) published a study of 29 patients with 44 liver metastases (size 1.3–5 cm) of colorectal, gastric, breast, and pancreatic carcinomas. Among them were 20 patients with solitary lesions. The operation took place using cooled systems, and a complete tumor ablation was achieved in 91% of cases. At the 3- and 6-month follow-up 66% of the treated lesions were still inactive. A survival rate of 100%, 94% and 86% after 6, 12, and 18 months was documented. Livraghi tried an approach using conventional systems and simultaneous irrigation with NaCl solution in 14 patients with 24 liver metastases (1.2–4.5 cm in size) but only 52% of the lesions were inactive after 6 months (Livraghi et al. 1997).

In 1999 Livraghi et al. presented a direct comparison of RF therapy (42 patients with 52 lesions) with percutaneous alcohol injection – PAI (44 patients with 60 tumors) – in treating HCC. This was the first direct comparison of these two different treatment techniques in similarly structured patient populations. Eighty percent of tumors were completely removed using PAI and 90% using RF (no statistical significance). The main advantage of the RF therapy proved to be the smaller number of treatment sessions (1.2 versus 4.8). On the other hand, a higher complication rate was documented (2% serious, 8% minor complications versus 0% for PAI) (Livraghi et al. 1999). Side-effects with regard to punctures are relevant, such as pneumothorax or hemothorax (2%), injury of the bile ducts and the gall bladder, intraperitoneal bleeding (8%) and also pleural effusions. Depending on the procedure some cases had to be upgraded from local to general anesthesia due to severe pain during the energy application.

Our data in a large population with liver metastases of different primary tumors, mainly colorectal carcinomas, show a very high local control rate (over 97% in 3- and 6-month control studies) and a very low local recurrence rate. LITT treatment can be performed easily under local anesthesia on an outpatient basis in metastases up to 5 cm in diameter with a 1-cm safety margin, which is very important for a low recurrence rate. Multiple applications can be performed simultaneously.

The wide range of the values of the applied energy to the metastases indicates that there is a high variance in heat distribution. Sometimes a couple of minutes are enough to treat a metastasis with a reliable safety margin and sometimes application times of 30 min and more are necessary to get the same necrosis in another metastasis of the same size. Therefore, reliable nearly online monitoring of treatment is absolutely necessary in order to avoid over- or undertreatment of the metastases. Due to the fact that laser ablation is fully compatible with MRI, which is the most reliable method for thermometry, MRI is very well suited for monitoring thermal ablation such as LITT.

The survival rates achieved, which represent the most relevant success criterion for a treatment, are comparable in patients with metastases of colorectal carcinoma or breast carcinoma to those in surgically resected patients. It must be considered, however, that a surgical resection was not or was no longer an option for most of the patients being treated due to metastatic relapse after surgical resection or a bilobular pattern of infestation. In spite of this it was possible to achieve survival rates comparable to surgical resection among these patients, who are actually in a group with a worse prognosis. Compared with the extensively published historic survival data after surgical metastatic resection, MR-guided LITT offers a very good further treatment option. Due to the survival data and local tumor control rates achieved so far, in our opinion randomized studies comparing LITT with chemotherapy solely in the case of patients who fulfill the inclusion criteria for LITT are no longer ethically tenable.

In the modern oncological concept of treatment the internationally defined terms of "clinical benefit", "performance status" and "quality of life" are of the utmost importance. This applies predominantly to patients suffering from local and generally advanced tumors that are no longer curative. Above all, however, intensive systemic or regional chemotherapy with marked toxic side-effects severely affects the quality of life in the majority of cases. Looking at it from this background all the more attention must be paid to the treatment concepts described here, because minimally invasive techniques are applied which adversely affect patients less and shorter-term (Vogl et al. 2001a-c, 2002a,b).

Consequently, the prerequisites are given to integrate these new procedures into oncological treatment programs which have been carried out up to now. LITT, which has been used for the past 8 years in the clinical routine, can play a great part in modern oncological treatment concepts.

References

Adson MA, Heerden van J, Adson MH, Wagner JS, Ilstrup DM (1984) Resection of hepatic metastases from colorectal cancer. Arch Surg 119:647–651

Amin Z, Lees WR, Bown SG (1993) Hepatocellular carcinoma: CT appearance after percutaneous ethanol ablation therapy. Radiology 188:882–883

Ardalan B, Sridhar KS, Benedetto P et al (1991) A phase I, II study of high-dose 5-fluorouracil and high-dose leucovorin with low-dose phosphonacetyl-L-aspartic acid in patients with advanced malignancies. Cancer 68:1242–1246

Bartolozzi C, Lencioni R (1996) Ethanol injection for the treatment of hepatic tumors. Eur Radiol 6:682–696

Bismuth H, Chiche L, Adam R, Castaing D, Diamond T, Dennison A (1993) Liver resection versus transplantation for hepatocellular carcinoma in cirrhotic patients. Ann Surg 218:145–151

Charnley RM, Doran J, Morris DL (1989) Cryotherapy for liver metastases: a new approach. Br J Surg 76:1040

Christophi C, Nikfarjam M, Malcontenti-Wilson C, Muralidharan V (2004) Long-term survival of patients with unresectable colorectal liver metastases treated by percutaneous interstitial laser thermotherapy. World J Surg 28:987–994

De Cobelli F, Castrucci M, Sironi S et al (1994) Role of magnetic resonance in the follow-up of hepatocarcinoma treated with percutaneous ethanol injection (PEI) or transarterial chemoembolization (TACE). Radiol Med Torino 88:806–817

Dodd GD 3rd, Soulen MC, Kane RA et al (2000) Minimally invasive treatment of malignant hepatic tumors: at the threshold of a major breakthrough. Radiographics 20:9–27

Douillard JY, Cunningham D, Roth AD et al (2000a) Irinotecan combined with fluorouracil compared with fluorouracil alone as first-line treatment for metastatic colorectal cancer: a multicentre randomised trial [published erratum appears in Lancet 2000 Apr 15;355(9212):1372]. Lancet 355:1041–1047

Douillard JY, Bennouna J, Vavasseur F et al (2000b) Phase I trial of interleukin-2 and high-dose arginine butyrate in metastatic colorectal cancer. Cancer Immunol Immunother 49:56–61

Finlay IG, Seifert JK, Stewart GJ, Morris DL (2000) Resection with cryotherapy of colorectal hepatic metastases has the same survival as hepatic resection alone. Eur J Surg Oncol 26:199–202

Fong Y, Blumgart LH (1998) Hepatic colorectal metastasis: current status of surgical therapy. Oncology (Huntingt) 12:1489–1498; discussion 1498–1500, 1503

Gillams AR (2005) The use of radiofrequency in cancer. Br J Cancer 92:1825–1829

Harrison LE, Brennan MF, Newman E et al (1997) Hepatic resection for noncolorectal, nonneuroendocrine metastases: a fifteen-year experience with ninety-six patients. Surgery 121:625–632

Hewitt PM, Dwerryhouse SJ, Zhao J, Morris DL (1998) Multiple bilobar liver metastases: cryotherapy for residual lesions after liver resection. J Surg Oncol 67:112–116

Hughes KS, Simon R, Songhorabodi S et al (1988) Resection of the liver for colorectal carcinoma metastases: a multi-institutional study of indications for resections. Surgery 103:278–288

Jenkins LT, Millikan KW, Bines SD, Staren ED, Doolas A (1997) Hepatic resection for metastatic colorectal cancer. Am J Surg 63:605–610

Kawai S, Tani M, Okumura J, Ogawa M et al (1997) Prospective and randomized clinical trial of lipiodol-transcatheter arterial chemoembolization for treatment of hepatocellular carcinoma: a comparison of epirubicin and doxorubicin (second cooperative study). Semin Oncol 24:38–45

Kemeny NE (1995) Regional chemotherapy of colorectal cancer. Eur J Cancer 31A:1271–1276
Kemeny NE, Atiq OT (1999) Non-surgical treatment for liver metastases. Baillieres Best Pract Res Clin Gastroenterol 13:593–610
Kemeny N, Huang Y, Cohen AM et al (1999) Hepatic arterial infusion of chemotherapy after resection of hepatic metastases from colorectal cancer. N Engl J Med 341:2039–2048
Livraghi T, Lazzaroni S, Vettori C (1990) Percutaneous ethanol injection of small hepatocellular carcinoma. Rays 15:405–410
Livraghi T, Lazzaroni S, Pellicano S, Ravasi S, Torzilli G, Vettori C (1993) Percutaneous ethanol injection of hepatic tumors: single-session therapy with general anesthesia. AJR Am J Roentgenol 161:1065–1069
Livraghi T, Goldberg SN, Monti F et al (1997) Saline-enhanced radiofrequency tissue ablation in the treatment of liver metastases. Radiology 202:205–210
Livraghi T, Goldberg SN, Lazzaroni S, Meloni F, Solbiati L, Gazelle GS (1999) Small hepatocellular carcinoma: treatment with radiofrequency ablation versus ethanol injection. Radiology 210:655–661
Lorenz M, Waldeyer M (1997) The resection of the liver metastases of primary colorectal tumors. The development of a scoring system to determine the individual prognosis based on an assessment of 1,568 patients. Strahlenther Onkol 173:118–119
Lorenz M, Waldeyer M, Muller HH (1996) Comparison of lipiodol-assisted chemoembolization versus only conservative therapy in patients with nonresectable hepatocellular carcinomas. Z Gastroenterol 34:205–206
Lorenz M, Heinrich S, Staib-Sebler E et al (2000) Relevance of locoregional chemotherapy in patients with liver metastases from colorectal primaries. Swiss Surg 6:11–22
Lubienski A (2005) Radiofrequency ablation in metastatic disease. Recent Result Cancer Res 165:268–276
Maksan SM, Lehnert T, Bastert G, Herfarth C (2000) Curative liver resection for metastatic breast cancer. Eur J Surg Oncol 26:209–212
Mariette D, Fagniez PL (1992) Hepatic metastasis of noncolorectal cancers. Results of surgical treatment. Rev Prat 42:1271–1275
Petrelli NJ, Nambisan RN, Herrera L, Mittelman A (1985) Hepatic resection for isolated metastasis from colorectal carcinoma. Am J Surg 149:205–208
Ramsey WH, Wu GY (1995) Hepatocellular carcinoma: update on diagnosis and treatment. Dig Dis 13:81–91
Rossi S, Di Stasi M, Buscarini E et al (1996) Percutaneous RF interstitial thermal ablation in the treatment of hepatic cancer. AJR Am J Roentgenol 167:759–768
Sato M, Watanabe Y, Tokui K, Kawachi K, Sugata S, Ikezoe J (2000) CT-guided treatment of ultrasonically invisible hepatocellular carcinoma. Am J Gastroenterol 95:2102–2106
Scheele J, Altendorf-Hofmann A, Stangl R, Schmidt K (1996) Surgical resection of colorectal liver metastases: gold standard for solitary and completely resectable lesions. Swiss Surg Suppl 4:4–17
Seifert JK, Achenbach T, Heintz A, Bottger TC, Junginger T (2000) Cryotherapy for liver metastases. Int J Colorectal Dis 15:161–166
Shapiro RS, Shafir M, Sung M, Warner R, Glajchen N (1998) Cryotherapy of metastatic carcinoid tumors. Abdom Imaging 23:314–317
Shiina S, Tagawa K, Unama T et al (1990) Percutaneous ethanol injection therapy of hepatocellular carcinoma: analysis of 77 patients. AJR Am J Roentgenol 155:1221–1226
Sironi S, Livraghi T, DelMaschio A (1991) Small hepatocellular carcinoma treated with percutaneous ethanol injection: MR imaging findings. Radiology 180:333–336
Solbiati L, Goldberg SN, Ierace T et al (1997) Hepatic metastases: percutaneous radiofrequency ablation with cooled-tip electrodes. Radiology 205:367–373
Stangl R, Altendorf Hofmann A, Charnley RM, Scheele J (1994) Factors influencing the natural history of colorectal liver metastases. Lancet 343:1405–1410
Vogl TJ, Mack M, Straub R, Zangos S et al (2001a) Perkutane Laserablation von malignen Lebertumoren. Zentralbl Chir 126:571–575
Vogl TJ, Eichler K, Straub R, Engelmann K et al (2001b) Laser-induced thermotherapy of malignant liver tumors: general principals, equipments, procedure – side effects, complications, and results. Eur J Ultrasound 13:117–127
Vogl TJ, Mack M, Straub R, Eichler K et al (2001c) MR-guided laser-induced thermotherapy (LITT) of malignant liver and soft tissue tumors. Med Laser Appl 16:91–102
Vogl TJ, Mack M, Straub R, Eichler K, Roggan A et al (2002a) Magnetic resonance (MR)-guided percutaneous laser-induced interstitial thermotherapy (LITT) for malignant liver tumors. Sur Technol Int 10:89–98
Vogl TJ, Engelmann K, Mack M, Straub R et al (2002b) CT-guided intratumoral administration of cisplatin/epinephrine gel for treatment of malignant liver tumors. Br J Cancer 12(86):524–529
Vogl TJ, Eichler K, Mack M, Straub R (2002c) MR-guided laser-induced thermotherapy of malignant liver tumors. Experience with complications in 899 patients. Radiology 225:367–377
Wang SS, VanderBrink BA, Regan J et al (2000) Microwave radiometric thermometry and its potential applicability to ablative therapy. J Interv Card Electrophysiol 4:295–300
Weiss L (1994) Inefficiency of metastasis from colorectal carcinomas. Kluwer, Boston, Mass.
Weiss L, Grundmann E, Torhorst J et al (1986) Haematogenous metastatic patterns in colonic carcinoma: an analysis of 1,541 necropsies. J Pathol 150:195–203
Yoon SS, Tanabe KK (1999) Surgical treatment and other regional treatments for colorectal cancer liver metastases. Oncologist 4:197–208
Zhou X, Strobel D, Haensler J, Bernatik T (2005) Hepatic transit time: indicator of the therapeutic response to radiofrequency ablation of liver tumours. Br J Radiol 78:433–436

Liver

Benign Tumors

3.7 Symptomatic Hemangiomas, Adenomas

Andreas Lubienski, Martin Simon, and Thomas K. Helmberger

CONTENTS

3.7.1 Introduction

Little has been published on the interventional treatment of benign liver tumors such as hemangiomas and adenomas. Hemangiomas have been reported to be present in as many as 7% of necropsies with women being affected predominantly (4:1 to 6:1) (Reddy et al. 2001). Incidental presentation is usually in the third or fourth decades. The majority of liver hemangiomas tend to be small with diameters less than 4 cm with no clinical symptoms. They are frequently discovered incidentally on routine ultrasound or computed tomography (CT). About 20% of hemangiomas are larger than 4 cm and 10%–29% are multiple. The latter are more likely to cause clinical symptoms with upper abdominal pain being the most common (Tait et al. 1992). Hemangiomas occasionally rupture spontaneously, resulting in hemoperitoneum or hemobilia. In children, Kasabach-Merritt syndrome with a large hemangioma combined with thrombocytopenia is a rare entity (Scribano et al. 1996). The therapeutic management of hemangiomas is still controversial. The vast majority of hemangiomas can safely be left untreated. Whereas surgical management in an acute or emergent situation seems mandatory, the most appropriate treatment of hemangiomas with just a few symptoms is debatable (Farges et al. 1995). The traditional approach to the treatment of a hemangioma has been surgical resection for the relief of disabling symptoms, disorders of coagulopathy and hemoperitoneum. The decision to operate depends on the balance of the operative risks and the severity of symptoms and complications associated with the hemangiomas. Conservative management can be performed safely, irrespective of the size of the hemangioma. Surgery is only advised in the case of severe complaints related to the tumor. To minimize the risks of surgical resection in basically healthy patients, interventional procedures seem to be attractive options (Zagoria et al. 2004).

In contrast adenomas are rare benign hepatic tumors that occur primarily in women, and that may be identified after life-threatening hemorrhage, or as an incidental radiology finding. Complete resection of the adenoma is the standard therapy. The standards for treatment of hepatic adenoma remain controversial. Usually adenoma is an indication for resection, due to its tendency to bleed and to degenerate (Foster and Berman 1994). The management of hepatic adenoma should be individualized based on their size and mode of presentation. Patients with tumors less than 3 cm and normal alpha-fetoprotein can be safely observed and followed by radiologic imaging. Tumors >3 cm are considered for resection by many hepatic surgeons due to the risk of malignancy (spontaneous hepatocellular carcinoma, HCC). Interventional procedures may be new options in the treatment of hepatic adenomas.

A. Lubienski, MD; M. Simon, MD
Institut für Radiologie, der Universität Lübeck, Ratzeburger Allee 160, 23538 Lübeck, Germany
T. K. Helmberger, MD
Professor, Department of Diagnostic and Interventional Radiology and Nuclear Medicine, Klinikum Bogenhausen, Engelschalkinger Strasse 77, 81925 Munich, Germany

3.7.2 Embolization

3.7.2.1 Hemangioma

Due to its favorable success in the treatment of non-resectable HCC, transarterial embolotherapy has been tried in several studies for symptomatic cavernous hemangiomas (Srivastava et al. 2001; Zeng et al. 2004). However, the hemodynamics of hemangiomas are different from those of HCC and the advantages of embolization have not been fully realized in the treatment of hemangiomas (Cui et al. 2003). But still the use of embolization provides a safe and effective treatment of patient's symptoms while avoiding operative intervention, extended hospitalization, and postoperative recuperation. This treatment modality should be considered for symptomatic hemangioma under elective conditions (Deutsch et al. 2001).

3.7.2.2 Adenoma

In contrast embolization does not play any role in the treatment of hepatic adenoma despite an acute hemorrhage due to adenoma rupture where transarterial embolization might be a therapeutic option (Terkivatan et al. 2001).

3.7.3 Radiofrequency Ablation (RFA)

3.7.3.1 Hemangioma

Because image-guided liver biopsies, even in hemangiomas, are low-risk procedures (Cui et al. 2003) and RFA has proven effective in malignant liver tumors with considerably low complication rates (Mulier et al. 2002), RFA has been tried for symptomatic cavernous hemangiomas with promising results (Cui et al. 2003; Tak et al. 2006). The mechanism of action of RFA in treating liver hemangiomas has yet to be determined, but it may involve its thrombogenic effect due to damage to the layer of the endothelial lining in the vascular structures (Cui et al. 2003).

3.7.3.2 Adenoma

In selected cases RFA can be safely used as an alternative to open surgical resection especially in cases with multiple adenomas, in order to reduce the amount of liver tissue to be resected (Fujita et al. 2006; Rocourt et al. 2006).

References

Cui Y, Zhou LY, Dong MK et al (2003) Ultrasonography guided percutaneous radiofrequency ablation for hepatic cavernous hemangioma. World J Gastroenterol 9:2132–2134

Deutsch GS, Yeh KA, Bates WB 3rd, Tannehill WB (2001) Embolization for management of hepatic hemangiomas. Am Surg 67:159–164

Farges O, Daradkeh S, Bismuth H (1995) Cavernous hemangioma of the liver: are there any indications for resection? World J Surg 19:19–24

Foster JH, Berman MM (1994) The malignant transformation of liver cell adenomas. Arch Surg 129:712–717

Fujita S, Kushihata F, Herrmann GE et al (2006) Combined hepatic resection and radiofrequency ablation for multiple hepatic adenomas. J Gastroenterol Hepatol 21:1351–1354

Mulier S, Mulier P, Ni Y, Miao Y, Dupas B, Marchal G, De Wever I, Michel L (2002) Complications of radiofrequency coagulation of liver tumours. Br J Surg 89:1206–1222

Reddy KR, Kligerman S, Levi J et al (2001) Benign and solid tumors of the liver: relationship to sex, age, size of tumors, and outcome. Am Surg 67:173–178

Rocourt DV, Shiles WE, Hammond S, Besner GE (2006) Contemporary management of benign hepatic adenoma using percutaneous radiofrequency ablation. J Pediatr Surg 41:1149–1152

Scribano E, Loria G, AscentiG et al (1996) Spontaneous hemoperitoneum from a giant multicystic hemangioma of the liver: a case report. Abdom Imaging 21:418–419

Srivastava DN, Gandhi D, Seith A, Pande GK, Sahni P (2001) Transcatheter arterial embolization in the treatment of symptomatic cavernous hemangiomas of the liver: a prospective study. Abdom Imaging 26:510–514

Tait N, Richardson AJ, Muguti G et al (1992) Hepatic cavernous haemangioma: a 10 year review. Aust N Z J Surg 62:521–524

Tak WY, Park SY, Jeon SW et al (2006) Ultrasonography-guided percutaneous radiofrequency ablation for treatment of a huge symptomatic hepatic cavernous hemangioma. J Clin Gastroenterol 40:167–170

Terkivatan T, de Wilt JH, de Man RA et al (2001) Indications and long-term outcome of treatment for benign hepatic tumors: a critical appraisal. Arch Surg 136:1033–1038

Zagoria RJ, Roth TJ, Levine EA, Kavanagh PV (2004) Radiofrequency ablation of a symptomatic hepatic cavernous hemangioma. AJR Am J Roentgenol 182:210–212

Zeng Q, Li Y, Chen Y et al (2004) Gigantic cavernous hemangioma of the liver treated by intra-arterial embolization with pingyangmycin-lipiodol emulsion: a multi-center study. Cardiovasc Intervent Radiol 27:481–485

Kidney – Radiofrequency Ablation (RFA)

4

Andreas H. Mahnken

CONTENTS

4.1 Introduction

Renal cancer is a large socioeconomic problem, accounting for 3% of the estimated new cancer cases in men. During 2004 the American Cancer Society reported 35,710 new cases and estimated 12,480 deaths from renal cancer (Jemal et al. 2004). Historically renal cell carcinoma (RCC) has been detected by flank pain and hematuria. The widespread availability of cross-sectional imaging techniques such as ultrasound (US) and computed tomography (CT) led to an increased detection rate of small renal tumors (Pantuck et al. 2001). Further advances in medical imaging with the introduction of multidetector row spiral CT (MDCT) and magnetic resonance (MR) imaging in clinical routine have resulted in even earlier tumor detection. About two-thirds of all RCCs are now discovered incidentally (Homma et al. 1995). However, the differentiation of small renal tumors remains a diagnostic dilemma (Zagoria and Dyer 1998).

The natural history of renal tumors varies but tumor stage and histological tumor type are relevant prognostic factors. The overall 5-year survival rate for patients with symptomatic tumors is 53% as opposed to 85% for incidentally detected lesions (Sweeney et al. 1996), indicating a survival advantage attributed to smaller tumors (Guinan et al. 1995). In addition, tumors less than 4 cm in diameter rarely metastasize.

The conventional treatment of RCC remains radical nephrectomy. The favorable prognostic indicators associated with small RCCs led to the development of less invasive operation techniques aiming at a preserved renal function. These nephron-sparing techniques were successfully established in clinical routine (Uzzo and Novick 2001), including partial nephrectomy via an open or laparoscopic approach. With 10-year tumor-free survival rates greater than 85% these results equaled nephrectomy (Fergany et al. 2000) and gave way to the development of new therapeutic concepts such as the introduction of even less invasive, energy-based treatment options. Several of these thermal ablation techniques are now used in clinical routine or are subject to clinical and experimental investigation, including radiofrequency (RF) ablation, cryotherapy, laser-induced thermotherapy (LITT), microwave ablation, and high intensity focused ultrasound. First applied in 1997 (Zlotta et al. 1997) renal RF ablation has gained most attention among these energy-based treatment modalities. This technique provides several advantages over surgical resection, including reduced morbidity and the ability to treat poor surgical candidates. Moreover, it can eventually be applied as an outpatient therapy.

4.2 Experimental Investigations

Several animal studies have assessed the immediate or short-term histopathological changes following

A. H. Mahnken, MD, MBA
Department of Diagnostic Radiology, University Hospital, RWTH Aachen University, Pauwelsstrasse 30, 52074 Aachen, Germany

RF ablation of normal porcine kidneys or of VX2 tumors implanted in rabbit kidneys. The animal's kidney demonstrated the zone of RF ablation as a sharply delineated area (Hsu et al. 2000). Immediately after the procedure increased cytoplasmic eosinophilia, loss of cell border integrity, blurring of nuclear chromatin, and interstitial hemorrhage are visible on microscopy. Typical coagulative necrosis develops by day 3. Inflammatory and fibroblastic changes separate ablated kidney from the adjacent healthy renal parenchyma. By day 14, nuclear degeneration is complete. Necrosis without features of renal parenchyma is complete by day 30. From the center to the periphery four different zones are described from histology: complete necrosis, inflammatory infiltrate, hemorrhage, fibrosis and regeneration (Crowley et al. 2000). In rabbits the renal medulla has been more sensitive to RF ablation than the renal cortex (Polascik et al. 1999). This is discussed to be caused by an increased ion concentration in the medulla with augmentation of frictional energy and heating. The same principle forms the basis of the instillation of saline into the area of ablation to increase the size of necrosis (Lee et al. 2005).

Induction of necrosis requires a temperature above 60°C. Thus, the size of RF-induced necrosis might be limited in well perfused tissue such as the renal parenchyma due to a heat sink. This potential limitation of RF ablation is caused by the cooling effect from the blood flow. To compensate for the cooling effect, temporary renal ischemia has been evaluated in animal experiments aiming on an increase of the lesion size. Immediate post-mortem analysis after transfemoral balloon occlusion of the renal artery as well as selective embolization using particles led to a significant enlargement in lesion size in the ischemic kidney (Aschoff et al. 2001; Chang et al. 2004). Another study with laparoscopic renal hilar occlusion showed greater lesion sizes in the ischemic kidneys than the non-ischemic kidneys at 2 and 4 weeks after ablation. At 4 weeks, however, the lesion sizes were not significantly different (Corwin et al. 2001). These results demonstrate potential strategies to modify the size of necrosis by modulation of the renal perfusion. Only recently, an ex-vivo study analyzed the effect of different RF devices on the size and shape of necrosis (Häcker et al. 2005). This information may also be used to design the ideal shape of necrosis by using different RF devices, depending on tumor size, shape, and location.

4.3 Indication

A comparison with the surgical reference standard of nephrectomy is not yet possible, as there are no substantial long-term follow-up data available yet on renal RF ablation. Only a single small study reports on a more than 4-year follow-up of renal RF ablation (McDougal et al. 2005). Until more data on long-term follow-up become available, renal RF ablation remains limited to selected patients. To provide all viable treatment options to a patient and to select the right patients for RF ablation close collaboration between urologists, oncologist, and interventional radiologist is essential.

As partial nephrectomy is not without morbidity, whether it is performed via the open or the laparoscopic approach, there is a need for nephron-sparing ablative techniques, which can eradicate the tumor without the attendant morbidity of surgery. Thus, RF ablation has to be considered as a treatment option for patients with contraindications for surgery especially comorbid conditions or those who refuse open surgery. Still, there are no uniform indications for renal RF ablation (Table 4.1). Patients without comorbid conditions and with life expectancies longer than 5–10 years are often excluded from RF ablation. Many investigators limit RF ablation to patients without metastatic disease and some centers even limit treatment with curative intent to patients with greater than 1-year life expectancy (Gervais et al. 2005a). Further indications include patients with a solitary kidney, multiple RCCs, von Hippel Lindau disease or limited renal function (Fig. 4.1). A potential palliative indication is treatment refractory

Table 4.1. Indications and contraindications for renal RF ablation. Extended indications and relative contraindications are given in parentheses

Indication	Contraindication
Unfit for surgery	Sepsis
Solitary kidney	Vascular invasion
Multiple renal tumors	Coagulopathy
von Hippel Lindau disease	
	(Life expectancy < 1 y or > 10 ys)
(Refractory hematuria)	(Severe debilitation)
(Tumor debulking)	(Central tumor location)
(Extrarenal tumor manifestation)	

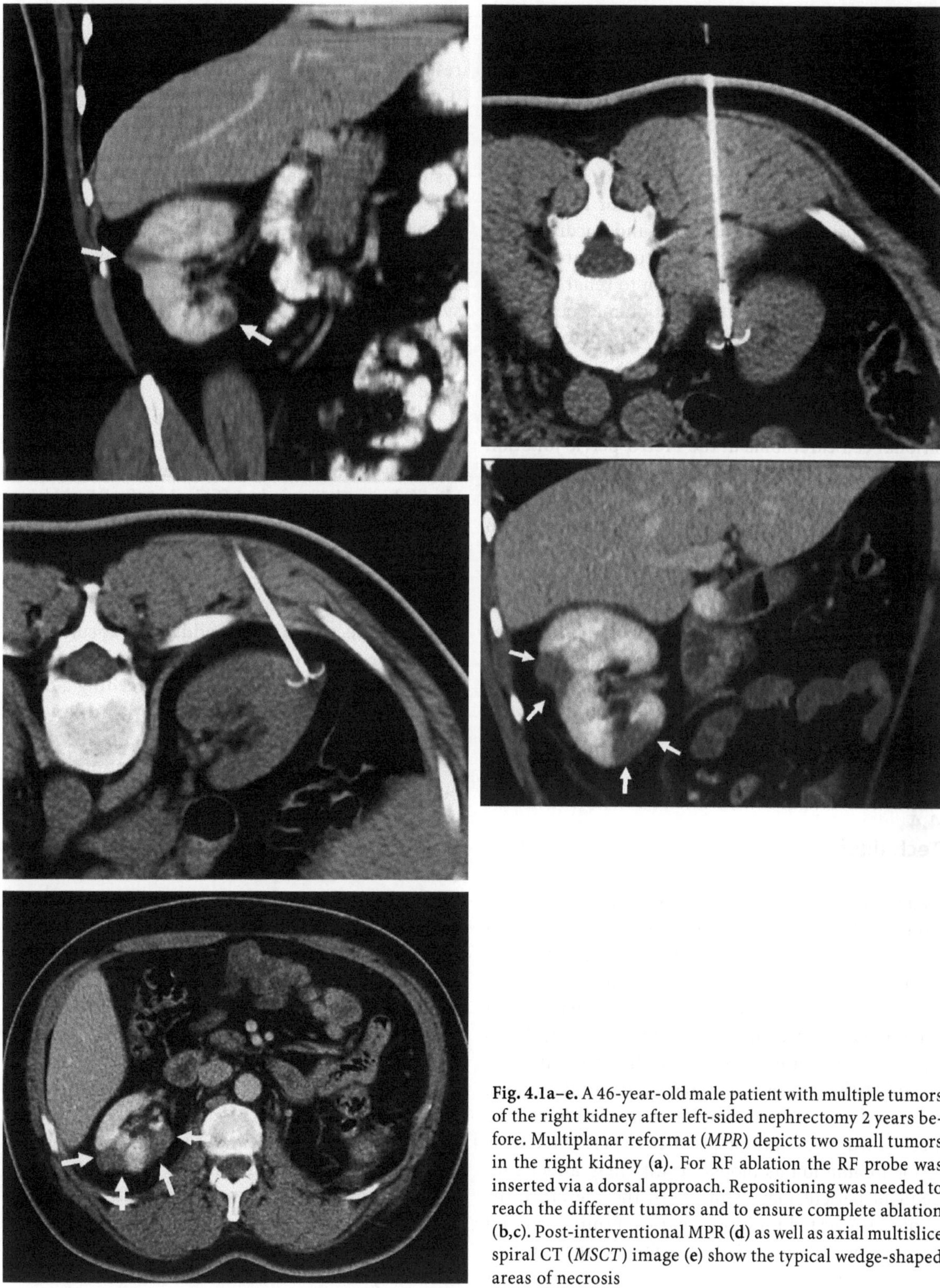

Fig. 4.1a–e. A 46-year-old male patient with multiple tumors of the right kidney after left-sided nephrectomy 2 years before. Multiplanar reformat (*MPR*) depicts two small tumors in the right kidney (**a**). For RF ablation the RF probe was inserted via a dorsal approach. Repositioning was needed to reach the different tumors and to ensure complete ablation (**b**,**c**). Post-interventional MPR (**d**) as well as axial multislice spiral CT (*MSCT*) image (**e**) show the typical wedge-shaped areas of necrosis

hematuria (Neeman et al. 2005). A rare indication is tumor debulking in conjunction with immunotherapy in patients with advanced stage of disease and tumor recurrence in the surgical bed after nephrectomy. Patients without a safe path for percutaneous treatment are excluded from image-guided RF ablation, but might be considered eligible for intraoperative RF ablation. Contraindications for RF ablation include sepsis, severe debilitation, and uncorrectable coagulopathies. The presence of a tumor thrombus is also considered a contraindication to renal RF ablation. In selected patients RF ablation may be considered as an innovative therapy. Thus successful RF ablation has been reported of a Wilms' tumor refractory to chemotherapy in a multimorbid child with a solitary kidney (Brown et al. 2005). Even in a transitional cell carcinoma at the uretro-pelvic junction this technique has profitably been applied for tumor reduction (Schultze et al. 2003). Some reports indicate that isolated foci of metastatic disease can also be treated successfully with RF ablation (Zagoria et al. 2001; Gervais et al. 2002) including the palliative treatment of painful osseous metastases (Goetz et al. 2004). Although these are sporadic reports, they clearly indicate the future potential of RF ablation as a treatment option in advanced stages of disease.

4.4 Technique

Renal RF ablation can be performed with intravenous analgo-sedation on an outpatient basis or, at most, requires overnight inpatient observation. In some centers the procedure is performed under general anesthesia. The latter ensures optimal patient compliance and comfort. Prophylactic antibiotics are generally not used, although their use might be useful if the procedure is expected to take a long time or if several repositioning maneuvers have to be performed. It is common practice to perform biopsy prior to ablation as biopsy results may affect subsequent patient management. In the literature the timing suggested for biopsy varies. From our point of view it is recommended to perform biopsy in combination with RF ablation in order to avoid tumor seeding along the puncture tract by tract ablation after the procedure.

Open surgical exposure, laparoscopic exposure and an entirely percutaneous approach have been reported as being used to apply RF to the kidney. Animal experiments showed no difference in the results using different approaches to the kidney (Crowley et al. 2000). In order to completely destroy the tumor, heat must exceed the tumor margin into healthy renal parenchyma. Although modern RF systems generate necrosis of 1.6–5 cm (Goldberg et al. 2000), many tumors need overlapping ablations as the tumor geometry and the shape of the ablation zone do not always match perfectly. As lesion size, volume, and shape depend on the selected RF system, procedure time, and electrode configuration, detailed knowledge of the specific characteristics of the used RF system is needed to assure complete and reliable ablation.

When planning the ablation procedure, tumor location, heat sink effect, and the probe characteristics have to be considered. Modulation of the local blood flow enhances the efficiency of a RF ablation. Tumor embolization with coils or particles prior to RF ablation reduces the blood flow in the parenchyma adjacent to the embolized tissue and therefore results in better and more homogeneous heat distribution. Furthermore, embolization adds a therapeutic effect on its own. As a consequence, devascularization of hypervascularized renal tumors exceeding a diameter of 3 cm can be recommended (Mahnken et al. 2005) (Fig. 4.2). To achieve optimal efficacy of such a combined procedure both interventions should be performed within 24 h. Moreover, large tumors need overlapping ablations to achieve a necrosis large enough to cover the entire tumor and to avoid remnants of viable tumor tissue in a treated lesion. Repositioning may involve simply pulling the RF probe to cover the length of the tumor parallel to the RF probe, or it may require withdrawal from the lesion and reinsertion at a different angle.

While a large area of necrosis is desirable to completely include the treated lesion, thermal damaging of the calices and renal pelvis has to be avoided in any case. Therefore, peripherally located tumors with exophytic growth are best suited for RF ablation, while centrally located tumors are considered a relative contraindication for RF ablation (Fig. 4.3). However, in selected cases even centrally located renal tumors may be ablated successfully. In these tumors the heat sink effect is particularly intense due to adjacent vessels in the renal hilum. Thus, the risk of incomplete coagulation necrosis increases, and the intensity of the heat sink effect has to be considered when planning the procedure (Gervais et al. 2003). To avoid damage to neighboring struc-

Fig. 4.2a–e. A 73-year-old male patient with renal cell carcinoma, diabetes mellitus and cardiovascular comorbidity. Multiplanar reformat (*MPR*) in the coronal plane from a pre-interventional multislice spiral CT depicts an eccentric 3.6-cm tumor of the right kidney (*arrows*) (**a**). The patient was considered to be at high risk for surgery. Because of the size of the hypervascularized tumor, a tumor embolization was performed prior to RF ablation (**b,c**). An umbrella-shaped RF probe was introduced percutaneously via a lateral approach (**d**). Four months after RFA the axial CT image shows no contrast enhancement in the tumor area (*arrows*), corresponding to complete tumor necrosis (**e**). A sufficient safety margin without contrast enhancement is visible

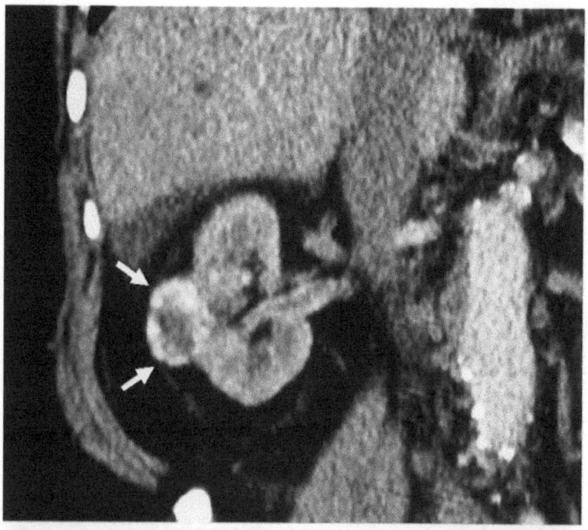

a

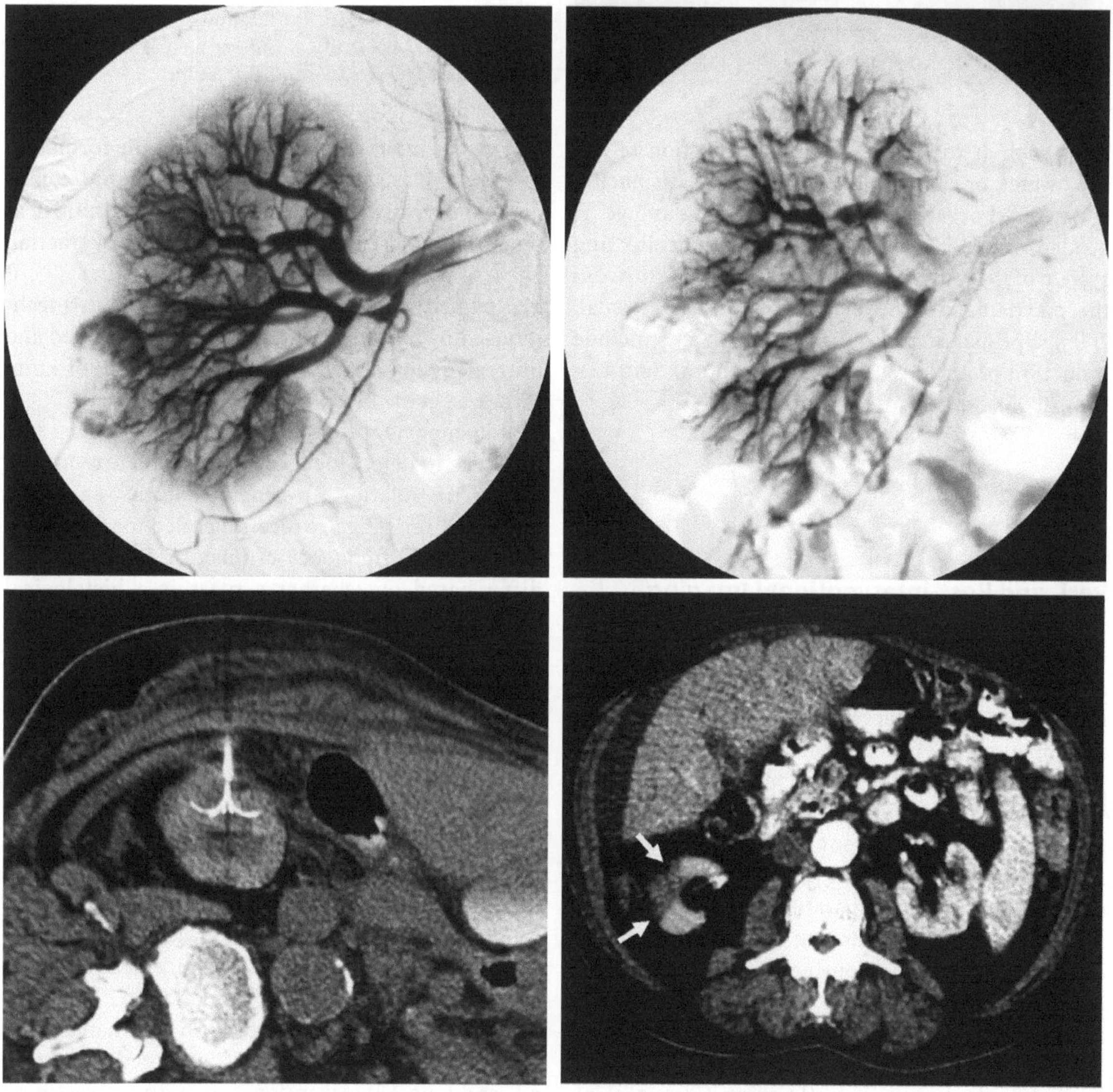

b c d e

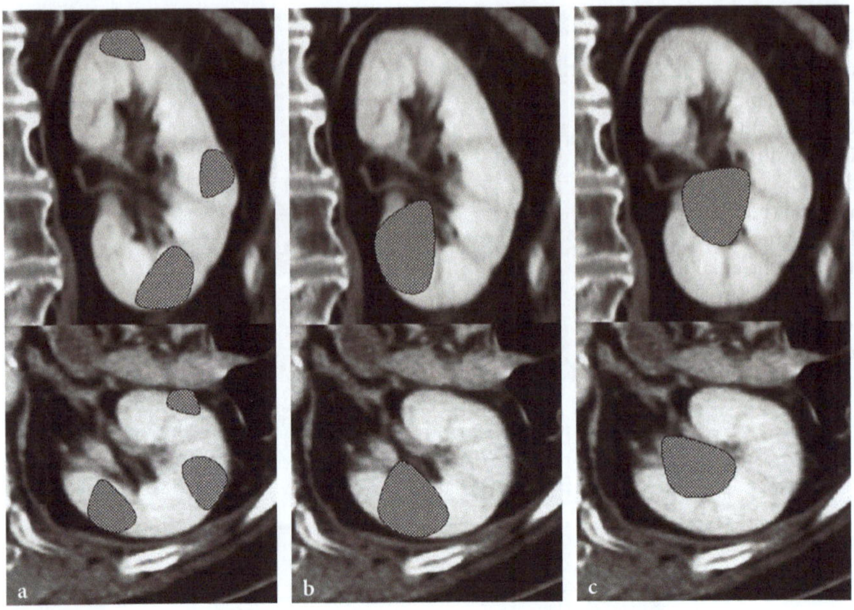

Fig. 4.3a–c. Tumor locations suited or not suited for percutaneous RF ablation. Exophytic and cortical tumors (**a**) are best suited for renal RF ablation. Parenchymal tumor location with contact to the renal hilum (**b**) might be considered for RF ablation, whereas central tumor location (**c**) is typically considered a contraindication for RF ablation

tures such as the colon, pararenal injection of air, CO_2, water, or saline might be useful for displacing endangered organs sensitive to thermal damage. If needed, infusion of cold saline into the collecting system of the kidney may also be considered to avoid thermal damage of the renal pelvis (Margulis et al. 2005). Optimal access to the tumor can also include induction of an iatrogenic pneumothorax (Ahrar et al. 2005).

4.5 Peri- and Post-interventional Imaging

Unlike open or laparoscopic surgery, thermal therapy allows no direct visualization of the critical structures during the intervention. Consequently, optimal imaging (US, CT or MR imaging) is mandatory. While placement of the RF probes is possible under US, CT, and MR guidance, none of these modalities permits real-time monitoring of the ablation results. Only MR-temperature mapping holds the potential for online temperature mapping and thus for instantaneous monitoring of the intervention's success. But, the technology needed for temperature mapping during RF ablation is not commercially available yet, although the basic principle of this technique even during application of RF pulses has been described previously (Lepetit-Coiffe et al. 2002). The use of US during and immediately following the intervention is limited by the formation of gas bubbles. As successfully treated and consequently necrotic tissue is not perfused, administration of contrast material before probe retraction helps to estimate the ablation result during CT- or MR-guided RF ablation. For MR imaging this technique allows for differentiation between treated and untreated renal parenchyma within a range of 2 mm (Merkle et al. 1999).

It is important to follow a stringent imaging surveillance to detect local or systemic recurrence following RF ablation. In general contrast-enhanced CT or MR imaging are recommended for follow-up. The need and frequency of imaging follow-up may differ based on whether a mass is a histological proven RCC or a benign tumor such as oncocytoma or angiomyolipoma (Tuncali et al. 2004). Typical imaging findings in successfully treated renal tumors include a wedge-shaped defect with a lack of contrast enhancement, shrinkage and occasional retraction from normal parenchyma by fat infiltration (Matsumoto et al. 2004). On MR imaging successfully treated lesions typically appear hypointense surrounded by a bright rim on T_2-weighted images, while these lesion are hyperintense on T_1-weighted images (Fig. 4.4). After administration of contrast material a thin rim enhancement might be seen (Merkle et al. 2005). Therefore, CT and MR imaging should be performed with unenhanced and enhanced imaging studies. It is agreed upon that an early post-interventional imaging assessment is needed to exclude residual tumor as this can be

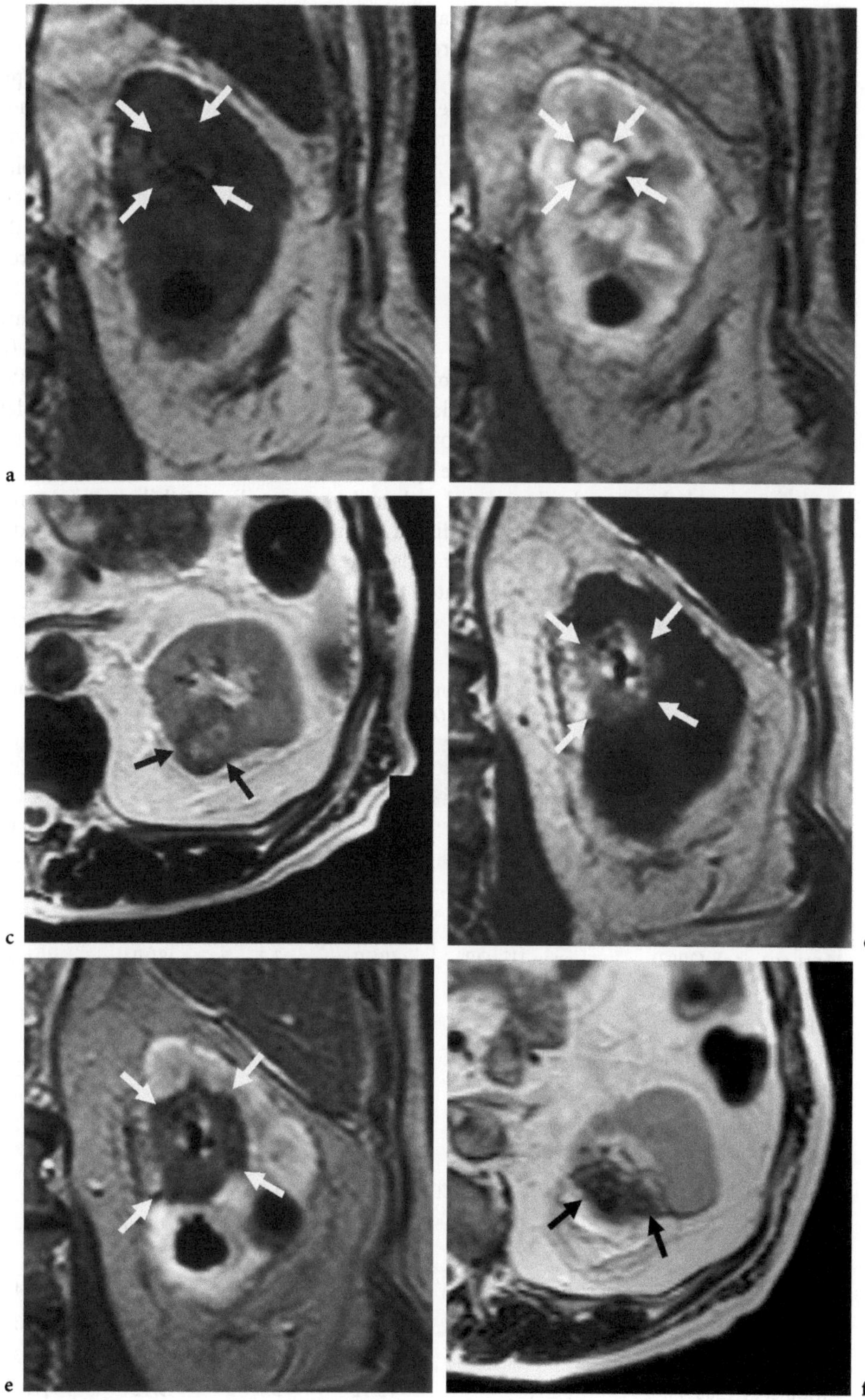

Fig. 4.4a–f. T_1-weighted pre-interventional MR images in this 72-year-old male patient with RCC show an isointense tumor on pre-contrast images (**a**) with marked contrast enhancement after administration contrast material (**b**). On T_2-weighted images the lesion appears inhomogeneous with hypodense areas (**c**). After RF ablation the tumor presents hyperintense on unenhanced T_1-weighted images (**d**) without contrast enhancement on post-contrast images (**e**). On T_2-weighted images the lesion appears hypointense with a bright rim (**f**). In addition, post-interventional MR imaging depicts central susceptibility artifacts, caused by metal abrasion from the RF probe

treated successfully by repeated percutaneous RF ablation. If no viable tumor is demonstrated, subsequent scans are generally performed at 3 months, 6 months and every 1 year. However, there is no uniform post-interventional imaging standard so far.

4.6 Results

The first case of percutaneous RF ablation prior to radical open nephrectomy of an exophytic RCC was reported by Zlotta et al. in 1997 (Zlotta et al. 1997). Histopathological evaluation of the operation specimen revealed stromal edema and pyknosis. The zones of ablation were correctly predicted from the needle deployment. No viable tumor cells were demonstrated in the percutaneously treated tumor. In 1999 the first case of RF ablation as sole treatment for a renal tumor with 3 months of follow-up was reported (McGovern et al. 1999). Since then, the increasing number of reports on percutaneous renal RF ablation outlines the potential of RF ablation for minimally invasive treatment of RCC. In addition percutaneous RF ablation proved to be less costly than open or laparoscopic partial nephrectomy (Lotan and Cadeddu 2005).

The first large series was reported by Gervais et al. in 2003 with 34 patients and 42 RCC undergoing 54 percutaneous RFA treatments (Gervais et al. 2003). The tumor size ranged from 1.1 to 8.9 cm with a mean diameter of 3.2 cm. With a mean follow-up period of 13.2 months RF ablation has been proven to be effective. Most important, this study firstly identified relevant factors for success of the ablation procedure. While parenchymal and central tumors recur more frequently if the diameter exceeds 3 cm, exophytic tumors can be treated effectively, even if they are bigger than 3 cm in diameter. So far there have been many studies confirming the short-

Table 4.2. Results of renal RF ablation. (*CT* Computed tomography, *lap.* laparoscopic, *MR* magnetic resonance, *n.a.* not applicable, *perc.* percutaneous, *OP* surgical, *US* ultrasound)

Author/Year	Technique	Patients/ Tumors	Mean size (cm)	Local tumor control (n)	Follow-Up (months)
Zlotta et al. (1997)	perc. US, OP	2/3	2–5	3/3	n.a.
Walther et al. (2000)	open	4/11	2.2	10/11	n.a.
Michaels et al. (2002)	open US, OP	15/20	2.4	1/20	n.a.
Ogan et al. (2002)	perc. CT	12/13	2.4	12/13	4.9
Matlaga et al. (2002)	open US, OP	10/10	3.2	8/10	n.a.
Pavlovich et al. (2002)	perc. US, CT	21/24	2.4	24/24	2
de Baere et al. (2002)	perc. US/CT	5/5	3–4	5/5	9
Rendon et al. (2002)	lap./perc., OP	10/11	2.4	4/11	n.a.
Jacomides et al. (2003)	lap. all, 5 OP	13/17	2.0	17/17	9.8
Su et al. (2003)	perc. CT	29/35	2.2	35/35	9
Mayo-Smith et al. (2003)	perc. US/CT	32/32	2.6	31/32	9
Farrell et al. (2003)	perc., OP US/CT	20/35	1.7	35/35	9
Lewin et al. (2004)	perc. MR	10/10	2.6	10/10	23
Zagoria et al. (2004)	perc. CT	22/24	3.5	20/24	7
Veltri et al. (2004)	perc. US	13/18	2.5	16/18	14
Hwang et al. (2004)	perc. CT, lap.	17/24	2.2	23/24	13
Mahnken et al. (2005)	perc CT	14/15	3.0	15/15	13.9
Chiou et al. (2005)	perc.	12/12	3.7	9/12	n.a.
Matsumoto et al. (2005)[a]	perc. CT, lap.	91/109	2.4	109/109	n.a.
Gervais et al. (2005a)	perc. CT/US	85/100	3.2	89/100	28
Boss et al. (2005)	perc. MR	8/8	2.3	8/8	13
all/mean		**445/536**	**2.6**	**90.3%**	**11.8**

[a] Includes 15 benign tumors

term effectiveness of RF ablation in small RCCs (Table 4.2).

Some investigators raised concern regarding the efficiency of renal RF ablation with respect to complete tumor necrosis. On histology MICHAELS et al. found viable tumor in all but one specimen of the tumors included in this study (MICHAELS et al. 2002). RENDON et al. found viable residual tumor in four of five tumors undergoing partial or radical nephrectomy immediately after RF ablation and in three of five tumors undergoing nephrectomy 1 week after RF ablation (RENDON et al. 2002). WALTHER et al. reported one tumor with residual viable cells in 11 RCCs treated with RF ablation prior to surgical resection, whereas the remaining 10 tumors were completely necrotic (WALTHER et al. 2000). These observations have to be taken seriously, but there are methodological problems with some of the studies. MICHAELS' study group omitted overlapping ablations and did not correlate the results with imaging findings. RENDON et al. based their conclusions on viability solely on hematoxylin and eosin staining instead of the required reference standard of NADHase stains. As a consequence, these studies are contradicted by the results of other investigators. JACOMIDES et al. performed tumor resection secondary to RF ablation in 5 of 17 laparascopically treated RCC and did not find residual tumor on histology (JACOMIDES et al. 2003). The latter is supported by recent 4-year results (MCDOUGAL et al. 2005). These observations, however, emphasize the need for a scrupulous RF ablation technique and strict imaging follow-up.

4.7 Complications

Complications may occur in about 7% of patients. The most common complication is self limiting hematuria. Severe complications are rare including hematoma, urinoma, renal infarction, ureteral obstruction, and cutaneous fistulas (RHIM et al. 2004). Although thermal damage to the urinary system is feared, urine leaks are rare. Direct thermal damage to the collecting system is more likely to cause stricture formation than perforation. In case a central tumor obscures the calyces, collecting system hemorrhage is a more relevant complication that may occur in up to 33% of these patients necessitating treatment (GERVAIS et al. 2005b). Most of these complications can be treated conservatively. In renal RF ablation a single 5-mm cutaneous metastasis along the puncture tract was reported, which was resected without any complications (MAYO-SMITH et al. 2003). This type of complication, however, can be avoided by coagulation of the puncture tract during RF probe withdrawal. When compared to other thermal ablation techniques, the ability to avoid tract bleeding and tumor seeding by coagulating the puncture channel is an important advantage of RF ablation. Consequently, the risk of extrarenal bleeding complications is low. Furthermore, animal experiments indicate an influence of tumor location on complication rate, with central tumors being prone to major complications including renal artery injury (LEE et al. 2003).

4.8 Summary

The introduction of minimally invasive thermal ablation techniques offers a safe and accurate alternative to open or laparoscopic surgery in the treatment of renal tumors. Experimental as well as clinical studies proved RF ablation to be a safe and effective treatment option for small RCCs. It is well tolerated in patients with percutaneously accessible lesions. However, the long-term outcome remains to be determined. Until then its use is limited to selected patients. Despite these limitations, published experience with renal RF ablation is continuously growing. As soon as its long-term effectiveness is proven, this technique holds the potential to replace surgery as first-line therapy in small RCCs.

References

Ahrar K, Matin S, Wallace MJ, Gupta S, Hicks EM (2005) Percutaneous transthoracic radiofrequency ablation of renal tumors using an iatrogenic pneumothorax. AJR Am J Roentgenol 185:86–88

Aschoff AJ, Sulman A, Martinez M, Duerk JL, Resnick MI, MacLennan GT, Lewin JS (2001) Perfusion-modulated MR imaging-guided radiofrequency ablation of the kidney in a porcine model. AJR Am J Roentgenol 177:151–158

de Baere T, Kuoch V, Smayra T, Dromain C, Cabrera T, Court B, Roche A (2002) Radiofrequency ablation of renal cell

carcinoma: preliminary clinical experience. Urology 167:1961–1964
Boss A, Clasen S, Kuczyk M, Anastasiadis A, Schmidt D, Claussen CD, Schick F, Pereira PL (2005) Radiofrequency ablation of renal cell carcinomas using MR-guidance: initial results. Rofo 177:1139–1145
Brown SD, Vansonnenberg E, Morrison PR, Diller L, Shamberger RC (2005) CT-guided radiofrequency ablation of pediatric Wilms tumor in a solitary kidney. Pediatr Radiol 35:923–928
Chang I, Mikityansky I, Wray-Cahen D, Pritchard WF, Karanian JW, Wood BJ (2004) Effects of perfusion on radiofrequency ablation in swine kidneys. Radiology 231:500–505
Chiou YY, Hwang JI, Chou YH, Wang JH, Chiang JH, Chang CY (2005) Percutaneous radiofrequency ablation of renal cell carcinoma. J Chin Med Assoc 68:221–225
Corwin TS, Lindberg G, Traxer O, Gettman MT, Smith TG, Pearle MS, Cadeddu JA (2001) Laparoscopic radiofrequency thermal ablation of renal tissue with and without hilar occlusion. J Urol 166:281–284
Crowley JD, Shelton J, Iverson AJ, Burton MP, Dalrymple NC, Bishoff JT (2000) Laparoscopic and computed tomography-guided percutaneous radiofrequency ablation of renal tissue: acute and chronic effects in an animal model. Urology 57:976–980
Farrell MA, Charboneau WJ, DiMarco DS, Chow GK, Zincke H, Callstrom MR, Lewis BD, Lee RA, Reading CC (2003) Imaging-guided radiofrequency ablation of solid renal tumors. AJR Am J Roentgenol 180:1509–1513
Fergany AF, Hafez KS, Novick AC (2000) Long-term results of nephron-sparing surgery for localized renal cell carcinoma: 10-year follow up. J Urol 163:442–445
Gervais DA, Arellano RS, Mueller PR (2002) Percutaneous radiofrequency ablation of nodal metastases. Cardiovasc Intervent Radiol 25:547–549
Gervais DA, McGovern FJ, Arellano RS, McDougal SW, Mueller PR (2003) Renal cell carcinoma: clinical experience and technical success with radio-frequency ablation of 42 tumors. Radiology 226:417–424
Gervais DA, McGovern FJ, Arellano RS, McDougal WS, Mueller PR (2005a) Radiofrequency ablation of renal cell carcinoma. Part 1: Indications, results, and role in patient management over a 6-year period and ablation of 100 tumors. AJR Am J Roentgenol 185:64–71
Gervais DA, Arellano RS, McGovern FJ, McDougal WS, Mueller PR (2005b) Radiofrequency ablation of renal cell carcinoma. Part 2: Lessons learned with ablation of 100 tumors. AJR Am J Roentgenol 185:72–80
Goetz MP, Callstrom MR, Charboneau JW, Farrell MA, Maus TP, Welch TJ, Wong GY, Sloan JA, Novotny PJ, Petersen IA, Beres RA, Regge D, Capanna R, Saker MB, Gronemeyer DH, Gevargez A, Ahrar K, Choti MA, de Baere TJ, Rubin J (2004) Percutaneous image-guided radiofrequency ablation of painful metastases involving bone: a multicenter study. J Clin Oncol 22:300–306
Goldberg SN, Gazelle GS, Mueller PR (2000) Thermal ablation therapy for focal malignancy: a unified approach to underlying principles, techniques, and diagnostic imaging guidance. AJR Am J Roentgenol 174:323–331
Guinan PD, Vogelzang NJ, Fremgen AM, Chmiel JS, Sylvester JL, Sener SF, Imperato JP (1995) Renal cell carcinoma: tumor size, stage and survival. Members of the Cancer Incidence and End Results Committee. J Urol 153:901–903
Häcker A, Vallo S, Weiss C, Grobholz R, Alken P, Knoll T, Michel MS (2005) Minimally invasive treatment of renal cell carcinoma: comparison of 4 different monopolar radiofrequency devices. Eur Urol 48:584–592
Homma Y, Kawabe K, Kitamura T, Nishimura Y, Shinohara M, Kondo Y, Saito I, Minowada S, Asakage Y (1995) Increased incidental detection and reduced mortality in renal cancer – recent retrospective analysis at eight institutions. Int J Urol 2:77–80
Hsu TH, Fidler ME, Gill IS (2000) Radiofrequency ablation of the kidney: acute and chronic histology in porcine model. Urology 56:872–875
Hwang JJ, Walther MM, Pautler SE, Coleman JA, Hvizda J, Peterson J, Linehan WM, Wood BJ (2004) Radio frequency ablation of small renal tumors: intermediate results. J Urol 171:1814–1818
Jacomides L, Ogan K, Watumull L, Cadeddu JA (2003) Laparoscopic application of radio frequency energy enables in situ renal tumor ablation and partial nephrectomy. J Urol 169:49–53
Jemal A, Tiwari R, Murray T, Ghafoor A, Samuels A, Ward E, Feuer EJ, Thun M (2004) Cancer statistics. CA Cancer J Clin 54:8–29
Lee JM, Kim SW, Chung GH, Lee SY, Han YM, Kim CS (2003) Open radio-frequency thermal ablation of renal VX2 tumors in a rabbit model using a cooled-tip electrode: feasibility, safety, and effectiveness. Eur Radiol 13:1324–1332
Lee JM, Han JK, Choi SH, Kim SH, Lee JY, Shin KS, Han CJ, Choi BI (2005) Comparison of renal ablation with monopolar radiofrequency and hypertonic-saline-augmented bipolar radiofrequency: in vitro and in vivo experimental studies. AJR Am J Roentgenol 184:897–905
Lepetit-Coiffe M, Quesson B, Seror O et al (2002) Real-time temperature control during RF induced local hyperthermia: a feasibility study. In: *Proceedings of the 19th Annual Scientific Meeting of the European Society for Magnetic Resonance in Medicine and Biology (ESMRMB 2002)*, August 2002, Cannes, France, p 251
Lewin JS, Nour SG, Connell CF, Sulman A, Duerk JL, Resnick MI, Haaga JR (2004) Phase II clinical trial of interactive MR imaging-guided interstitial radiofrequency thermal ablation of primary kidney tumors: initial experience. Radiology 232:835–845
Lotan Y, Cadeddu JA (2005) A cost comparison of nephron-sparing surgical techniques for renal tumour. BJU Int 95:1039–1042
Mahnken A, Rohde D, Brkovic D, Günther RW, Tacke J (2005) Percutaneous radiofrequency ablation of renal cell carcinoma: preliminary results. Acta Radiol 46:208–214
Margulis V, Matsumoto ED, Taylor G, Shaffer S, Kabbani W, Cadeddu JA (2005) Retrograde renal cooling during radiofrequency ablation to protect from renal collecting system injury. J Urol 174:350–352
Matlaga BR, Zagoria RJ, Woodruff RD, Torti FM, Hall MC (2002) Phase II trial of radio frequency ablation of renal cancer: evaluation of the kill zone. J Urol 168:2401–2405
Matsumoto ED, Watumull L, Johnson DB, Ogan K, Taylor GD, Josephs S, Cadeddu JA (2004) The radiographic evolution of radio frequency ablated renal tumors. J Urol 172:45–48

Matsumoto ED, Johnson DB, Ogan K, Trimmer C, Sagalowsky A, Margulis V, Cadeddu JA (2005) Short-term efficacy of temperature-based radiofrequency ablation of small renal tumors. Urology 65:877–881

Mayo-Smith WW, Dupuy DE, Parikh PM, Pezzullo JA, Cronan JJ (2003) Imaging-guided percutaneous radiofrequency ablation of solid renal masses: techniques and outcomes of 38 treatment sessions in 32 consecutive patients. AJR Am J Roentgenol 180:1503–1508

McDougal WS, Gervais DA, MCGovern FJ, Mueller PS (2005) Long-term follow-up of patients with renal cell carcinoma treated with radiofrequency ablation with curative intent. J Urol 174:61–63

McGovern FJ, Goldberg SN, Wood BJ, Mueller PR (1999) Radiofrequency ablation of renal cell carcinoma via image guided needle electrodes. J Urol 161:599–600

Merkle EM, Shonk JR, Duerk JL, Jacobs GH, Lewin JS (1999) MR-guided RF thermal ablation of the kidney in a porcine model. AJR Am J Roentgenol 173:645–651

Merkle EM, Nour SG, Lewin JS (2005) MR imaging follow-up after percutaneous Radiofrequency ablation of renal cell carcinoma: findings in 18 patients during first 6 months. Radiology 235:1065–1071

Michaels MJ, Rhee HK, Mourtzinos AP, Summerhayes IC, Silverman ML, Libertino JA (2002) Incomplete renal tumor destruction using radio frequency interstitial ablation. J Urol 168:2406–2410

Neeman Z, Sarin S, Coleman J, Fojo T, Wood BJ (2005) Radiofrequency ablation for tumor-related massive hematuria. J Vasc Interv Radiol 16:417–421

Ogan K, Jacomides L, Dolmatch BL, Rivera FJ, Dellaria MF, Josephs SC, Cadeddu JA (2002) Percutaneous radiofrequency ablation of renal tumors: technique, limitations, and morbidity. Urology 60:954–958

Pantuck AJ, Zisman A, Belldegrun AS (2001) The changing natural history of renal cell carcinoma. J Urol 166:297–301

Pavlovich CP, Walther MM, Choyke PL, Pautler SE, Chang R, Linehan WM, Wood BJ (2002) Percutaneous radio frequency ablation of small renal tumors: initial results. J Urol 167:10–15

Polascik TJ, Hamper U, Lee BR, Dai Y, Hilton J, Magee CA, Crone JK, Shue MJ, Ferrell M, Trapanotto V, Adiletta M, Partin AW (1999) Ablation of renal tumors in a rabbit model with interstitial saline-augmented radiofrequency energy: preliminary report of a new technology. Urology 53:465–472

Rendon RA, Kachura JR, Sweet JM, Gertner MR, Sherar MD, Robinette M, Trachtenberg JTJ, Sampson H, Jewett MAS (2002) The uncertainty of radiofrequency treatment of renal cell carcinoma: findings at immediate and delayed nephrectomy. J Urol 167:1587–1592

Rhim H, Dodd GD, Chintapalli KN, Wood BJ, Dupuy DE, Hvizda JL, Sewell PE, Goldberg SN (2004) Radiofrequency thermal ablation of abdominal tumors: lessons learned from complications. Radiographics 24:41–52

Schultze D, Morris CS, Bhave AD, Worgan BA, Najarian KE (2003) Radiofrequency ablation of renal transitional cell carcinoma with protective cold saline infusion. J Vasc Interv Radiol 14:489–492

Su LM, Jarrett TW, Chan DY, Kavoussi LR, Solomon SB (2003) Percutaneous computed tomography-guided radiofrequency ablation of renal masses in high surgical risk patients: preliminary results. Urology 61 [Suppl 4A]:26–33

Sweeney JP, Thornhill JA, Graiger R, McDermott TE, Butler MR (1996) Incidentally detected renal cell carcinoma: pathological features, survival trends and implications for treatment. Br J Urol 78:351–353

Tuncali K, vanSonnenberg E, Shankar S, Mortele KJ, Cibas ES, Silverman SG (2004) Evaluation of patients referred for percutaneous ablation of renal tumors: importance of a preprocedural diagnosis. AJR Am J Roentgenol 183:575–582

Uzzo RG, Novick AC (2001) Nephron sparing surgery for renal tumors: indications techniques and outcomes. J Urol 166:6–18

Veltri A, De Fazio G, Malfitana V, Isolato G, Fontana D, Tizzani A, Gandini G (2004) Percutaneous US-guided RF thermal ablation for malignant renal tumors: preliminary results in 13 patients. Eur Radiol 14:2303–2310

Walther MM, Shawker TH, Libutti SK, Lubensky I, Choyke PL, Venzon D, Linehan WM (2000) A phase 2 study of radio frequency interstitial tissue ablation of localized renal tumors. J Urol 163:1424–1427

Zagoria RJ, Dyer RB (1998) The small renal mass: detection, characterization, and management. Abdom Imaging 23:256–265

Zagoria RJ, Chen MY, Kavanagh PV, Torti FM (2001) Radio frequency ablation of lung metastases from renal cell carcinoma. J Urol 166:1827–1828

Zagoria RJ, Hawkins AD, Clark PE, Hall MC, Matlaga BR, Dyer RB, Chen MY (2004) Percutaneous CT-guided radiofrequency ablation of renal neoplasms: factors influencing success. AJR Am J Roentgenol 183:201–207

Zlotta AR, Wildschutz T, Raviv G, Peny MO, van Gansbeke D, Noel JC, Schulman CC (1997) Radiofrequency interstitial tumor ablation (RITA) is a possible new modality for treatment of renal cancer: ex vivo and in vivo experience. J Endourol 11:251–258

Lung

5

5.1 Radiofrequency Ablation (RFA)

Karin Steinke

CONTENTS

K. Steinke, MD
Associate Professor, Medical Imaging, Royal Brisbane and Womens Hospital, Herston, 4029 QLD, Australia

5.1.1 Introduction

5.1.1.1 Lung Neoplasms

Primary lung cancer is a severe worldwide health problem causing a greater death toll than breast, prostate, and colorectal cancer combined (Brescia 2001). Non-small cell lung cancer (NSCLC) accounts for 80% of primary lung cancer. Unresectability represents the poorest prognostic factor for survival outcome (Strauss 1997). Less than one in five patients can be resected with a curative intent at the time of presentation. Even those patients able to have a complete resection often relapse, making lung cancer one of the most biologically aggressive cancers known with a 5-year mortality rate of nearly 90% (Salgia and Skarin 1998).

Pulmonary metastases can arise from virtually any primary source. Lung metastases have been found at autopsy in 25%–30% of all patients with malignant disease (Ollila and Morton 1998). Despite nearly a third of cancer patients dying with evidence of pulmonary metastases, those patients satisfying criteria for surgical resection represent a much smaller subgroup.

In a retrospective study of 5206 cases undergoing pulmonary metastasectomy, 42% had sarcoma, 14% colorectal cancer, 9% breast cancer, 8% renal cancer, 7% germ cell tumor, 6% melanoma, and 5% head and neck cancer (Friedel et al. 1999).

Tumors exhibiting preferential spread to the lungs as the only site of metastasis include sarcoma, renal cell cancer, and head and neck cancer. In contrast, tumors such as breast, melanoma, and colorectal carcinoma typically metastasize to multiple organ sites (Davidson et al. 2001).

Several studies on metastasectomies have recently been published using heterogeneous patient populations (Friedel et al. 2002; Pastorino 2002; Pfannschmidt et al. 2002) demonstrating that metastasectomy is safe and provides extended survival. Completeness of resection was of prognostic significance with respect to survival in all analyses. Less agreement is over disease-free interval (DFI), tumor type, number and size of metastases.

Pulmonary metastases from colorectal cancer (CRC) occupy a special position. CRC is the second most common visceral malignancy in industrialized countries, the highest incidences being encountered in North America, Australia, New Zealand, Europe, and Japan (Faivre et al. 2002). An increasing incidence of CRC has been observed in most areas of the world recently (Faivre et al. 2002). Although the recurrence of disease is mainly loco-regional, in 20% of patients it will recur at distant sites (Davidson et al. 2001). The lung is the most common site of extra-abdominal disease, although isolated pulmonary metastases are rare with an incidence of 2%–4% (McCormack and Ginsberg 1998). Unlike many other cancers, the presence of distant metastases from CRC does not preclude curative treatment (Penna and Nordlinger 2002).

The type of resection was shown not to significantly affect survival following 85 patients who underwent pulmonary metastasectomy by either conventional resections with diathermy dissection or stapler suture lines, lobectomy or laser ablation with an Nd:YAG laser (Mineo et al. 2001).

The well-established data on survival after pulmonary surgery of CRC-metastases lead to the conclusion that if we are able to completely ablate the lung tumors by RFA we may achieve comparable survival rates to surgical tumor removal. Lower morbidity and mortality, as well as a better life quality additionally accompany this treatment with the possibility that the patients may be treated on an overnight or even outpatient base.

5.1.1.2 Local Tumor Destruction of Lung Tumors

5.1.1.2.1 Overview of Methods

The different options for local tumor ablation in medical radiology together with their clinical indication have been detailed in Chapters 2 and 3.

The methods for local ablation of lung tumors include hyperthermia [RFA, laser-induced thermotherapy (LITT), microwave coagulation, high intensity focused ultrasound (HIFU)], cryotherapy, ionizing irradiation (internal, external), photodynamic therapy and electrochemotherapy.

Some methods, such as RFA and LITT (Vogl et al. 2004), within the hyperthermia modalities have been used more extensively than the other methods listed.

Microwave-induced coagulation can produce the ablation of a relatively large volume within a few minutes; in liver the results are at least as good as those achieved with percutaneous alcohol injection (PEI) (Seki et al. 1999). It may become attractive for percutaneous use in lung tumors if clinically relevant lesions can be produced with a probe size of less than 2 mm.

In HIFU the working principle is the transformation of energy into heat, a principle that it shares with RFA, LITT, and microwave coagulation. The attraction of this method is of course its complete lack of invasiveness. Frequencies in the range 0.5–4.0 MHz are used to provide a treatment which allows thermal ablation of pre-selected soft tissue targets at depth, whilst sparing the more superficial layers. Potential sites for HIFU treatment are limited by the fact that megahertz ultrasound is not transmitted through air or bone. A fluid or soft tissue path is required for sound wave propagation (Visioli et al. 1999).

Cryotherapy, an effective method for liver tumor destruction despite a higher morbidity rate than RFA, was not successfully developed for lung ablation, probably because of its bigger probe diameter (Wang et al. 2004).

Methods such as ionizing irradiation and photodynamic therapy have rarely been used in patients, electrochemotherapy has not progressed beyond the experimental level, while local tumor destruction by chemical means, extensively used in liver, is not an option in lung due to the special tissue properties.

5.1.1.2.2 Indications for Local Tumor Destruction

The indications for local destruction of lung tumor are similar to those established for resection, although with some modifications. It is usually felt that the number of lesions per hemithorax should not be more than five and that the largest lesion diameter should be less than 5 cm. Most authors think that the treatment should be offered only to patients with no evident extrapulmonary disease, however there is a role for RFA in pain palliation, a topic covered later in this chapter. Ideally tumors should be smaller than 3.5 cm in diameter and completely surrounded by non-tumorous lung. Tumors abutting the pleura can be efficiently treated, but this is associated with increased pain during and after treatment.

5.1.1.2.3 Advantages as Compared to Lung Resection

As compared to lung resection local ablative methods bear indisputable advantages. The surgical trauma may contribute to recurrence, growth of metastases, and metastatic spread. These unwanted consequences of surgery depend on factors such as immunosuppression (Colacchio et al. 1994), shedding of tumor cells into the wounded area and the circulation (Hansen et al. 1995) and the production and release of growth factors for wound healing, which influence tumor cell adhesion and growth (Brown et al. 1999).

The potential advantages of local tumor destruction methods might include: (1) selective damage which leads to less immunosuppression and release of less growth factors, (2) minimal treatment morbidity and mortality, (3) less breathing impairment in patients with borderline lung function through sparing healthy lung tissue, (4) repeatability, (5) fairly low costs, (6) excellent imaging during the procedure and for follow-up and last but not least (7) the gain in quality of life with less pain, much shorter hospitalization times with the interventions performed on an outpatient base or with overnight stays and thus a quicker re-access to social life.

Following hyperthermic treatment there are a number of events inducing favorable immunological effects, such as heat shock protein (HSP) expression within tumors (Srivastava 2002), increased expression of cancer antigens (Gromkowski et al. 1989) and increased lymphocyte adhesion to endothelial cells (Lefor et al. 1994).

5.1.1.2.4 Requirements for Curative Treatment

5.1.1.2.4.1 Biopsy and Treatment Without Seeding

The nature of a tumor is often evident from the appearance of new lesions, or the growth of existing lesions, or an increase in tumor markers, such as CEA in CRC disease. However, without a biopsy one cannot always be certain that a nodule in the lung, especially when it is relatively small, is indeed a malignant tumor of a specific origin. It would thus be preferable in some instances to obtain biopsy proof.

Implantation metastases along the needle track following fine-needle biopsy of lung tumors have often been reported. This is a disastrous complication, especially in patients who undergo a curative lung resection. A solution to this problem is the double needle technique (Wales et al. 1981), additionally allowing a single needle pass through the pleura and taking multiple samples of the lesion without increasing the risk of pneumothorax.

Seeding along the needle track with percutaneous minimally invasive tumor treatment modalities has not yet been reported in lung; data for liver therapy report seeding to occur along the track in 0.7%–2.3% of hepatocellular carcinoma patients treated with PEI (Ishii et al. 1998).

Corresponding figures for electrode track seeding after percutaneous liver RFA vary from 0.3% (Mulier et al. 2002) to 12.5% (Llovet et al. 2001).

It is likely that the incidence of electrode track seeding is underestimated because many patients have had advanced disease and/or disease recurrence and a short survival or follow-up.

The risk appears to be substantially reduced by carefully coagulating the tissue immediately surrounding the probe track at the end of treatment.

5.1.1.2.4.2 Imaging and Real-Time Monitoring

Percutaneous treatment relies on accurate description of the spread of tumors by imaging techniques.

In contrast to solid organs, lung parenchyma is not visible on ultrasound. Computed tomography (CT) and positron emission tomography (PET) for pre-operative imaging, CT and magnetic resonance imaging (MRI) for intra-operative monitoring and CT, PET and MRI for follow-up are the imaging techniques in use.

Although CT is not ideal for real-time monitoring because thermal tissue changes are not visible within 24 h, in lung a reproducible ovoid opacification (ground-glass attenuation) can be seen around the adequately ablated lesion, which is equivalent to the heat-damaged area and is sharply demarcated from the surrounding healthy tissue. Accordingly, technical success can be defined as the emergence of the surrounding GGA on a CT scan immediately after RF ablation (Yasui et al. 2004).

MRI appears to be the ideal tool for temperature mapping. A particular advantage of MRI for guiding thermal procedures is that it not only allows temperature mapping but can be used as well for target definition, and it may provide an early evaluation of the therapeutic efficacy (Quesson et al. 2000). However, availability is low and costs are high.

Fluorine 18-fluorodeoxyglucose (FDG), an analogue of glucose, accumulates in most tumors in a greater amount than it does in normal tissue. FDG PET is being used in diagnosis and follow-up of several malignancies, lung cancer above all (Rohren et al. 2004). CT scanners are now being combined with PET scanners. The combined PET/CT devices offer several potential advantages over PET scanner alone: better quality PET images because of the more accurate correction for attenuation provided by CT, automatic registration of CT (anatomic) and PET (metabolic) information, and shorter imaging times.

5.1.1.2.4.3 Comparison of Local Destruction Methods

There are no prospective, randomized studies comparing the various local destruction methods in lung with each other. RFA and LITT are the only two really competitive minimally invasive treatment methods, however there are far more data available on lung RFA with LITT restricted to German groups (Vogl et al. 2004). Short-term follow-up seems to be comparable to RFA, in that LITT lesion size is restricted to a maximal diameter of 3 cm; however, the pneumothorax rate is much lower with LITT (10%) than with RFA (30%–40%).

5.1.1.2.4.4 Comparison with Surgical Resection

The minimally invasive local treatment options for lung malignancy are too new to allow for a direct comparison to surgical resection with follow-up data not surpassing the 2-year threshold. There will definitely be a patient bias to consider, as the patient population so far referred to RFA consists of nonresectable candidates.

In primary lung cancer, the most favorable numbers with radical surgery of stage IA NSCLC showed overall 1-, 3- and 5-year survival rates of 89%, 76%, and 66% (Campione et al. 2004). With higher stages surgically approached (up to selected IIIB cases), the figures for survival and recurrence considerably worsen. A direct comparison would be again very difficult, as most patients receive adjuvant or neoadjuvant therapy, be it chemotherapy, radiation, or chemoradiation (Okawara et al. 2004).

As far as resection of lung metastases is concerned, numbers again vary considerably. The International Registry of Lung Metastases assessed the long-term results of lung metastasectomy with prognostic analyses based on 5206 cases. The actuarial survival after complete metastasectomy was 36% at 5 years, 26% at 10 years, and 22% at 15 years (median 35 months); the corresponding values for incomplete resection were 13% at 5 years and 7% at 10 years (median 15 months). Among complete resections, the 5-year survival was 33% for patients with a disease-free interval of 0–11 months and 45% for those with a disease-free interval of more than 36 months; 43% for single lesions and 27% for four or more lesions.

5.1.1.3 Radiofrequency Ablation

Heat has been used clinically for thousands of years dating back to ancient Hindu and Greek healers who used it for hemostasis. In fact, Hippocrates is reported as saying that those diseases that medicine cannot cure, the knife cures; those which the knife cannot cure, fire cures (Adams 1886).

More recently, heat has been utilized in the surgical setting as electrocautery to control bleeding and to cut tissue.

RFA has been used for the last 30 years to treat cardiac arrhythmia (Luderitz 2003). It has been used over many years for the treatment of trigeminal neuralgia (Oturai et al. 1996) and osteoid osteomas (Rosenthal et al. 1998).

The application of RFA for the treatment of tumors in solid organs other than the lung is detailed elsewhere in this volume. However, the most promising and most common clinical application so far has been for liver tumors and seems to be evolving similarly for lung tumors.

A range of electrode designs is available ranging in caliber from 14 to 17 G. Various design features have been put forward, such as water cooling, saline perfusion, monopolar or bipolar, straight needle, coil or expandable design, all aimed at increasing the volume of necrosis that can be achieved per time unit. The systems vary in the amount of generator power (50–250 W), generator cost (12,000–30,000 USD), electrode cost (500–1500 USD), parameters monitored, algorithm used and the amount of operator input. All electrodes are currently nonreusable.

The procedure details and outcomes reported in this chapter represent our experience with the RITA system (RITA Medical Systems, Mountain View, Calif., USA) and the RITA® StarBurst™ XL electrode. The electrode deployment is adjustable for the creation of ablation from 3 to 5 cm. This device has nine active electrodes (five with thermocouples), and an active trocar tip. We have opted for this system because of its expandable hooks, which cling to the tissue and thus are not subject to breathing-related dislocation. The system is user-friendly, and data from the generator (power, impedance, temperature, time, etc.) can be collected and displayed on a computer.

5.1.2 Animal Experiments

5.1.2.1 Effect of Vessel Diameter on Ovine Lung Radiofrequency Lesion in Vivo

Experimental studies have evaluated the feasibility and safety of percutaneous RFA of normal pulmonary tissue in rabbits (Goldberg et al. 1995) and have assessed its effectiveness in the destruction of experimentally induced lung malignancies (Goldberg et al. 1996; Miao et al. 2001; Ahrar et al. 2003). Nevertheless lung RFA in patients was started before much experience was obtained with in vivo animal lung RFA. The few animal experiments published have been performed in rodents and rabbits; no large animal data have been reported.

One of the important issues was to evaluate whether the heat sink effect applies to lung in this same way as it does to liver (Lu et al. 2002).

Using an in vivo sheep model we macroscopically evaluated the effect of vessel size on the radiofrequency lesion creation in the lung with respect to the potential for a perfusion-mediated heat-sink effect and vascular injury, with histological correlation and assessing the type and severity of complications.

Radiofrequency ablations in predetermined locations – in the hilus of the lung, surrounding the hilar region and in the outer third of the lung – were sequentially performed. Acute (immediate euthanasia), subacute (euthanasia 72 h post ablation), and chronic (euthanasia 28 days post ablation) ablations were carried out.

Gross and histological analysis of all radiofrequency lesions was performed to determine the extent of both vascular injury and the heat sink effect and to assess for complications.

Representative gross sections of all lesions were photographed. Selected representative pulmonary lesions were submitted for histological examination.

Gross pathology typically revealed a central discolored necrotic zone, surrounded by two concentric rims, the inner pale rim consistent with eosinophilic coagulative necrosis, the outer dark red consistent with hemorrhage. On the acute samples a further outer concentric layer was identified, containing edema and blood cells.

There was a sharp cut-off between ablated lesions and normal lung (Fig. 5.1.1), as previously shown in an ablate-resect model (Steinke et al. 2002). The final appearance was of a nodule comprised of central coagulation necrosis surrounded by a fibrous capsule (Fig. 5.1.1c).

In the acute, subacute, and chronic setting, the heat sink effect, indicated by invagination of the tissue between the vessel and the ablated region, is only observed in vessels greater than 3 mm in diameter. Thrombus is seen in 20% of vessels smaller than 3 mm. On histopathology, vessels smaller than 3 mm show at least partial vessel wall injury, characterized by endothelial cell necrosis and luminal thrombus. In vessels greater than 3 mm the extent of vessel wall injury decreases with increasing vessel diameter (Steinke et al. 2005).

5.1.2.2 Safety of Radiofrequency Ablation of Myocardium and Lung Adjacent to the Heart

To assess the feasibility and safety of applying RFA to lung parenchyma adjacent to the heart and to evaluate the clinical impact and the histopathological damage to the heart caused by RF electrodes penetrating the pericardium and the myocardium we have sequentially performed RFA in predetermined locations related to these structures.

Ventricular tachycardia was noted in all ablations adjacent to the heart. Tachycardia was most severe in the ablation where one of the electrodes had deeply penetrated the myocardium of the left ventricle (Fig. 5.1.2) with heart rates up to 180/min, but no effect other than transient ventricular tachycardia was noted.

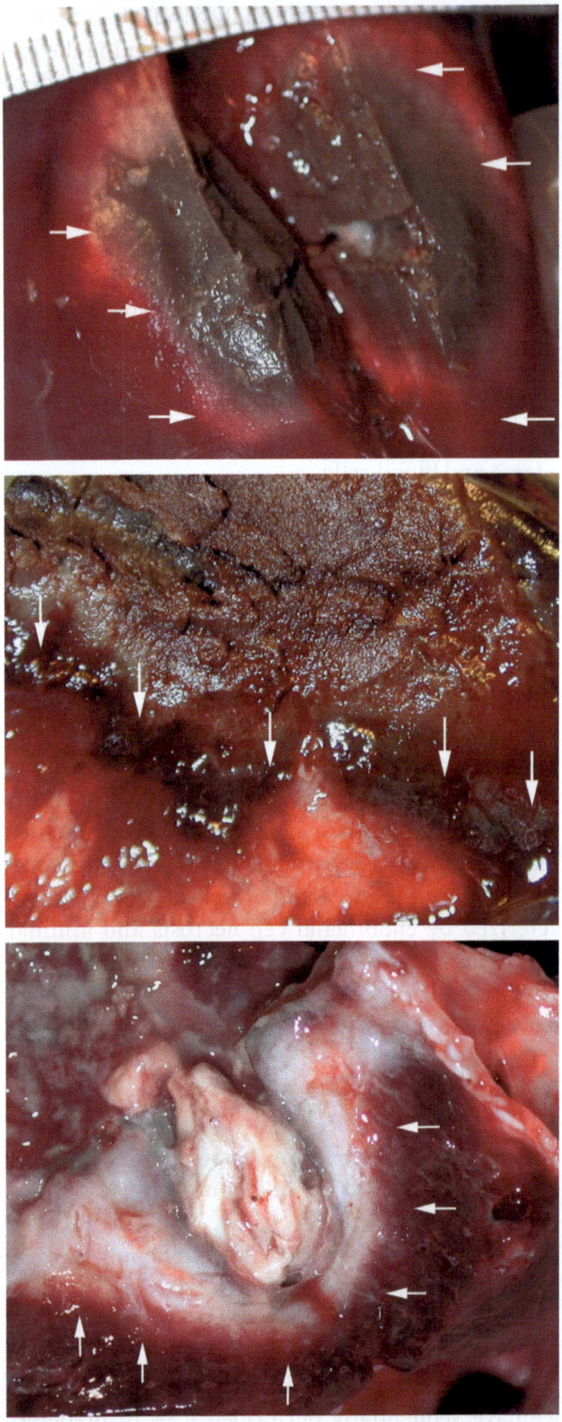

a b c

Fig. 5.1.1a–c. Gross pathology of acute (**a**), subacute (**b**), and chronic (**c**) RF ovine lung lesions with clearly demarcated concentric rims surrounding the necrotic center

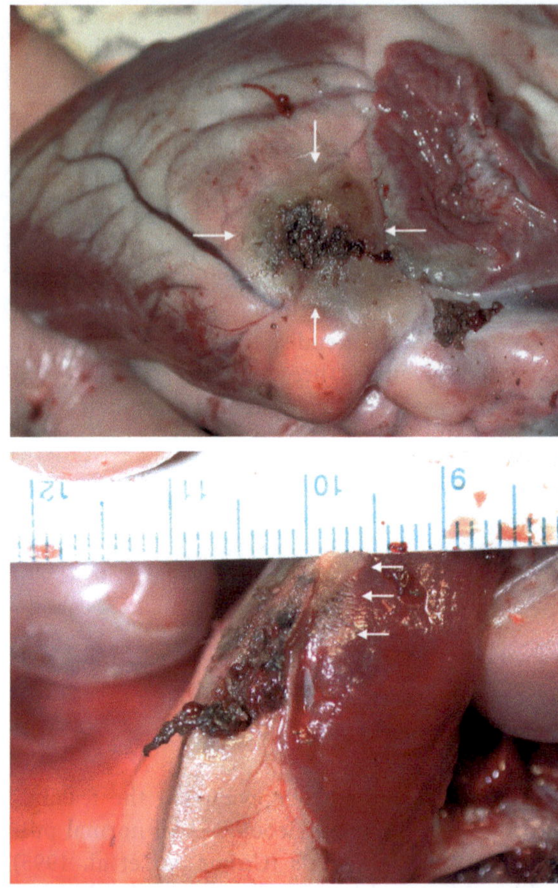

a b

Fig. 5.1.2. a Overview of the left ventricle with RF-caused thermal lesion (*white arrows*). **b** Cut-through myocardium of the left ventricle along the electrode track macroscopically showing the thermal injury to the heart muscle (*white arrows*)

Due to the muscular strength of the continuously beating myocardium there appears to be an occasional deviation of the probe tines from the heart.

Temperature around the tip of the electrode closest to the heart did not exceed 47°C, even if maximum power was administered. This may be explained by the cooling effect of the circulating blood, preventing thermal injury to the vessel/heart, while also preventing the tissue from being lethally damaged and thus allowing for tumor recurrence.

We obviously do not advocate intended RFA of tumors where the myocardium would be damaged by RFA or where thermal damage to coronary arteries could occur.

It seems that lung tumors adjacent to the heart or even abutting the heart can safely be ablated; it is of more concern that incomplete tumor ablation can occur in the vicinity of the heart and large vessels due to the cooling effect of the circulating blood.

5.1.3 Patient Handling

5.1.3.1 Patient Selection and Pretreatment Assessment

Patients are selected by a joint tumor board. Patients amenable for RFA treatment are judged not suitable for surgery because of the site and distribution of their lung tumors or because of their limited cardiorespiratory function. Occasional refusal of the patient to undergo major surgery despite qualification for it, opting for the less invasive alternative, does occur.

Bilateral metastases are treated, but for safety reasons only one lung a time should be ablated.

In lesions >3.5 cm in largest diameter overlapping ablations are required.

Our only exclusion criteria are an uncorrectable coagulopathy and more than five metastases per hemithorax. Patients who had previously undergone pneumonectomy must be considered at very high risk for RFA; the intervention should only be performed with the option of thoracic surgeons, anesthetist on stand-by and intensive care unit facilities.

Before treatment, a careful clinical evaluation has to be performed, along with any relevant laboratory, imaging, and pulmonary function tests.

Pretreatment CT of the chest is a key examination for determining the number, size, and location of the lesions. Their relationship to the heart, major bronchi and vessels has to be evaluated, as well as the status of the surrounding pulmonary parenchyma. Furthermore it constitutes the term of reference for post-treatment follow-up studies.

Our ongoing protocol considers candidates with no more than five lesions per hemithorax suitable for RF, and maximum lesion diameter should not exceed 4 cm. Individual exceptions are being made.

5.1.3.2 Procedure

Written informed consent is obtained from all patients.

The patient is positioned on the CT table according to the location of the lesion(s). Mindful that the ablation procedure takes at least 15 min per lesion at target temperature, the patient should be positioned as comfortable as possible, preferably supine or prone.

Patient's blood pressure, pulse rate and blood oxygen saturation via a pulse oximeter are monitored and recorded. Continuous oxygen administration (usually 2–4 l/min) is advisable.

The patient is made into an electrical circuit by placing two grounding pads on the back muscles or one on each thigh (Fig. 5.1.3) with the longer edge facing the coagulation site, therefore providing a large "leading edge" of the pad to lessen the risk of skin burns. In procedures where a large amount of RF energy is delivered to the patient, repeated checking of the grounding pad temperature is advisable to avoid skin burns.

The skin entry site allowing the shortest, most vertical path that avoids bullae, interlobar fissures or pulmonary vessels and bronchi is chosen, allowing for a minimum depth of the electrode inside the thoracic cage to reduce displacement due to breathing, motion or generator cable weight.

After cleansing the needle entry site the tissue down to the pleura is anesthetized with local anesthetic. Sedation/analgesia generally consists of conscious sedation, usually a combination of a hypnotic drug and a ultrashort half-life analgesic – that can be given and increased on demand and modulated in relation to the individual patient's compliance and to the different phases of the procedure. Very occasional agitation despite (or due to) profound sedation is sometimes observed, but mostly does not require any anesthetist intervention. Anesthetic service non-dependence allows greater flexibility in RF procedures/CT room management and is cost-

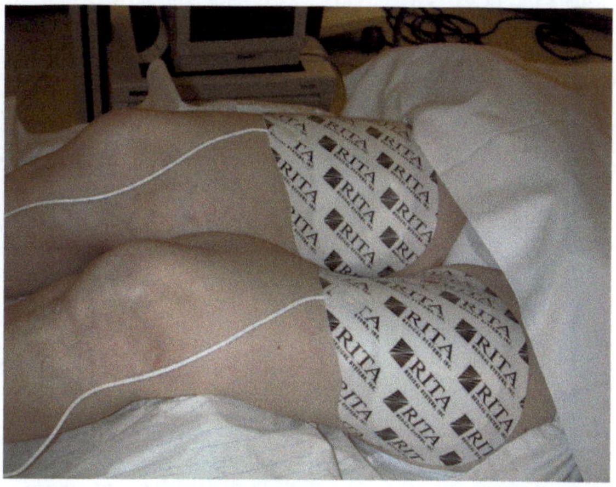

Fig. 5.1.3. Grounding pads properly attached to the patient's thighs, equidistant to the RF site

effective. General anesthesia could be necessary, in procedures that are foreseeably long or painful, with broad pleural tumor contact and where the patient is likely to be agitated and to move.

The electrode is positioned under CT guidance (Fig. 5.1.4); CT fluoroscopy is preferred. Guidance without fluoroscopy is more complicated and thus less precise due to the breathing-related motion. With CT fluoroscopy the radiation exposure for the patient is decreased due to faster electrode placement into the tumor with real-time visual control (Carlson et al. 2001). Clinicians performing the procedure can minimize their radiation exposure by using a tool, such as an artery clamp, to grasp and move the device during scanning.

Once the needle tip is in the right place, preferably assessed in all three planes (Fig. 5.1.4b), the tines are deployed to a 2-cm array and the probe is connected to the generator. One should be alert to the risk of "push back," in that instead of forwarding the electrodes from the device's trocar and into the tumor, the trocar is pushed backwards exposing the electrodes proximal to the tumor and not penetrating the tumor, as intended.

The protocol we use is temperature-based; it recommends a power setting at 50 W, adjustable to 150 W, and an average temperature setting at 90°C. The aim is a gradual heating leading to coagulation necrosis. We attempt to avoid charring with subsequent loss of heat dissipation by starting with a lower power setting.

Intermittent radiological confirmation of the position of the probe should be performed especially after changing deployment size or if the patient has moved significantly. When the average temperature has been maintained for the required duration, the generator automatically switches off and the automatic, 20-s cool-down cycle starts. After completion of the cool-down-cycle, provided the tissue temperature does not fall below 60°C, the electrodes are retracted into the trocar and the "track ablation" can be started. This procedure allows for coagulating the needle track and thus minimizing the risk of bleeding or tumor cell dissemination. Should one or more of the thermocouples indicate temperatures below 60°C after completion of the cool-down cycle, an incomplete ablation has to be assumed and a second ablation cycle added.

5.1.3.3 Post-treatment Assessment and Patient Follow-Up

After completion of the procedure, the patient should be under standard cardiac, blood pressure, and oxygen monitoring for another 3–4 h. The patient should lie preferably on the puncture site, which helps reduce air leak and post-procedural pneumothorax. We perform an erect chest radiograph after these 3–4 h to exclude a new or increased pneumothorax. Small, asymptomatic

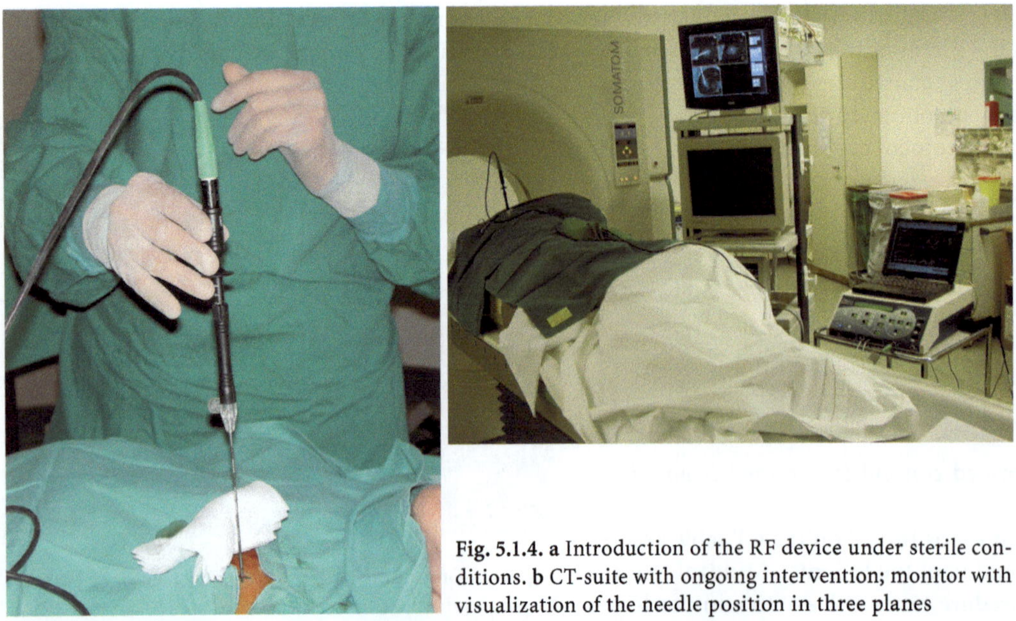

a b

Fig. 5.1.4. a Introduction of the RF device under sterile conditions. **b** CT-suite with ongoing intervention; monitor with visualization of the needle position in three planes pneumothoraces are conservatively managed with follow-up radiographs to confirm stability. Large symptomatic pneumothoraces usually require the placement of a small-bore catheter. It is generally accepted that a pneumothorax exceeding 30% of the ipsilateral lung volume requires drainage, even in asymptomatic patients; however, the decision to drain a pneumothorax must be determined on an individual basis.

Follow-up studies include clinical evaluation, laboratory and lung function test; if the ablations are being performed as part of a study quality of life is also assessed. As far as follow-up imaging is concerned, CT is so far the modality of choice, being the best available option. We perform follow-up chest CT at 1 month, then at 3-month intervals post ablation within the first year followed by 6-monthly intervals thereafter. The size of the ablated lesions and their contrast uptake is assessed. The 1-month follow-up CT scan measurement is obtained as a post-RF reference measurement with any further increase in size or in attenuation raising suspicious of recurrence.

MRI and PET are also a very good and sensitive procedures for follow-up (MacManus and Hicks 2003), providing a better discrimination between residual granulation tissue and recurrent tumor, but to many institutions access is limited by availability and cost.

5.1.4 Radiomorphological Appearance of CT-Guided Percutaneously RF-Ablated Lung Lesions

Lung is not visible on US or MR, therefore CT remains the only image-guidance modality for percutaneous diagnostic and therapeutic interventions.

During the ablation procedure the typical feature of the RF-ablated site is a bulb-shaped opacification

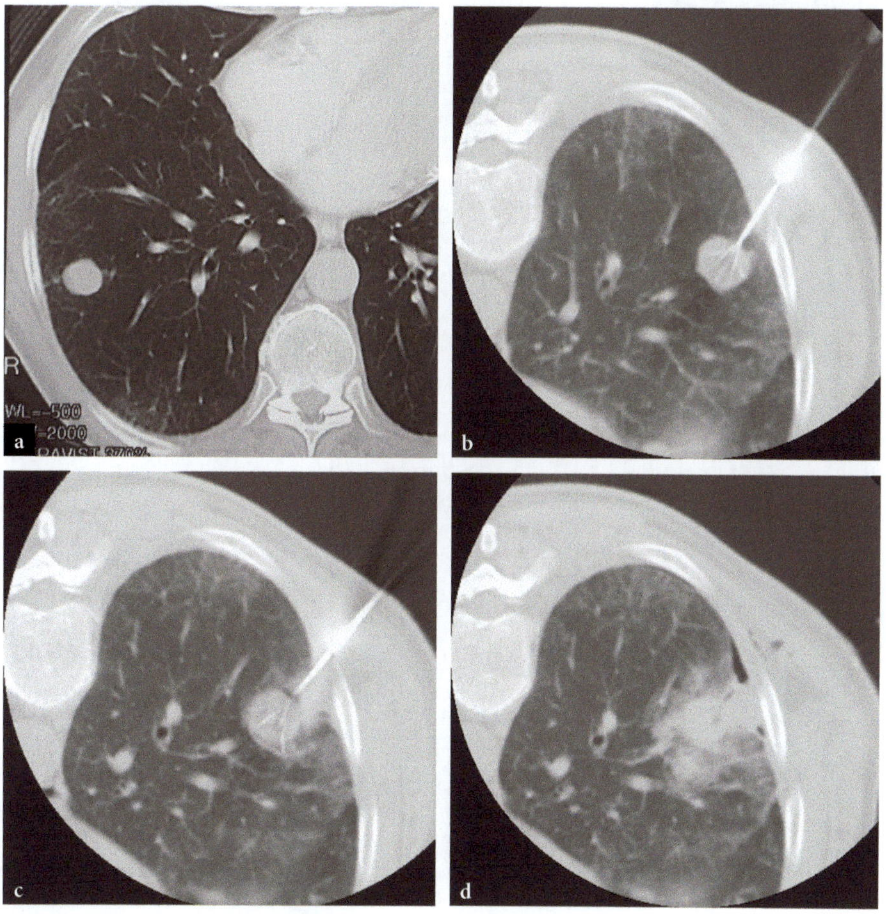

Fig. 5.1.5a–d. Continuous increase in density during RF procedure. **a** Lesion pre RFA. **b** beginning of RFA session. **c** Halfway through RF procedure. **d** Immediately post RFA

surrounding the probe, continuously increasing in density (Fig. 5.1.5).

The size of the ablated lesion is increased at 1 week from baseline in all lesions, provided there was a preceding technically successful ablation, not only encompassing the tumor, but also a circumferentiall surrounding safety margin. At 1 month 95% of the lesions are still larger than baseline, at 3 months 76% are still larger than baseline, at 6 months the majority of the lesions should be smaller or equaling baseline (Fig. 5.1.6). Every solid lesion larger than baseline at 6 months should be considered suspect for local incomplete ablation and recurrence. A residual scar is the usual feature that remains, a complete resolution is sometimes seen in small ablations < 3 cm in diameter.

5.1.5 Difficulty Achieving Complete Ablations in Big Lung Lesions

The size of both primary and metastatic lung tumors often exceeds 3 cm in diameter at the time of diagnosis. The RF electrodes of the three leading companies currently in use are designed for a maximum ablation diameter of 5 cm. Therefore, the tumor to be ablated should not exceed 3 cm in maximum diameter, as a 1-cm safety ablation margin surrounding the tumor should ideally be achieved.

A possible solution in treating larger tumors is to create overlapping ablations, a method successfully used in the RFA of liver tumors (Curley 2001; Livraghi et al. 2000). Local recurrences usually

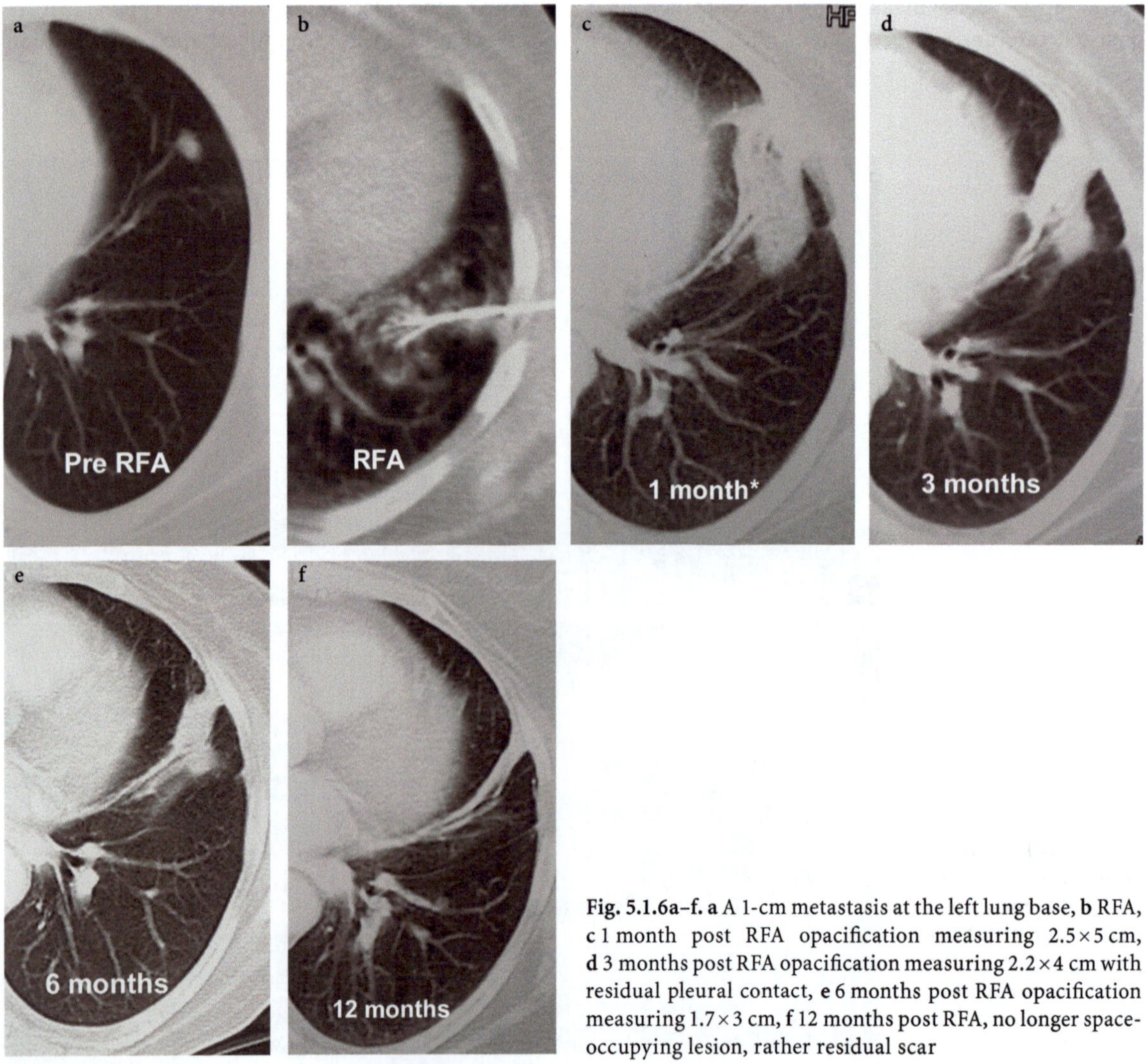

Fig. 5.1.6a–f. **a** A 1-cm metastasis at the left lung base, **b** RFA, **c** 1 month post RFA opacification measuring 2.5 × 5 cm, **d** 3 months post RFA opacification measuring 2.2 × 4 cm with residual pleural contact, **e** 6 months post RFA opacification measuring 1.7 × 3 cm, **f** 12 months post RFA, no longer space-occupying lesion, rather residual scar

become evident on CT within the first 3–6 months post ablation and in some cases very early evidence of recurrence is given after a few weeks post ablation (Fig. 5.1.7); however, the risk of false-positive findings due to surrounding enhancing granulation tissue has to be borne in mind.

Exact probe placement into the tumor is crucial for successful ablations. Ideally, tumors measuring 3–5 cm in diameter should be treated with six overlapping ablations, four in the axial plane and two along the *y*-axis, with all ablations positioned to touch the centre of the tumor (Dodd et al. 2002).

The lesion, part of a breathing patient, is a moving target. The extent of the ablation is limited by large vessels adjacent to the tumors, which prevent a complete ablation because of the so-called heat-sink effect, caused by the circulating blood (Lu et al. 2002).

Nevertheless the advantage of RFA is that it can be repeated with multiple repeat ablations to destroy residual tumor. Furthermore RFA, even if it achieves less than 100% tumor necrosis, may prove complementary to chemotherapy and radiation therapy in the treatment of lung tumors.

5.1.6 Limitations and Complications of CT-Guided Percutaneously RF-Ablated Lung Lesions

Technical problems occur in <5% and consist of hard tumors bouncing off the electrode tip, desiccated tissue that adheres to the electrode tines and

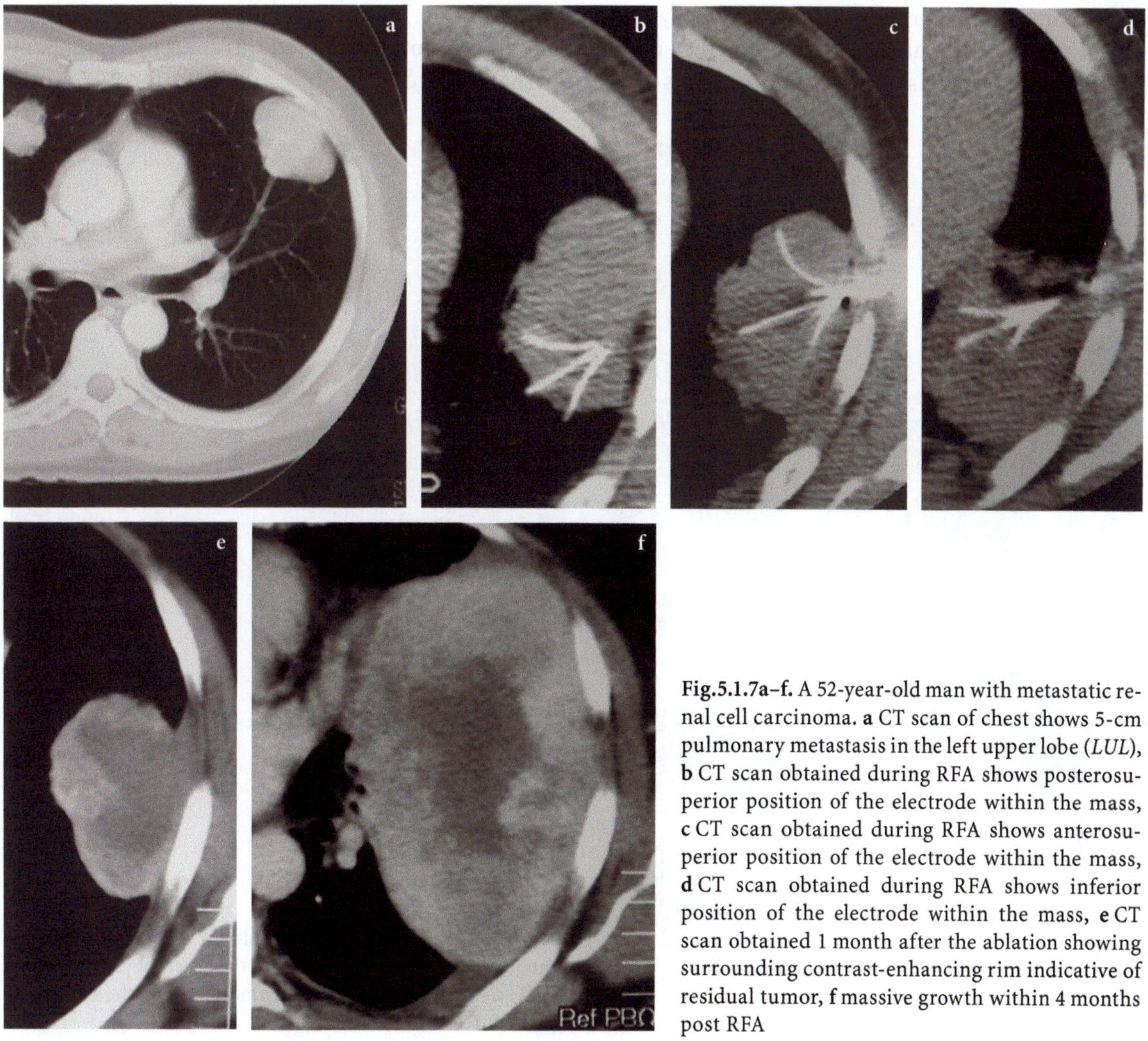

Fig.5.1.7a–f. A 52-year-old man with metastatic renal cell carcinoma. **a** CT scan of chest shows 5-cm pulmonary metastasis in the left upper lobe (*LUL*), **b** CT scan obtained during RFA shows posterosuperior position of the electrode within the mass, **c** CT scan obtained during RFA shows anterosuperior position of the electrode within the mass, **d** CT scan obtained during RFA shows inferior position of the electrode within the mass, **e** CT scan obtained 1 month after the ablation showing surrounding contrast-enhancing rim indicative of residual tumor, **f** massive growth within 4 months post RFA

possibly preventing the easy withdrawal of the electrodes into the trocar, and failure to reach target temperature.

Lesions abutting the heart or major bronchi and vessels also constitute a technical challenge, both for spiking the tumor without harming these structures, but mainly for a successful and complete ablation due to cooling effects of the circulating blood.

5.1.6.1 Pneumothorax and Intraparenchymal Hemorrhage

Pneumothorax occurs fairly commonly; approximately one-third of the patients with metastatic lung disease of extrapulmonary origin and approximately half of the patients with primary lung cancer (not abutting the pleural surface) develop a pneumothorax during the ablation procedure (Fig. 5.1.8). In patients with prior lung surgery or biopsy at the target site the pleural sheets stick together and as a consequence the risk for pneumothorax is lower. Pneumothorax occurs more often with multiple procedures. In patients who developed a pneumothorax an average of 2.6 lesions were treated compared with 1.4 lesions treated in those without pneumothorax (Steinke et al. 2003).

The pneumothorax rate for lung biopsies reported in the literature ranges from 19% to 60% (Richardson et al. 2002) with requirement for chest drain ranging between 3% (Saji et al. 2002) and 50% (Richardson et al. 2002).

Hemorrhage is a known complication in lung RFA, and results from the positioning of the device rather than from the ablative procedure (Fig. 5.1.9). While the reported percentage of infection (< 1%) and bronchopleural fistula formation (< 1%) in the literature (Dupuy et al. 2002) accords with our experience, the occurrence of pneumothorax, reported as 20% (Dupuy et al. 2002; Vaughn et al. 2002), and the incidence of hemorrhage, reported as < 1%, seem to be underestimates.

Data in the literature for percutaneous biopsy-related pneumothoraces and intraparenchymal hemorrhage range from 8.2% and 1.4% for fine needle

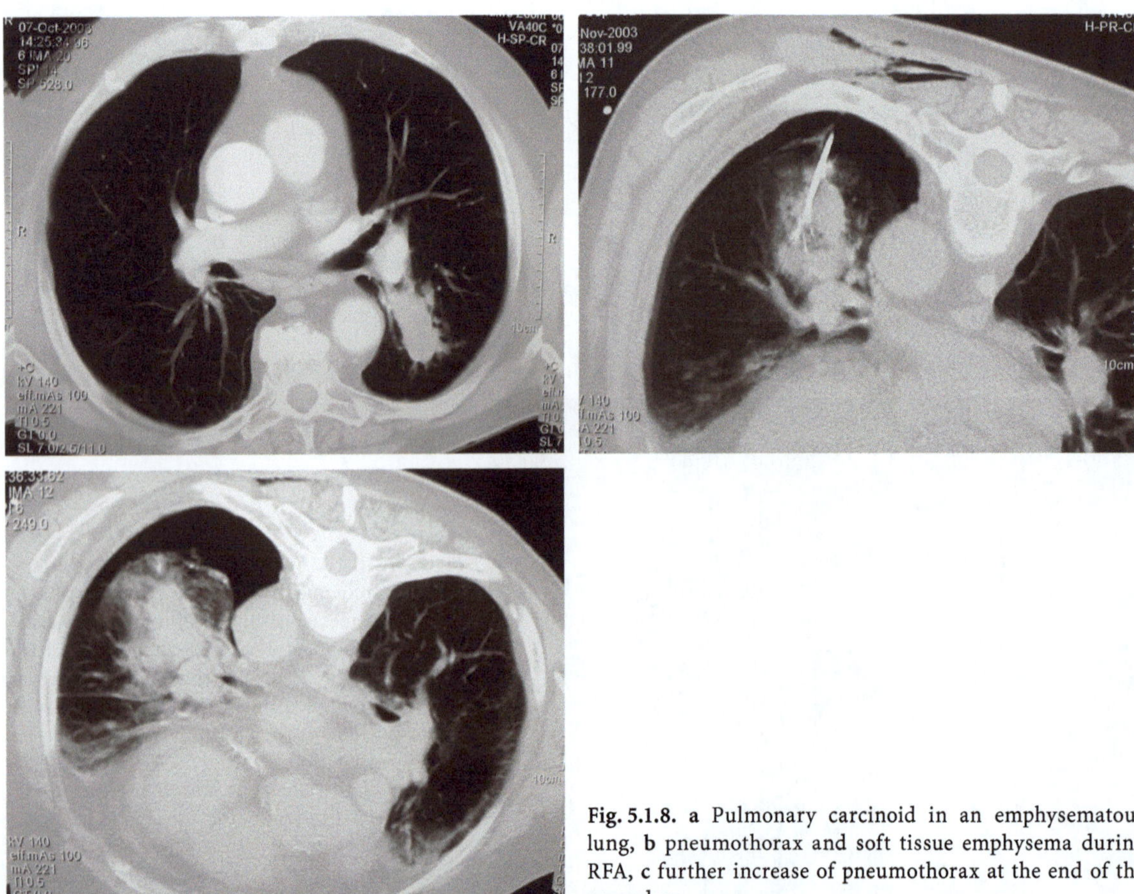

Fig. 5.1.8. **a** Pulmonary carcinoid in an emphysematous lung, **b** pneumothorax and soft tissue emphysema during RFA, **c** further increase of pneumothorax at the end of the procedure

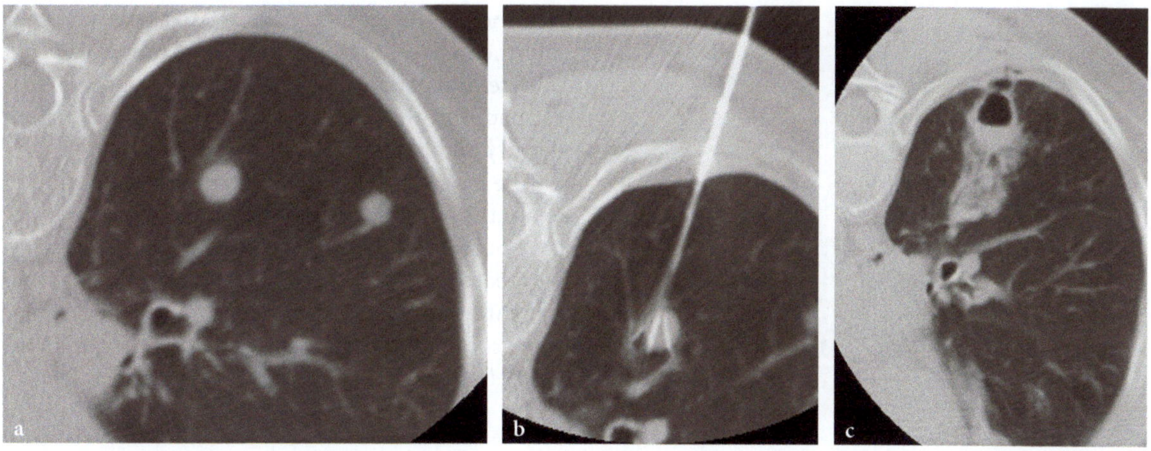

Fig. 5.1.9a–c. Hemorrhage and cavitation during RFA. **a** Two metastases of colorectal carcinoma (*CRC*) in the LLL; **b** start of RFA of the medially located metastasis; **c** hemorrhage upon further hook deployment and cavitation post track ablation

aspirations (FNA) with a 22-gauge needle (Arslan et al. 2002) to 24% and 29% for core biopsies with a 20 gauge needle (Arslan et al. 2002). The largest study published is a survey of UK practice of 5444 biopsies, which reports a pneumothorax rate of 20.5% and a rate of hemoptysis of 5.3% (Lopez Hanninen et al. 2001). The hemoptysis rate does not allow a conclusion to be made on the rate of intraparenchymal hemorrhage, as none of the 29% with lung hemorrhage in Richardson's work has been reported as having had hemoptysis. Taking into account the thicker RF device (14 gauge) and that we perform multiple ablations, this can explain our higher pneumothorax rate than that seen with simple diagnostic biopsy. The discrepancy between the reported data and our results may be explained by a bias in patient inclusion and management. We ablate up to six metastases per hemithorax. The size and central lesions' location close to major vessels and bronchi are not a contraindication to treating multiple lesions, as it was earlier in our experience.

Practitioners of RFA should be aware of the risk of peri-procedural intrapulmonary hemorrhage, which is usually self-limiting, but according to the literature (Dupuy et al. 2002; Vaughn et al. 2002) can also be massive and lead to death.

For patients with poor respiratory reserve, as often encountered in heavy smokers, severe parenchymal hemorrhage may lead to a sudden deterioration of oxygen saturation, which could be even more difficult to manage than in the setting of open resection.

A careful medication history should be taken, including the use of anticoagulants or anti-platelet drugs use, which, if considered necessary, should be discontinued for the appropriate period before ablation. When evaluating patients for RFA treatment pulmonary artery hypertension (PAH) should be taken into account and echocardiographic evaluation of tricuspid regurgitation should be undertaken prior to treatment, especially when targeting central lesions such as that shown in this case report.

5.1.6.2 Skin Burns

First-, second- and third-degree burns at the grounding pad site during and after RFA do occasionally occur. We have experienced two severe skin burns after open liver RFA and one after percutaneous liver RFA (Fig. 5.1.10). All dispersive pads are believed to have been placed correctly; none of the pads have been noticed to be improperly attached at the end of the ablation procedures. The use of higher currents for a longer period of time in RFA of tumors has led to an increased incidence of pad burns in our experience as well as that of others.

We have delivered the maximum power (150 W) in a stepwise progression for relatively prolonged times (121, 72, and 45 min) in all three patients with severe pad burns.

Further factors that may constitute a risk for skin burns are vascular disease with poor peripheral circulation, artery bypass grafts, diabetes, and a history of peripheral neuropathy.

The complication of skin burns seems to be underestimated; especially, the rate of mild skin irritations seems to get lost to follow-up, as the patients

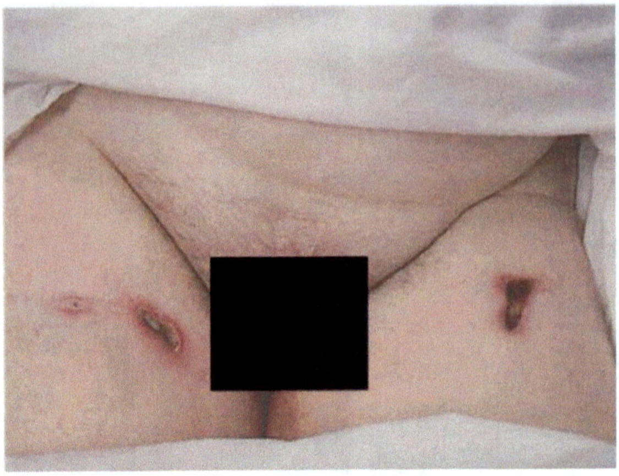

Fig. 5.1.10. Skin burns at grounding pad site on both thighs

are usually discharged the same day or the day after the (percutaneous) procedure and they probably do not consider the pad burns a serious problem.

There are reports that a threshold temperature required to produce thermal injury at the pad site is between 45°C and 47°C (Berber et al. 2000). Whilst rapidly advancing RFA technology allows a large ablation diameter, the factors that control the ablation size on the active electrodes also play an equally important role in the dispersive electrodes site, as the same current flows through both these electrodes. These factors include the current density, the amount of power delivered and the factors that affect heat distribution such as blood flow and conduction and convection of heat.

The current density at the dispersive pad site is intended to be small due to the large surface area of the grounding pad. Mitchell et al. determined the minimum area of the pad for the diathermy units (Pearce et al. 1997). They suggest a maximum safe power density of approximately 1.5 W/cm^2. Therefore, for a maximum power output of 200 W the minimum required surface area of the dispersive pad is 133 cm^2.

The orientation of the dispersive pads was shown by Goldberg et al. to be an important factor in the maximum temperature that is reached in the skin at the pad site (Goldberg et al. 2001). The leading edge is the site of maximum power concentration and therefore the side of the pad with the largest edge should face the active electrode. Proper pad placement is critical to the avoidance of burns. Skin preparation with shaving of the area the pads are to be placed on and proper cleansing of the skin are essential to avoid poor contact. The placement of multiple pads needs close attention in that the level and the distance of the pads relative to each other and the active electrode should be similar to avoid preferential path of current return through the closest pad and therefore result in too high a current density and burns.

The burns noted had occurred within a period of 5 months and no further burns except one first-degree burn in a lung patient with multiple metastases treated and an ablation time over 2 h were noted thereafter, although we have not changed the ablation protocol – thus malfunctioning of the pads cannot definitely be ruled out.

5.1.6.3
Pleural Effusion

A small amount of pleural effusion is usually seen during the RFA procedure, increasing in size with ablation duration and number of lesions treated. On the control erect chest radiograph post intervention the lateral costophrenic angle is obliterated. These effusions, sympathetic in character, do not require tapping. They usually resolve within a couple of days and are asymptomatic.

5.1.6.4
Cavitation and Infection

Cavitation at the ablation site occurs in about 25% of lesions, but it usually resolves uneventfully. Cavitation is seen significantly more frequently when the size of the lesion at 1 week after treatment exceeds the size of the pretreatment lesion by 200% or more, $p=0.0001$ (Steinke et al. 2003).

Expectoration of ablated lung particles occasionally is observed, without any clinical signs of pneumonia or abscess.

It should be mandatory for the treatment and patient care that the clinical status of the patient is more important than the radiological features. If a slight fever for a few days following the RF procedure does not increase, or is accompanied by chills, malaise, and pain that is more than the usually encountered mild pleuritic pain and thus possibly indicating pneumonia or abscess formation, the patient can be discharged with non-opioid analgesics.

The typical course of a cavitating lesion is shown in (Fig. 5.1.11).

Some centers performing RFA apply prophylactic intravenous antibiotics on the day of the interven-

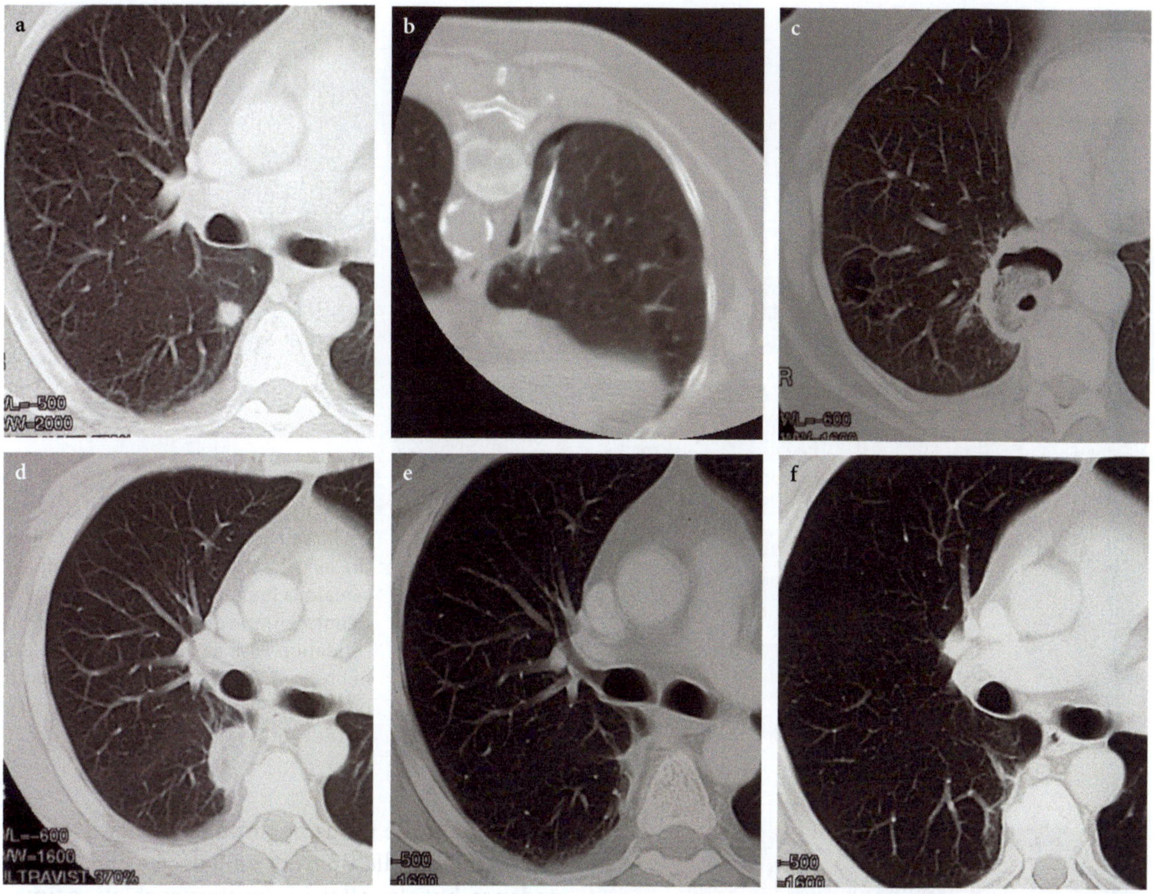

Fig. 5.1.11a–f. Typical course of a cavitating lesion. **a** Small initial lesion, **b** RFA, **c** central cavitation within the ablated area, exceeding the initial lesion volume by at least 200% 1 month post RFA, **d** resorption of cavitation at 3 months post RFA, **e** residual pleural-based thickening 6 months post RFA, **f** complete resolution

tion prior to the ablation; others even cover the day before and the day after ablation.

Abscess formation may be delayed by as long as 3 weeks (Fig. 5.1.12), may require drainage or even surgical intervention and, in patients with poor health and marginal cardiopulmonary function, may even be fatal.

5.1.6.5 Other Complications

A most unusual technical problem upon trying to withdraw the electrode hooks into the shaft following lung RFA may occur if charred ablated tissue caught in the space between the hooks and the shaft or sticking to the hooks subsequently hinders the hooks from being withdrawn into the shaft.

Charred tissue sticking to the electrodes is very often observed and usually can be overcome by redeploying and retracting the hooks a few times. In our experience a considerable amount of charred tissue sticking to the tines is seen if the impedance rises above 200 Ω associated with low power requirements <20 W to maintain the target temperature. In impedance-based systems this is the end-point of the ablation cycle; however, in temperature-based systems the ablation cycle may proceed despite the so-called roll-off if the set time has not been reached yet. If the impedance does not rise above 900 Ω, which would lead to automatic switch-off of the generator, the charring advances as the heat cannot further dissipate into the surrounding tissue. To prevent or minimize tissue charring in the setting of rising impedance, it may be useful to pause the delivery of RF energy, fully retract the electrode arrays, rotate and re-deploy the arrays and then resume delivery of RF energy.

Compared to the liver, which is a homogeneous solid organ, the lung seems to be predisposed more

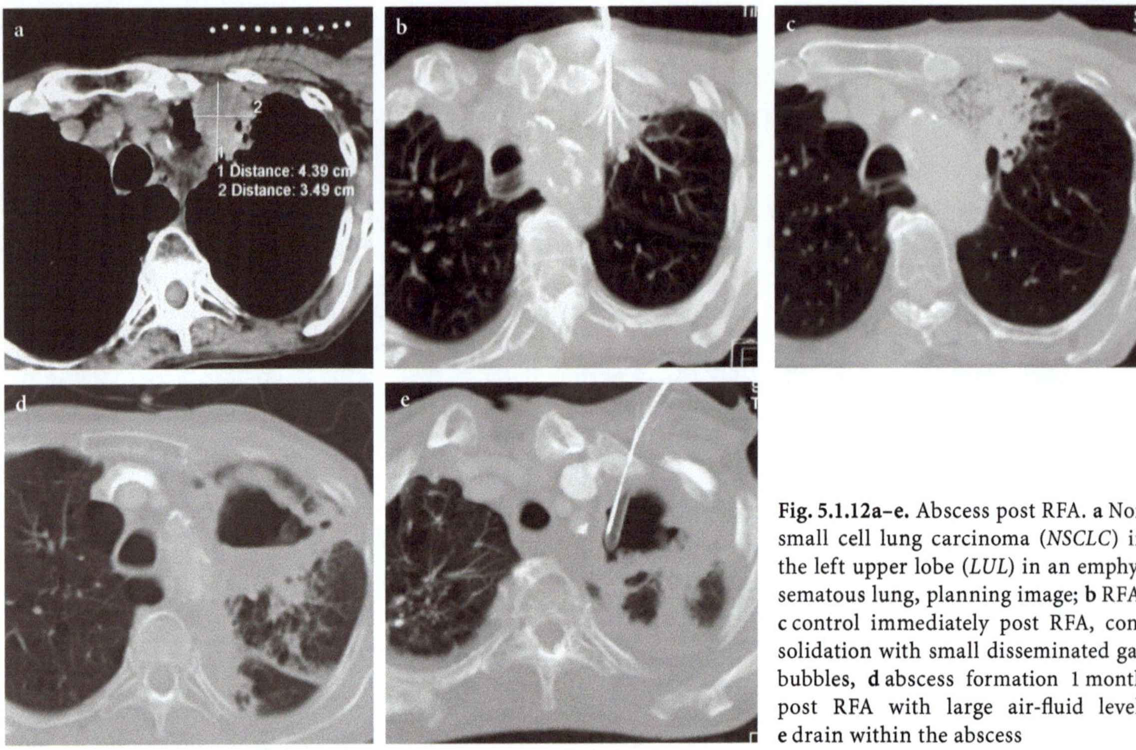

Fig. 5.1.12a–e. Abscess post RFA. **a** Non small cell lung carcinoma (*NSCLC*) in the left upper lobe (*LUL*) in an emphysematous lung, planning image; **b** RFA, **c** control immediately post RFA, consolidation with small disseminated gas bubbles, **d** abscess formation 1 month post RFA with large air-fluid level, **e** drain within the abscess

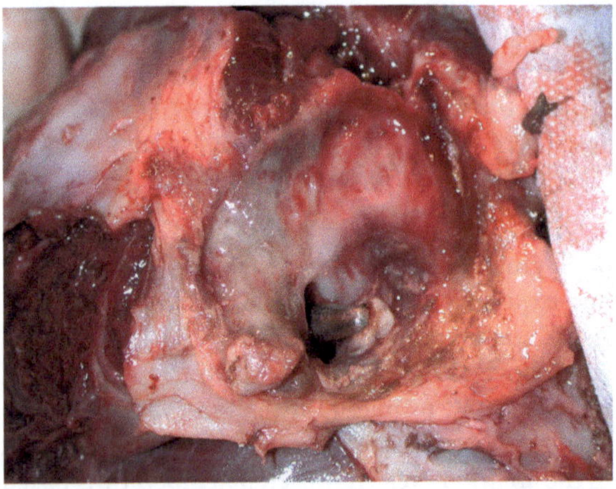

Fig. 5.1.13. Bronchopleural fistula, marked by the tip of the forceps

to charring due to its tissue composition with alternating air-filled spaces and bronchovascular bundles. As the aim of the RFA is not only to ablate the solid tumor, but also a 1-cm safety margin surrounding the tumor, this safety margin consists of normal healthy air-filled lung tissue that may lead to charring.

A possible solution to this problem might be injection of saline, either through a central access provided on the probe or through holes within the retractable needle tips, not only decreasing the impedance, but also allowing for shorter ablation times and significantly larger ablation lesions (Miao et al. 2001; Ahmed and Lobo 2002).

Bronchopleural fistula has been reported as a complication after lung RFA (Jungraithmayr et al. 2005), we have observed and documented it after the ablation of sheep lung (Fig. 5.1.13).

As for CT-guided biopsy the risk for air embolism applies similarly for RFA, especially if a coaxial technique is used.

5.1.7 Conclusion and Future Outlook

Local ablation of pulmonary disease is used for unresectable tumors. The advantages of local tumor destruction include selective tissue damage with less immunosuppression and less release of growth factors, minimal treatment morbidity and mortality, lower costs compared to open surgery, and a considerable gain in quality of life. Nevertheless, as the procedure is not free of complications, a careful assessment of risks and benefits has to be made in each patient by a multidisciplinary team.

The ultimate goal of local ablation treatment is to prolong survival. Presently, however, influence on survival is difficult to estimate because of the heterogeneity of indications and treatments and short follow-up times. There are no prospective, randomized studies comparing local destruction methods. RFA seems to be by far the best treatment option.

Successful RFA can be divided into technical and clinical success. The aim is to achieve local tumor control. The advantage of RFA is its repeatability with multiple possible repeat ablations, either to destroy residual tumor or to treat recurrent disease. Furthermore, even if RFA achieves less than 100% tumor destruction, it may prove to be complementary to chemotherapy and radiation therapy in the treatment of lung tumors.

Lower morbidity and mortality, as well as a better life quality accompany this treatment with the additional possibility for patients to be treated on an overnight or outpatient base.

References

Adams F (1886) Translator. Genuine works of Hippocrates. William Wood, New York

Ahmed M, Lobo SM (2002) Improved coagulation with saline solution pretreatment during radiofrequency tumor ablation in a canine model. J Vasc Interv Radiol 13:717–724

Ahrar K, Price RE, Wallace MJ, Madoff DC, Gupta S, Morello FA Jr, Wright KC (2003) Percutaneous radiofrequency ablation of lung tumors in a large animal model. J Vasc Interv Radiol 14(8):1037–1043

Arslan S, Yilmaz A, Bayramgurler B, Uzman O, Nver E, Akkaya E (2002) CT-guided transthoracic fine needle aspiration of pulmonary lesions: accuracy and complications in 294 patients. Med Sci Monit 8:493–497

Berber E, Flesher NL, Siperstein AE (2000) Initial clinical evaluation of the RITA 5-centimeter radiofrequency thermal ablation catheter in the treatment of liver tumors. Cancer J 6:319–329

Brescia FJ (2001) Lung cancer – a philosophical, ethical, and personal perspective. Crit Rev Oncol Hematol 40(2):139–148

Brown LM, Malkinson AM, Rannels DE, Rannels SR (1999) Compensatory lung growth after partial pneumonectomy enhances lung tumorigenesis induced by 3-methylcholanthrene. Cancer Res 59(20):5089–5092

Campione A, Ligabue T, Luzzi L, Ghiribelli C, Paladini P, Voltolini L, Di Bisceglie M, Lonzi M, Gotti G (2004) Impact of size, histology, and gender on stage IA non-small cell lung cancer. Asian Cardiovasc Thorac Ann 12(2):149–153

Carlson SK, Bender CE, Classic KL, Zink FE, Quam JP, Ward EM, Oberg AL (2001) Benefits and safety of CT fluoroscopy in interventional radiologic procedures. Radiology 219(2):515–520

Colacchio TA, Yeager MP, Hildebrandt LW (1994) Perioperative immunomodulation in cancer surgery. Am J Surg 167(1):174–179

Curley SA (2001) Radiofrequency ablation of malignant liver tumors. Oncologist 6:14–23

Davidson RS, Nwogu CE, Brentjens MJ, Anderson TM (2001) The surgical management of pulmonary metastasis: current concepts. Surg Oncol 10(1-2):35–42

Dodd GD 3rd, Soulen MC, Kane RA, Livraghi T, Lees WR, Yamashita Y, Gillams AR, Karahan OI, Rhim H (2000) Minimally invasive treatment of malignant hepatic tumors: at the threshold of a major breakthrough. Radiographics 20(1):9–27

Dupuy DE, Mayo-Smith WW, Abbott GF, DiPetrillo T (2002) Clinical applications of radio-frequency tumor ablation in the thorax. Radiographics 22:259–269

Faivre J, Bouvier AM, Bonithon-Kopp C (2002) Epidemiology and screening of colorectal cancer. Best Pract Res Clin Gastroenterol 16(2):187–199

Friedel G, Pastorino U, Buyse M, Ginsberg RJ, Girard P, Goldstraw P, Johnston M, McCormack P, Pass H, Putnam JB, Toomes H (1999) Resection of lung metastases: long-term results and prognostic analysis based on 5206 cases – the International Registry of Lung Metastases. Zentralbl Chir 124(2):96–103

Friedel G, Pastorino U, Ginsberg RJ, Goldstraw P, Johnston M, Pass H, Putnam JB, Toomes H (2002) Results of lung metastasectomy from breast cancer: prognostic criteria on the basis of 467 cases of the International Registry of Lung Metastases. Eur J Cardiothorac Surg 22(3):335–344

Goldberg SN, Gazelle GS, Compton CC, McLoud TC (1995) Radiofrequency tissue ablation in the rabbit lung: efficacy and complications. Acad Radiol. 2(9):776–784

Goldberg SN, Gazelle GS, Compton CC, Mueller PR, McLoud TC (1996) Radio-frequency tissue ablation of VX2 tumor nodules in the rabbit lung. Acad Radiol 3(11):929–935

Goldberg SN, Ahmed M, Gazelle GS, Kruskal JB, Huertas JC, Halpern EF, Oliver BS, Lenkinski RE (2001) Radiofrequency thermal ablation with NaCl solution injection: effect of electrical conductivity on tissue heating and coagulation-phantom and porcine liver study. Radiology 219(1):157–165

Gromkowski SH, Yagi J, Janeway CA Jr (1989) Elevated temperature regulates tumor necrosis factor-mediated immune killing. Eur J Immunol 19(9):1709–1714

Hansen E, Wolff N, Knuechel R, Ruschoff J, Hofstaedter F, Taeger K (1995) Tumor cells in blood shed from the surgical field. Arch Surg 130(4):387–393

Ishii H, Okada S, Okusaka T, Yoshimori M, Nakasuka H, Shimada K, Yamasaki S, Nakanishi Y, Sakamoto M (1998) Needle tract implantation of hepatocellular carcinoma after percutaneous ethanol injection. Cancer 82(9):1638–1642

Jungraithmayr W, Schafer O, Stoelben E, Hasse J, Passlick B (2005) Radiofrequency ablation of malignant lung tumours. Judicious approach? Chirurg 76(9):887–893

Lefor AT, Foster CE 3rd, Sartor W, Engbrecht B, Fabian DF, Silverman D (1994) Hyperthermia increases intercellular adhesion molecule-1 expression and lymphocyte adhesion to endothelial cells. Surgery 116(2):214–220; discussion 220–221

Livraghi T, Goldberg SN, Lazzaroni S, Meloni F, Ierace T, Solbiati L, Gazelle GS (2000) Hepatocellular carcinoma: radio-frequency ablation of medium and large lesions. Radiology 214:761–768

Llovet JM, Vilana R, Bru C, Bianchi L, Salmeron JM, Boix L, Ganau S, Sala M, Pages M, Ayuso C, Sole M, Rodes J, Bruix J (2001) Increased risk of tumor seeding after percutaneous radiofrequency ablation for single hepatocellular carcinoma. Hepatology 33(5):1124–1129

Lopez Hanninen E, Vogl TJ, Ricke J, Felix R (2001) CT-guided percutaneous core biopsies of pulmonary lesions. Diagnostic accuracy, complications and therapeutic impact. Acta Radiol 42:151–155

Lu DS, Raman SS, Vodopich DJ, Wang M, Sayre J, Lassman C (2002) Effect of vessel size on creation of hepatic radiofrequency lesions in pigs: assessment of the "heat sink" effect. AJR Am J Roentgenol 178(1):47–51

Luderitz B (2003) Historical perspectives on interventional electrophysiology. J Interv Card Electrophysiol 9(2):75–83

MacManus MP, Hicks RJ (2003) PET scanning in lung cancer: current status and future directions. Semin Surg Oncol 21(3):149–155

McCormack PM, Ginsberg RJ (1998) Current management of colorectal metastases to lung. Chest Surg Clin N Am 8(1):119–126

Miao Y, Ni Y, Bosmans H, Yu J, Vaninbroukx J, Dymarkowski S, Zhang H, Marchal G (2001) Radiofrequency ablation for eradication of pulmonary tumor in rabbits. J Surg Res 99(2):265–271

Mineo TC, Ambrogi V, Tonini G, Nofroni I (2001) Pulmonary metastasectomy: might the type of resection affect survival? J Surg Oncol 76:47–52

Mulier S, Mulier P, Ni Y, Miao Y, Dupas B, Marchal G, De Wever I, Michel L (2002) Complications of radiofrequency coagulation of liver tumours. Br J Surg 89(10):1206–1222

Okawara G, Ung YC, Markman BR, Mackay JA, Evans WK (2004) Postoperative radiotherapy in stage II or IIIA completely resected non-small cell lung cancer: a systematic review and practice guideline. Lung Cancer 44(1):1–11

Ollila DW, Morton DL (1998) Surgical resection as the treatment of choice for melanoma metastatic to the lung. Chest Surg Clin N Am 8(1):183–196

Oturai AB, Jensen K, Eriksen J, Madsen F (1996) Neurosurgery for trigeminal neuralgia: comparison of alcohol block, neurectomy and radiofrequency coagulation. Clin J Pain 12:311–315

Pastorino U (2002) History of the surgical management of pulmonary metastases and development of the International Registry. Semin Thorac Cardiovasc Surg 14(1):18–28

Pearce JA, Geddes LA, Bourland JD, Silva LF (1979) The thermal behaviour of electrolyte-coated metal-foil dispersive electrodes. Med Instrum 13:298–300

Penna C, Nordlinger B (2002) Colorectal metastasis (liver and lung). Surg Clin North Am 82(5):1075–1090

Pfannschmidt J, Hoffmann H, Muley T, Krysa S, Trainer C, Dienemann H (2002) Prognostic factors for survival after pulmonary resection of metastatic renal cell carcinoma. Ann Thorac Surg 74(5):1653–1657

Quesson B, de Zwart JA, Moonen CT (2000) Magnetic resonance temperature imaging for guidance of thermotherapy. J Magn Reson Imaging 12(4):525–533

Richardson CM, Pointon KS, Manhire AR, MacFarlane JT (2002) Percutaneous lung biopsies: a survey of UK practice based on 5444 biopsies. Br J Radiol 75:731–735

Rohren EM, Turkington TG, Coleman RE (2004) Clinical applications of PET in oncology. Radiology 231(2):305–332

Rosenthal DI, Hornicek FJ, Wolfe MW, Jennings LC, Gebhardt MC, Mankin HJ (1998) Percutaneous radiofrequency coagulation of osteoid osteoma compared with operative treatment. J Bone Joint Surg Am 80:815–821

Saji H, Nakamura H, Tsuchida T et al (2002) The incidence and the risk of pneumothorax and chest tube placement after percutaneous CT-guided lung biopsy: the angle of the needle trajectory is a novel predictor. Chest 121(5):1521–1526

Salgia R, Skarin AT (1998) Molecular abnormalities in lung cancer. J Clin Oncol 16(3):1207–1217

Seki T, Wakabayashi M, Nakagawa T, Imamura M, Tamai T, Nishimura A, Yamashiki N, Okamura A, Inoue K (1999) Percutaneous microwave coagulation therapy for patients with small hepatocellular carcinoma: comparison with percutaneous ethanol injection therapy. Cancer 85(8):1694–1702

Srivastava P (2002) Roles of heat-shock proteins in innate and adaptive immunity. Nat Rev Immunol 2(3):185–194

Steinke K, Habicht J, Thomsen S, Jacob LA (2002) CT-guided radiofrequency ablation of a pulmonary metastasis followed by surgical resection: a case report. Cardiovasc Intervent Radiol 25:543–546

Steinke K, King J, Glenn D, Morris DL (2003) Radiologic appearance and complications of percutaneous computed tomography-guided radiofrequency-ablated pulmonary metastases from colorectal carcinoma. J Comput Assist Tomogr 27:750–757

Steinke K, Haghighi KS, Wulf S, Morris DL (2005) Effect of vessel diameter on the creation of ovine lung radiofrequency lesions in vivo: preliminary results. J Surg Res 124(1):85–91

Strauss GM (1997) Prognostic markers in resectable non-small cell lung cancer. Hematol Oncol Clin North Am 11(3):409–434

Vaughn C, Mychaskiw G, Sewell P (2002) Massive hemorrhage during radiofrequency ablation of a pulmonary neoplasm. Anesth Analg 94:1149–1151

Visioli AG, Rivens IH, ter Haar GR, Horwich A, Huddart RA, Moskovic E et al (1999) Preliminary results of a phase I dose escalation clinical trial using focused ultrasound in the treatment of localized tumours. Eur J Ultrasound 9(1):11–18

Vogl TJ, Fieguth HG, Eichler K, Straub R, Lehnert T, Zangos S, Mack M (2004) Laser-induced thermotherapy of lung metastases and primary lung tumors. Radiologe 44(7):693–699

Wales LR, Stark P, Morishima MS (1981) Percutaneous aspiration biopsy of the lung. The double needle technique. Radiologe 21(3):150–154

Wang HW, Zhang YQ, Luo J, Yan X, Lu HY (2004) Percutaneous lung cancer cryotherapy guided by computer tomography. Zhonghua Jie He He Hu Xi Za Zhi 27(5):311–314

Yasui K, Kanazawa S, Sano Y, Fujiwara T, Kagawa S, Mimura H, Dendo S, Mukai T, Fujiwara H, Iguchi T, Hyodo T, Shimizu N, Tanaka N, Hiraki Y (2004) Thoracic tumors treated with CT-guided radiofrequency ablation: initial experience. Radiology 231(3):850–857

Lung

5

5.2 Laser-Induced Thermotherapy (LITT) in the Treatment of Lung Metastases

Thomas J. Vogl, Martin G. Mack, and Mohammed Nabil

CONTENTS

5.2.1 Introduction

Pulmonary metastases are very common, being more frequently associated with tumors that have a rich systemic venous drainage, such as bone sarcomas, choriocarcinomas, melanomas, testicular teratomas, and renal and thyroid carcinomas. The detection of pulmonary metastases is crucial in the treatment of patients with cancer.

Tumor metastases reach the lung via the systemic veins and pulmonary arteries and subsequently lodge in the small pulmonary arteries or arterioles and extend into adjacent lung tissue forming multiple, spherical, and variably sized pulmonary nodules. Metastases that occur via bronchial arteries, pulmonary lymphatics, transbronchial aspiration, and across the pleural cavity are less common (Isaac Hassan, Lung metastases, at http://www.emedicine.com/radio/topic404.htm).

Metastasectomy, at present, is considered to be the gold standard of local tumor therapy for lung metastases just as it is in the liver, although the lung lacks the liver's high regenerative ability. A 5-year survival of 20%–62% and a long-term survival of up to 10 years were reported (Vogl et al. 2004). The chances of curative success depend upon different variables, which are as follows: more favorable in solitary rather than multiple metastases, in metachronous rather than synchronous metastases, and in colorectal rather than other primary tumors. The decision of metastasectomy usually requires the patient to be free from extrapulmonary metastases. Moreover, appropriate therapy of extrapulmonary metastases needs to be available (Diederich and Hosten 2004; Weigel et al. 2004). The cardiopulmonary reserve of the patient should permit a radical resection. R0-resection should be technically possible and no other superior less-invasive therapy option such as systemic therapy should be available. An advantage of the latter was unacceptably high parenchymal loss with resection compared to thermal ablation. Nevertheless, new parenchymal-sparing surgical techniques can overcome this problem (Diederich and Hosten 2004). The video-assisted thoracoscopy operation is one of the less invasive surgical procedures which are increasingly accepted. This procedure is possible only in up to 20% of all patients, since the lesion must be located in the outer third of the lung or in the interlobar fissures. The proportion of patients treatable by this procedure could be increased, if it were to be complemented by another procedure such as percutaneous ablation.

T. J. Vogl, MD, Professor; M. G. Mack, MD, PD;
M. Nabil, MD
Institute for Diagnostic and Interventional Radiology, University Hospital, Johann Wolfgang Goethe University, Theodor-Stern-Kai 7, 60590 Frankfurt, Germany

Minimally invasive interventional management of lung metastases can be categorized into percutaneous thermal ablation and the recently developed transarterial chemoembolization. All these methods are relatively new and almost all are widely regarded as experimental.

Radiofrequency is the most widespread percutaneous thermal ablation technique used in liver tumors. In the few studies in which it was used in lung tumors it achieved a morphological response of up to 100% with a mean survival of up to 19.7 months (Lee et al. 2004).

One of the image-guided percutaneous modalities is microwave ablation in lung cancer showing marked effect with minimum tissue trauma. The overall response rate in one of the studies reached 57.1% without sideeffects or complications (Feng et al. 2002). Complete tumor necrosis was proven by biopsy.

Laser-induced thermotherapy (LITT) has been performed in several centers with different devices and applications showing promising results.

Transarterial chemoembolization was performed using an endovascular balloon catheter introduced into the segmental pulmonary arteries for superselective injection of the chemotherapeutic drugs lipiodol and microspheres, while the inflated balloon prevented backflow of embolic material into the main pulmonary artery. A mean decrease in tumor volume of 56.8% was found as a response to treatment. It might well be a promising treatment modality in the future after it has been adequately developed to provide maximum effectiveness (Vogl et al. 2005).

5.2.2 Physical Principles

The physical mechanism of tumor destruction using laser ablation is temperature elevation within the tumor core by the laser fiber high enough to induce coagulation necrosis. Laser coagulation is performed by using neodymium–yttrium aluminium garnet (Nd:YAG) laser light (Dornier mediLas 5060, Dornier mediLas 5100; Dornier Medizintechnik, Germering, Germany) with a wavelength of 1064 nm. The light is delivered through 400-mm-long fibers terminated by a specially developed diffuser which emits laser light to an effective distance of up to 12–15 mm (Knappe and Mols 2004; Vogl et al. 2004b; Weigel et al. 2004).

The water content was estimated to be 83.7% of human lung parenchyma. This relatively high water content (water content being only 71.5% in the liver) leads to good thermal conduction and high thermal capacity. Thus, induced warmth is stored, and the heat front spreads only slowly into the periphery. Hence, in comparison to the liver, higher temperatures yet longer exposure times are required ranging between 10 and 30 min for clinically relevant lesion sizes. An effective rise in temperature leads to thermal change and tissue damage. Since a part of the energy as a function of the temperature gradient diffuses into the colder environment, thermally induced necroses can reach sizes that exceed the optical penetration depth (Knappe and Mols 2004).

The lung has a complex structure of ventilated alveoli and bronchi in addition to blood vessels. The air-filled cavities work as heat insulators, while the enclosing capillary beds function as heat dissipaters. Air in the bronchial system is continually exchanged by ventilation, and, similarly, the high blood circulation carries away heat. The location-dependent variability of these structures can lead to a variation in thermal parameters. In addition, the metastatic lesions vary in their optical and thermal characteristics depending upon the histology of the primary tumor (Knappe and Mols 2004).

Energy propagation from radiofrequency ablation is focused on the solid tumor portions due to the insulating effects of the surrounding lung tissue. However, the same effect limits further energy deposition, and the impedance rise at the zone of transition between tumor and lung parenchyma leads to a break of current flow (roll off). In contrast to RFA, the laser functions with the irradiation of coherent monochromatic light, which is appropriately absorbed by the tissue and works independently of the impedance rise (Knappe and Mols 2004; Vogl et al. 2004c).

5.2.3 Animal Experiments

5.2.3.1 Effect of LITT Ablation on Immunity Stimulation

A relation between ablation and stimulation of the immunity response was considered. This relation was proven through an experimental animal study.

The aim of the study was to compare the effects of LITT and hepatic resection on the immune response to residual intrahepatic tumor tissue and the growth of untreated liver metastases. Adenocarcinoma cells were implanted into both lobes of 60 Wistar Albino Glaxo (WAG) rats. The left lobe tumor was treated either by LITT or partial hepatectomy. The control right lobe tumor was subjected to further investigation at regular intervals after treatment. The expression of several immunity factors was significantly enhanced at the invasion front of untreated control tumors after LITT compared to hepatic resection, which can then lead to reduced tumor growth (Isbert et al. 2004).

A study designed to evaluate the same effect of LITT in lung tumors is being conducted in our department.

5.2.3.2 Effect of LITT Ablation on Tumor Growth

The effect of laser ablation on the stimulation of tumor growth and the relation of this effect to tumor size was studied in an animal model. Colorectal carcinoma liver metastases of various sizes were implanted in 20 WAG rats. The animals were divided into two groups with regard to the measured tumor size. After 14 days, the tumors were exposed to a 1064-nm Nd:YAG laser. The tumor volumes before and after treatment were determined by MRI and the mean tumor growth ratio was calculated. The mean volume of the induced necrosis was the same for both groups. The interventional treatment of large hepatic tumors with LITT led to faster tumor growth compared to smaller lesions (Maataoui et al. 2005).

5.2.4 Pre-interventional Protocol

5.2.4.1 Patient Selection

The indications of LITT in lung metastases, like any other regional treatment of metastases in any organ, can be classified into neoadjuvant, and palliative and/or symptomatic. The curative potential of LITT can be defined as the achievement of long-term survival associated with effective local control. In a patient whose condition is so serious this can be a goal worth achieving. The nature of disseminated malignancies limits the chances of a complete cure because the development of new metastases in the same or another organ is always possible. Besides, there is always the risk of recurrence at the treated location due to incomplete ablation (Fig. 5.2.1). Thus, cure should not always be the primary intention of LITT application in patients with metastases although complete remission can be achieved in some cases.

Neoadjuvant LITT treatment associated with surgery aims mainly at converting inoperable conditions, due to the tumor extent, into operable ones. An example of this is a patient with bilateral involvement of both lung lobes. The ablation of a solitary lesion in one of these lobes would spare this lobe from resection and hence preserve lung tissue which otherwise could not be totally resected surgically. This approach can also spare a whole lung from being surgically molested. In other words, neoadjuvant LITT can minimize the extent of surgical resection by changing the option of pneumonectomy into a lobectomy and lobectomy to segmentectomy or localized resection. LITT can be used as a neoadjuvant measure to systemic chemotherapy especially in the presence of extrapulmonary spread.

On the other hand, it can be used as a palliative measure in cases of inoperability, post-surgical recurrence, or failed systemic chemotherapy leading to symptomatic relief, and hence a better life quality in this group of patients.

Oncological inclusion criteria for LITT vary between different centers. The maximum lesion size to be treated is dependent on the maximum necrosis size attainable which, in turn, depends upon the type and size of needle used. The size ranges from 3.0 to 4.0 cm. Regarding the maximum number of metastases per lung to be treated in one or several settings, the data vary between 3, 6 and 12. No fixed recommendations exist yet. In our experience up to three lesions per lung should be maximum whith a maximum size of 3 cm. The distance of the lesion from vital structures such a major bronchi shout be at least 1 cm. In case of bilateral involvement it is recommended that only one lung is treated in a single session. The contralateral side can be treated after at least 3–4 weeks in another session (Diederich and Hosten 2004; Vogl et al. 2004a).

The same conditions that favor surgical curative success also apply for percutaneous ablation of lung

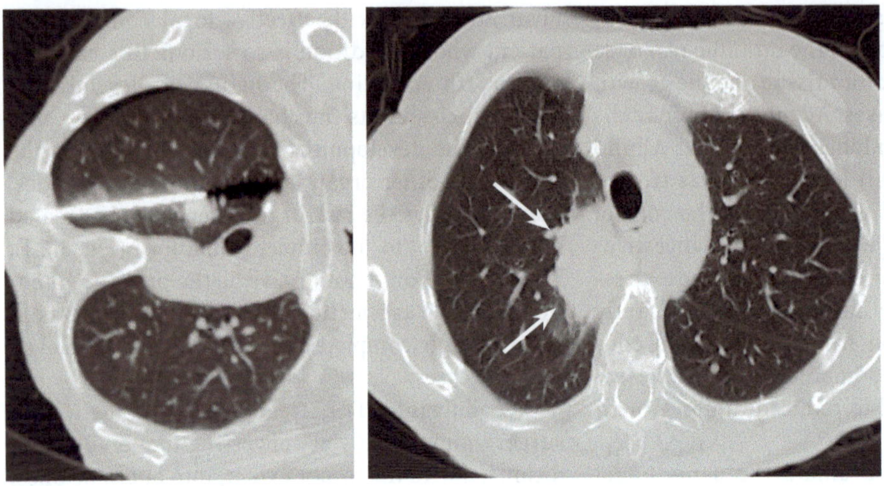
a b

Fig. 5.2.1. **a** A 2-cm upper lobe metastatic lesion during laser-induced thermotherapy (*LITT*) ablation in the left lateral decubitus position. **b** Follow-up CT after 1 year showing a residual lesion in the ablated zone with progression in size (*arrows*)

metastases. However, percutaneous ablation can be applied to patients indicated for operative resection if they have a medical contraindication for surgery or general anesthesia, or if they simply refuse surgery. However, it should be considered that in case of complications of percutaneous tumor ablations, surgical therapy is occasionally necessary (Diederich and Hosten 2004).

5.2.4.2
Pre-treatment Assessment

Preliminary investigations that could be employed are staging computed tomography, laboratory evaluation of tumor markers, bleeding profile, pulmonary function tests, and electrocardiogram (Vogl et al. 2004a).

5.2.5
Equipment and Procedure

5.2.5.1
Laser Applicators

The standard laser application set (SOMATEX, Berlin, Germany) consists of a cannulation needle, a guide wire, a sheath system, and a special double-lumen protective catheter closed at the distal end. Power applicators are 9 F in diameter and internally cooled with a room-temperature sodium chloride solution that circulates within the double-lumen catheter. Cooling the surface of the laser applicator modifies the radial temperature distribution so that the maximum temperature shifts in deeper tissue layers and avoids the carbonization, allowing the use of higher laser power up to 35 W. These parameters result in a more homogeneous tissue penetration of laser radiation. These laser systems are fully compatible with magnetic resonance imaging (MRI) units (Knappe and Mols 2004; Vogl et al. 2004b).

A special "one step system" applicator (Somatex, Berlin, Germany) was developed for more practical and less traumatic lung ablation. It consists of a 9-F Teflon sheath, provided with a sharp end and a stable dilator (Vogl et al. 2004a).

The laser fibers Mikrodom and Mikroflexx (Trumpf Medical Systems) have diffusers of 1, 2, 2.5 or 3 cm in length. For the thermal therapy of lung metastases both flexible and rigid diffusers can be used. The length of the diffuser dome should cover the diameter of the lesion in the access direction with an additional 1 cm safety margin (Weigel et al. 2004).

5.2.5.2
Puncture

The procedure can be performed under CT or MRI guidance. Only local anesthesia and intravenous sedation are usually sufficient. For analgesia and sedation, piritramid (Dipidolor, Janssen Cilaq, Germany) is injected intravenously in a dose dependent on the body weight. All patients are supervised by means of pulse oximeter and electrocardiogram online monitoring. After skin disinfection the optimal entrance to the lesion is selected. It is possible to perform the puncture in supine, decubitus or prone position according to the location of the lesion and puncture access (Fig. 5.2.2). The criteria for optimal entrance planning are based on the location of the lesion and its relation to the pleura, major bronchi, and pulmonary blood vessels. In each case it should be attempted to obtain as acute an angle as possible for entrance through the pleura and to obtain the broadest plane of contact of the laser applicators to the tumor (Vogl et al. 2004a). With small pleural-related lesions, the diffuser length and puncture access should be selected in such a way as to avoid painful heating of the pleura as much as possible, without concessions regarding the safety margin of ablation (Fig. 5.2.3) (Hosten et al. 2003).

First, 10 ml of 0.5% mepivacaine (Scandicain) is injected for local anesthesia. The "one-step system" applicator is advanced under CT fluoroscopy (Care vision, Siemens, Erlangen) directly in the planned route. CT fluoroscopy facilitates near real-time control of the applicator position and its relationship to the vital structures. After verified intratumoral positioning of the system, the inner mandrin is removed and a thermostable catheter is introduced. The flexible laser fiber (Medilas Dornier, Sunnydale, Calif., USA) is then inserted within (Vogl et al. 2004a).

Miniature applicators of 5.5 F facilitate the entrance to the lung, increase cooling efficiency, and minimize complications. This can more appro-

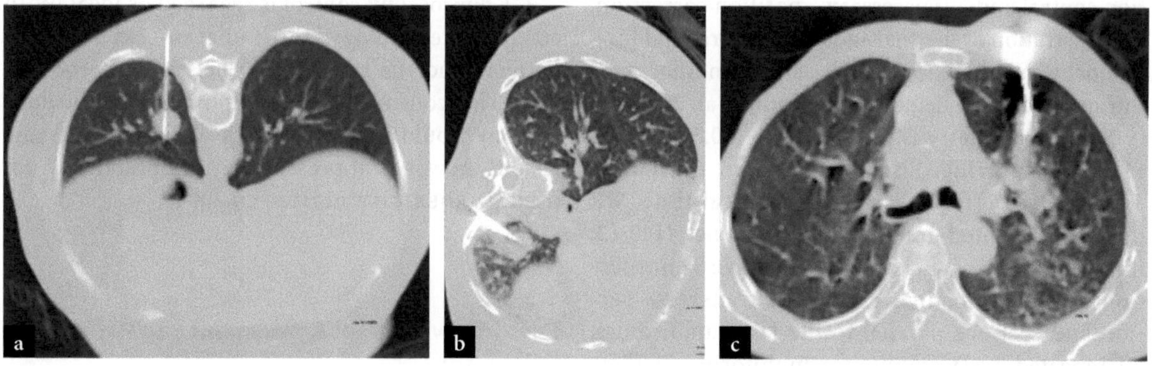

Fig. 5.2.2a–c. Different approaches and patient positions. **a** Prone position for posterior access to treat a posteriorly located lesion. **b** Decubitus position for a similarly located lesion. Posterior approach while the patient lies on the same side of the lesion. This limits the respiratory movements on this side thus facilitating accurate positioning of the applicator. **c** Supine position. An anterior lesion simply treated by anterior access

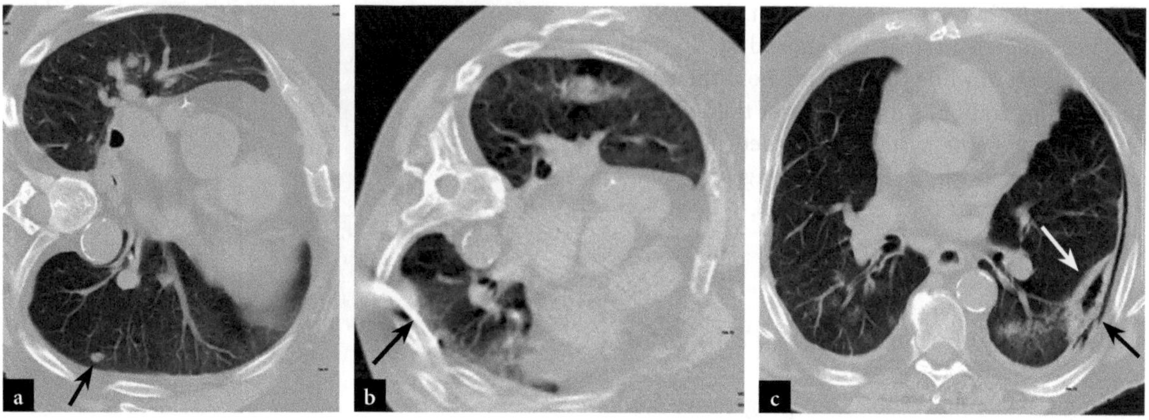

Fig. 5.2.3. a Peripheral subpleural lesion (*arrow*). Lateral decubitus position with the patient lying on the same side of the lesion. **b** Posterior access to reach the lesion in a shorter distance. The applicator (*arrow*) is placed with an acute angle relative to the lesion and pleural surface. **c** Follow-up non-contrast CT in the supine position. The lesion is completely ablated leaving a gaseous collection in place and overlying minimal pneumothorax (*arrows*)

priately fulfill the minimal invasive concept of the treatment (Weigel et al. 2004).

Applicators are available for simultaneous multiple application (Dornier Medizintechnik, Germering, Germany). Each of these fibers can be used with a beam splitter TT SWITCH 3 (Trumpf Medical Systems), so that up to six applicators can operate together (Weigel et al. 2004).

5.2.5.3 Image-Monitored Laser Ablation

The energy application starts with 10–12 W/cm of applicator length. The average duration of the application is about 15–20 min according to the tumor size. During the laser application, CT monitoring is performed at 3-min intervals. This serves for the position control and – if necessary – position correction, demonstration of thermal-induced tumoral and lung parenchymal changes, as well as pneumothorax or intraparenchymal hemorrhage (Vogl et al. 2004a).

MR thermometry is performed in a 0.5-T closed MRI unit (Privilig; Elscint, Frankfurt, Germany). Ablation is performed under near real-time MR using T_1-weighted gradient-echo sequence (140/12, flip angle of 80°, matrix of 128 × 256, five 8-mm sections, acquisition time of 15 s) in transverse section and sections parallel to the laser applicators, all repeated every minute for monitoring of thermal ablation. The pull-back technique involves the retraction of the fiber optic bundle at the end of the first laser cycle by a distance of 2 cm, followed by a second laser cycle, to enlarge the area of coagulation necrosis. Necrosis manifests as a progressively deepening T_1 hypointensity (Vogl et al. 2004b).

The complete system is removed at the end of the application while the patients hold their breath in deep inspiration. During each of these steps, air entry through the system is avoided using saline injection. To finish, a plaster bandage is applied at the puncture site (Vogl et al. 2004a).

5.2.5.4 Radiological Appearance After LITT Ablation

During CT-monitored ablation, progressive formation of air vesicles is observed within the lesion around the laser applicator. This phenomenon can be observed 3 min after starting laser application with maximum expansion documented after 10 min. The average size of this hypodense area is between 7 and 22 mm. The lung parenchyma directly bordering the ablation range shows increasing ground-glass opacity due to edema and/or parenchymal hemorrhage (Vogl et al. 2004a) (Figs. 5.2.3–5.2.5).

During MRI-monitored ablation, increasing energy deposition can be documented as signal reduction of the isointense lung lesion in the T_1-weighted sequences. As a function of the applied energy and duration, a complete signal loss of the lung lesion results, merging with the low signal of the surrounding lung tissue. The MR thermometry proved useful with lesions in the proximity of the thorax wall or in large blood vessels where the retarded signal loss could result from the heat dissipation over the neighboring vessels and, hence, an MR-coordinated compensatory increase in ablation time (Vogl et al. 2004a).

CT fluoroscopy control is regarded as ideal. With adequate technology, the radiation exposure for patients and the treating physician is unproblematic. The control by sonography and X-ray fluoroscopy would be feasible, in principle, with some lesions; however, at present they are practically not used (Diederich and Hosten 2004).

5.2.5.5 Post-interventional Assessment and Patient Follow-Up

A spiral control CT of the thorax immediately following the intervention serves directly for the final

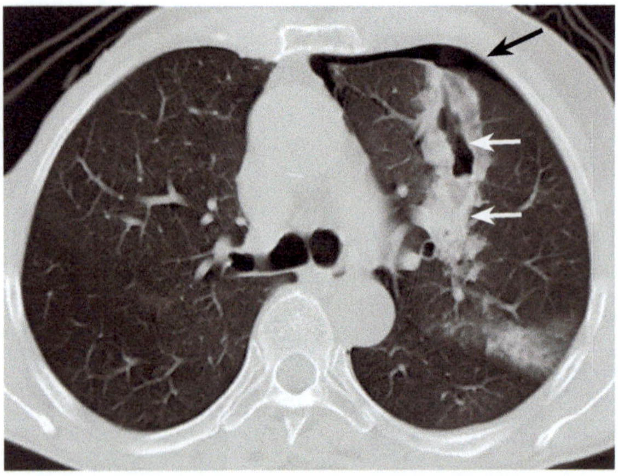

Fig. 5.2.4. Post LITT non-contrast CT showing the ablated lesion as an air vesicle surrounded by a hyperdense zone of edema/hemorrhage (*short arrows*). Overlying mild pneumothorax (*long arrow*)

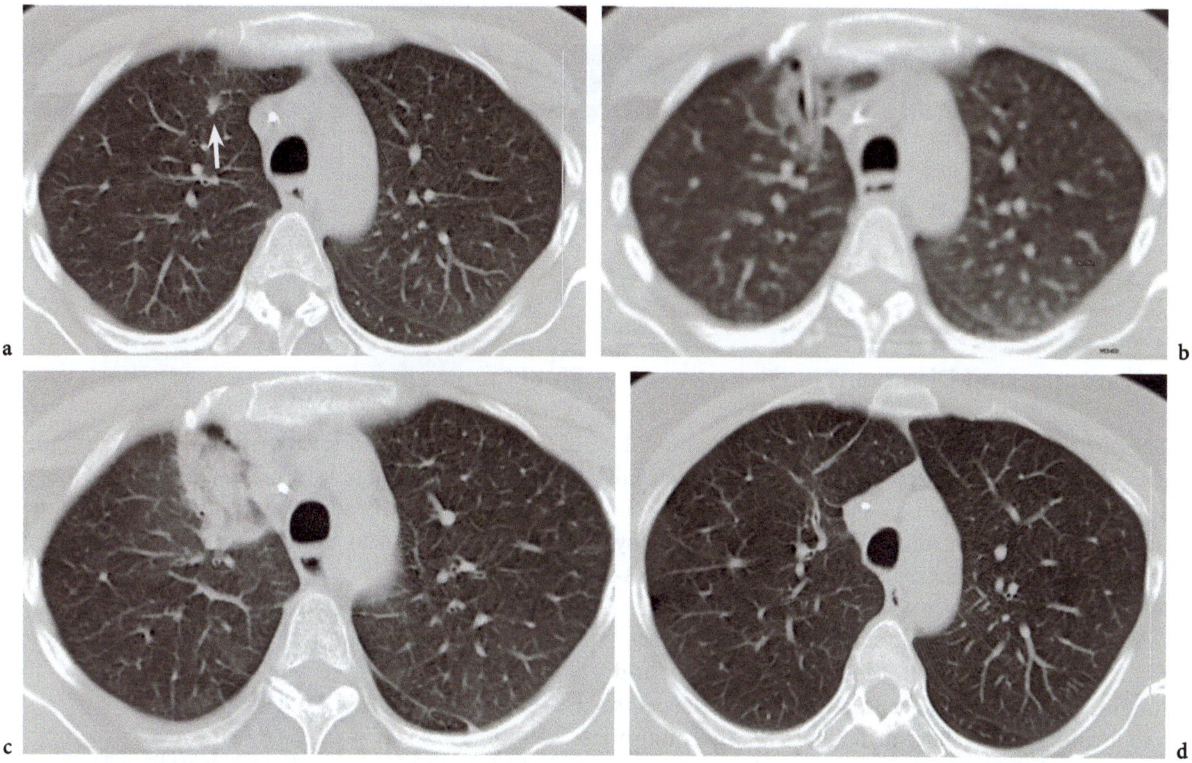

Fig. 5.2.5a–d. **a** A 6-mm upper lobe metastatic lesion (*arrow*). **b** During ablation the necrosis manifested by gaseous transformation in the lesion. **c** Control CT on the following day shows a hyperdense lesion at the ablation site suggestive of a hematoma. **d** Follow-up CT after 8 months showing complete resolution of the hematoma and no residual or recurrent lesions in the ablated zone

evaluation and for the detection of possible complications. A thorax radiograph in two positions is performed 6 h after the procedure. This is followed by control noncontrast CT and MRI (Symphony Quantum, Siemens, Germany) with and without gadolinium DTPA contrast medium (Magnevist, Schering, Germany) within the following 24 h. After 3 months control imaging is performed (Vogl et al. 2004a).

5.2.6 Limitations and Complications

Most of the patients tolerate the procedure without major side-effects or restrictions. The analgesia described above proved sufficient as a routine measure. Nevertheless, some centers use full narcosis and intubation for some of their patients. A minority of patients (2%) experience a longer persistent pain, which can be controlled by means of intravenous analgesics and subsequent oral medication (Diederich and Hosten 2004; Vogl et al. 2004a).

The pneumothorax rate in our study using 9-F applicators amounted to 3% of the number of patients and 9.8% of the number of procedures (Fig. 5.2.4). A thorax drainage catheter was necessary in only two patients to prevent progression of pneumothorax. Computer tomographic documentation of complete resolution was followed by careful removal of the catheter (Vogl et al. 2004a). Using miniature 5.5-F applicators the pneumothorax rate was 48% (Weigel et al. 2004).

Hemorrhage amounted to 21% while hemoptysis was noted in 9% of the cases treated using 5.5-F applicators (Weigel et al. 2004), while it was only 3% with 9-F applicators (Vogl et al. 2004a) (Table 5.2.1; Fig. 5.2.5). These results signify that the larger applicator sizes may actually not be related to the incidence of complications. However, this issue must be addressed in a dedicated, preferably randomized, study in which both applicator sizes can be compared.

Table 5.2.1. Complication (% relative to patient number)

Complication	Pneumothorax (%)	Pleural drainage (%)	Intrapulmonary hemorrhage (%)	Hemoptysis (%)	Pleural effusion (%)	Pericardial effusion (%)
Weigel et al. (2005)	48	21	21	9		
Vogl et al. (2004b)	9.8	6.6	3			
Hosten et al. (2003)	30	10	20		40	10

5.2.7 Advantages and Disadvantages

The position of LITT among other treatment modalities is not yet settled. It is one of several thermal ablation techniques which share broadly the same indications and contraindications. These can play the same complementary role to surgery, and systemic chemotherapy as well as transarterial chemotherapy in the near future. These ablation techniques differ, however, in their physical nature and this leads to some differences in technical aspects and local effects. If these differences are thoroughly evaluated, the actual effectiveness can be compared. Still, the lack of adequate patient series does not allow the final results of these modalities to be demonstrated in a way to favor one of them completely above the rest.

In a comparative evaluation of LITT versus radiofrequency of the lung, the lower cooling effect by neighboring vessels and the absence of impedance problem induction of larger ablation volumes, and higher rate of complete ablation are in favor of LITT compared to radiofrequency ablation. The disadvantages of LITT are difficult puncture with less precise positioning of the application system, and the limitation of the thermal ablation due to carbonization. In contrast, RF allows a direct puncture of the lesion with simple manipulation (Vogl et al. 2004c).

The pros and cons of RFA versus LITT of lung tumors are shown in Table 5.2.2.

Table 5.2.2. Pros and cons of LITT and RFA

Modality	Advantages	Disadvantages
LITT	Lower cooling effect Absence of impedance problem Induction of larger ablation volumes Possible thermometry	Difficult puncture Larger applicator diameter Tissue carbonization
RF	Direct puncture of the lesion with simple manipulation	Impedance problem Smaller ablation volumes Thermometry is not possible

5.2.8 Final Comment

LITT represents an innovative promising technique for thermal ablation of lung metastases and primary lung cancers. Still, some methodical and physical problems have to be tackled to achieve better results.

References

Diederich S, Hosten N (2004) Percutaneous ablation of pulmonary tumours: state-of-the-art 2004. Radiologe 44(7):658–662

Feng W, Liu W, Li C, Li Z, Li R, Liu F, Zhai B, Shi J, Shi G (2002) Percutaneous microwave coagulation therapy for lung cancer. Zhonghua Zhong Liu Za Zhi 24:388–390

Hassan I. Lung, Metastases. http://www.emedicine.com/radio/topic404.htm

Hosten N, Stier A, Weigel C, Kirsch M, Puls R, Nerger U, Jahn D, Stroszczynski C, Heidecke CD, Speck U (2003) Laser-induced thermotherapy (LITT) of lung metastases: description of a miniaturized applicator, optimization, and initial treatment of patients. Rofo 175(3):393–400

Isbert C, Ritz JP, Roggan A, Schuppan D, Ruhl M, Buhr HJ, Germer CT (2004) Enhancement of the immune response to residual intrahepatic tumor tissue by laser-induced thermotherapy (LITT) compared to hepatic resection. Lasers Surg Med 35(4):284–292

Knappe V, Mols A (2004) Laser therapy of the lung: biophysical background. Radiologe 44(7):677–683

Lee JM, Jin GY, Goldberg SN, Lee YC, Chung GH, Han YM, Lee SY, Kim CS (2004) Percutaneous radiofrequency abla-

tion for inoperable non-small cell lung cancer and metastases: preliminary report. Radiology 230(1):125–134
Maataoui A, Qian J, Mack MG, Straub R, Oppermann E, Khan MF, Knappe V, Vogl TJ (2005) Laser-induced interstitial thermotherapy (LITT) in hepatic metastases of various sizes in an animal model. Rofo 177(3):405–410
Vogl TJ, Fieguth HG, Eichler K, Straub R, Lehnert T, Zangos S, Mack M (2004a) Laser-induced thermotherapy of lung metastases and primary lung tumors. Radiologe 44(7):693–699
Vogl TJ, Straub R, Eichler K, Sollner O, Mack MG (2004b) Colorectal carcinoma metastases in liver: laser-induced interstitial thermotherapy – local tumor control rate and survival data. Radiology 230(2):450–458
Vogl TJ, Straub R, Lehnert T, Eichler K, Luder-Luhr T, Peters J, Zangos S, Sollner O, Mack M (2004c) Percutaneous thermoablation of pulmonary metastases. Experience with the application of laser-induced thermotherapy (LITT) and radiofrequency ablation (RFA), and a literature review. Rofo 176(11):1658–1666
Vogl TJ, Wetter A, Lindemayr S, Zangos S (2005) Treatment of unresectable lung metastases with transpulmonary chemoembolization: preliminary experience. Radiology 234(3):917–922
Weigel C, Kirsch M, Mensel B, Nerger U, Hosten N (2004) Percutaneous laser-induced thermotherapy of lung metastases: experience gained during 4 years. Radiologe 44(7):700–707

Soft Tissue and Musculoskeletal – Radiofrequency Ablation in Bone Metastases

6

Dirk Proschek, Martin G. Mack, and Thomas J. Vogl

CONTENTS

6.1 Introduction

The radiologist has emerged as a consultant with increased interaction with patients. In fact, the interventional radiologist has assumed the role of the surgeon for many conditions; for example, minimally invasive therapy of bone metastases using radiofrequency techniques. Recent advances in imaging and interventional techniques have had an impact on medical diagnosis. Interventional imaging-based procedures include percutaneous biopsy, which has decreased the need for open surgical procedures. Due to the advent of system hardware and improvements in different technical systems and instruments, interventional radiology is now an upcoming special field in radiology.

Bone metastases are common in many advanced cancers and are a clinically relevant source of skeletal morbidity. Nearly 30% of all malignant tumors induce bone metastases (Jemal et al. 2004; Thomas et al. 1996). Most often, the spinal column (80%) and the femur (40%) are affected. In particular, breast, lung and bronchus, prostate and kidney cancer types have a high rate of inducing bone metastases. Prostate cancer in males and breast cancer in females are the most common cancer types (Jemal et al. 2004). In the US 33% of the estimated new cases of cancer in males are induced by prostate cancer (230,110 cases of new prostate cancer per year). Of the new cases in females, 32% are induced by breast cancer (215,990 cases of new breast cancer per year) (Jemal et al. 2004; Thomas et al. 1996). Of all patients with breast and prostate cancer, 60%–80% develop bone metastases. Pain is the most frequent complication in metastatic bone disease. More than 80% of patients suffer from pain with a reduction of mobility and life quality; therefore they have a high risk of concomitant complications. Therapy of bone metastases has three main goals:

1. Pain relief
2. Improvement in mobility and quality of life
3. Improvement of life time

Therapeutic possibilities comprise local strategies such as radiation, surgical therapy and systemic therapy. A new and upcoming, minimally invasive therapy option is thermal ablation of bone tumors. For this procedure, ultrasound, computed tomography (CT) scanning, or magnetic resonance imaging (MRI) is used by the radiologist to guide percutaneous placement of long, thin (usually less than 18-gauge), insulated needles into the tumor. Electrodes are attached to a generator and the electrical energy

D. Proschek, MD
Orthopedic University Hospital, Johann Wolfgang Goethe University, Marienburgstrasse 2, 60528 Frankfurt am Main, Germany
M. G. Mack, MD, PD; T. J. Vogl, MD, Professor
Institute for Diagnostic and Interventional Radiology, University Hospital, Johann Wolfgang Goethe University, Theodor-Stern-Kai 7, 60590 Frankfurt am Main, Germany

is converted to heat, which kills cells through coagulation necrosis.

6.2 Interventional Imaging

Recent years have seen remarkable advances in imaging technology. This is particularly true in the field of CT, where the introduction of multidetector CT, continued improvement in 3D imaging capabilities, and greater sophistication in interventional CT techniques have strengthened CT's central role in diagnostic radiology. Multidetecor CT in particular significantly reduces room use time for interventional procedures (Kataoka et al. 2006). CT- and MR-guided interventional procedures are divided into diagnostic and therapeutic techniques. Diagnostic procedures in bone include biopsy and aspiration (Haaga 2005). Therapeutic procedures are more varied, including local cancer treatment, guided surgery, and vascular techniques. In bone, interventional techniques comprise thermal or chemical tumor ablation in particular.

6.3 Image-Guided Radiofrequency Ablation

In early thermal ablation therapy, electrode placement was typically performed under direct visualization using preoperative CT data. Variations in ablation size and shape during therapy could not be predicted and were not recognized during therapy, and had to wait until follow-up image scans were performed.

CT guidance affords the best available visualization of needle and probe placement in the lesion nidus. Helical CT with low-dose and CT fluoroscopy makes for a quicker procedure and a lower patient dose (Silverman et al. 1999; Teeuwisse et al. 2001). Lesion size and the configuration of the thermal lesion in particular can be controlled directly during the procedure. Therapy strategy can be adjusted by the operator during the procedure and provides an effective thermal ablation and therapy result. However, the complication rate is reduced significantly using image-guided radiofrequency ablation (RFA).

Other possibilities for image-guided thermoablation include ultrasound and MR guidance. MR-guided therapy has been limited by the inability to actively monitor the size and shape of the lesions. New software and hardware provide excellent ability to monitor tissue destruction during the procedure. MR is well suited because of its excellent soft-tissue discrimination; however, in the therapy of bone metastases, CT guidance actually affords the best available visualization.

6.4 Radiofrequency Therapy

Heat has always been used in medicine. Ancient Hindu medicine used heated metal bars and the Greeks used heated stones to stop bleeding. Electrocautery has been used for decades in surgery to stop bleeding, to cauterize and cut tissue. RFA has been used especially in the field of neurosurgery. In former times, electrode placement was typically performed under direct visualization using preoperative CT data. Indications included cordotomy, pallidotomy and thalamotomy (Hitchcock 1981; Laitinen and Hariz 1992; Sweet and Hamlin 1960).

The radiofrequency generator forms an electric current. Resistance of biologic structures causes local ions to vibrate. This ionic agitation results in friction around the electrode tip as ions attempt to pursue changes in direction of the alternating current and create heat to the point of desiccation (Dupuy 1999). Radiofrequency thermal ablation differs from electrocautery in that the tissue around the electrode, rather than the electrode itself, is the primary source of heat. RFA depends upon the transfer of electrical energy to tissue (Aronow 1960). This is achieved by passing radiofrequency energy from a generator through an electrode with an exposed tip of variable length which has been placed within the abnormal tissue. The energy at the needle tip causes ionic agitation and frictional heat in the surrounding tissue, which, when hot enough, leads to cell death and coagulation necrosis (Fig. 6.1). Generator applicator systems can be divided into monopolar and bipolar systems. When using monopolar systems, the patient is made into an electrical circuit by

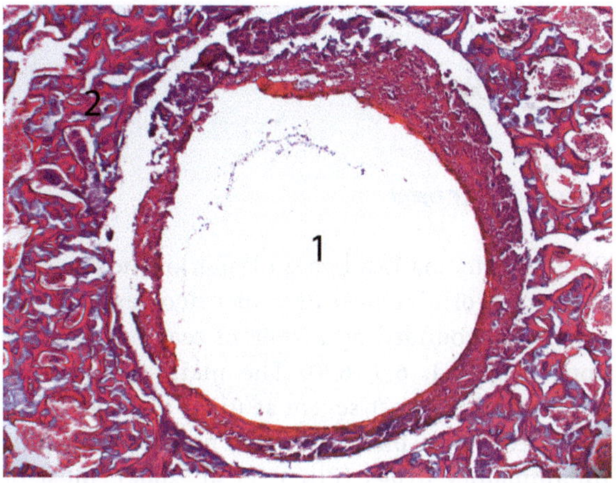

Fig. 6.1. Histopathologic imaging of the remaining channel (*1*) of the RF electrode after thermal ablation. See the massive cell destruction and necrosis around the channel (*2*)

placing grounding pads on the thighs. With bipolar systems, no grounding pads are necessary.

RFA has several advantages:

- Long history of use
- Major complications are uncommon
- Relatively inexpensive technique compared to laser light procedures
- Thermal lesion size and shape can be controlled using different applicator designs
- Energy application can be controlled through the applicator and generator design throughout the whole procedure
- Impedance measurements allow exact thermal ablation of pathologic tissue without destroying healthy tissue
- Repeated therapy is possible without concern about the cumulative dose
- Image-guided RFA using MRI or CT provides a safe and efficient therapy

6.4.1 The Procedure

All patients should undergo physical examination before entering treatment. A complete blood count and coagulation laboratory is necessary at least 24 h before treatment. Pretreatment radiographics, including CT scans, MRI and radiographs, need to be evaluated. All procedures are performed in a strictly sterile manner in the CT room or a similar intervention room. The procedure may be performed on an outpatient basis under general anesthesia or conscious sedation. Local anesthesia/conscious sedation is possible in most cases. Most authors use a combination of local anesthesia and intravenous analgesia and sedation therapy, for example a combination of mepivacaine, piritramid and midazolam to provide conscious sedation. Routine cardiovascular and respiratory monitoring ensures patient safety during the procedure. Under continuous CT, fluoroscopy, ultrasound or MR guidance, and after a small skin incision, a cannula (e.g., 14-G vertebroplasty cannula) is used to gain access to the affected bone (Fig. 6.2). The positioning of the instruments should be controlled precisely by fluoroscopy, CT, MR, or a combination of techniques (Fig. 6.3). In our institution, we use a combination of CT guidance and fluoroscopy. The radiofrequency applicator is introduced, using a variety of techniques; for example, a vertebroplasty cannula as a gateway (Fig. 6.3). The length of the radiofrequency applicator depends on tumor size, varying between 20 and 30 mm.

Radiofrequency energy is generated by a power generator system. The application power depends on tumor size and is 10 W per centimeter of active length of the electrode. Tumor coagulation is finished when the continuing energy flow is stopped because of impedance increase. Each treatment session has about 10–15 min of active ablation. Postprocedural CT should be performed to confirm the lack of soft tissue swelling and hematoma.

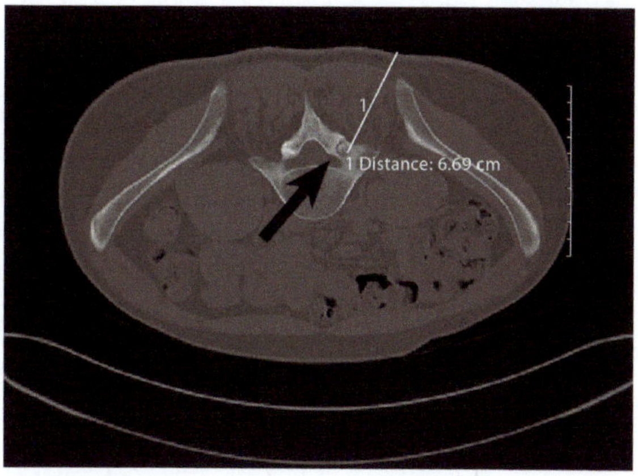

Fig. 6.2. A 64-year-old female patient with breast cancer and bone metastases. Pre-interventional axial CT scan shows an osteolytic metastasis in the left pedicle of the fifth lumbar vertebra (*arrow*). Note the pre-interventional planning

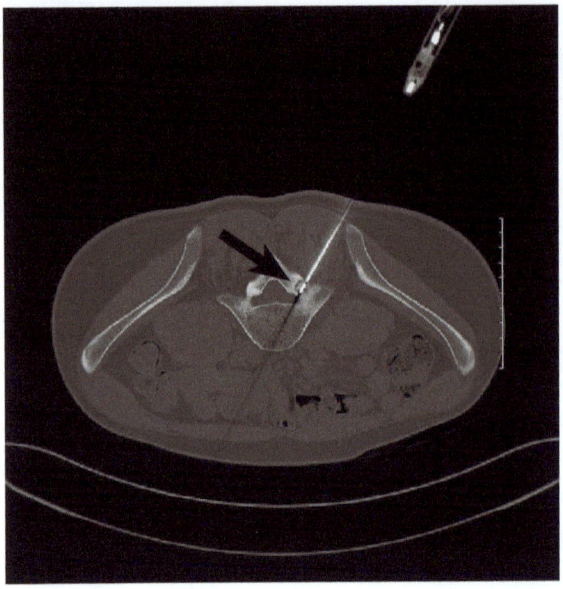

Fig. 6.3. A 64-year-old female patient with breast cancer and bone metastases. Axial CT scan shows the approach to the metastasis in the left pedicle of the fifth lumbar vertebra using a bipolar radiofrequency electrode (*arrow*). The CT scan shows the positioning of the bipolar radiofrequency probe within the metastasis. Note the insulation between the electrodes of the bipolar radiofrequency probe

6.5 Complications

RFA is a safe method. The reported complication rate is about 1%–2%, with most of the complications characterized as minor and not life threatening. In the literature, the mortality rate is reported to be <0.1% (Jakobs et al. 2004; Livraghi et al. 2003). Major complication are absolutely rare and comprise acute bleeding, tumoral abscess, vascular and nerve injuries (Albisinni et al. 2004; Dupuy 1999; Livraghi et al. 2003). Minor complications are rare and comprise self-limiting bleeding and hematoma, skin burn and especially transient pain. Although this technique is minimally invasive, potential complications that may occur during needle passage include bleeding and nerve injury. These can be avoided by knowledge of anatomic structures in the region of needle passage.

6.6 Clinical Experience

6.6.1 Osteoid Osteoma

Osteoid osteoma is a benign lesion of the skeleton consisting of a central area of osteoplastic tissue (nidus) surrounded by a zone of reactive sclerotic bone (Figs. 6.4, 6.5, 6.6). The main symptom is pain, which is most severe at night and can often be relieved by aspirin and other nonsteroidal anti-inflammatory drugs (Pinto et al. 2002). Most of

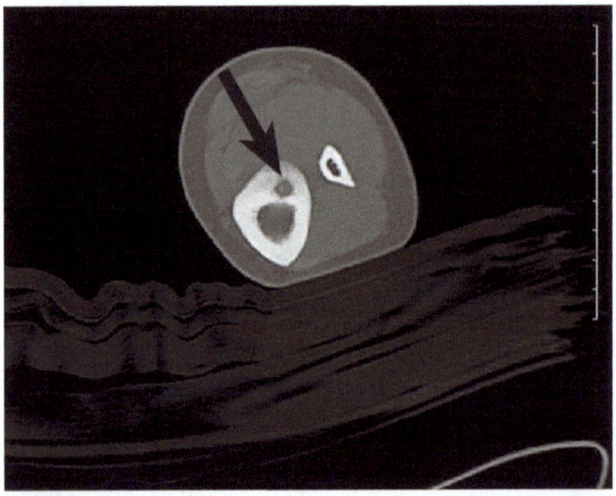

Fig. 6.4. A 17-year-old female patient with osteoid osteoma in the left tibia. Note the nidus (*arrow*)

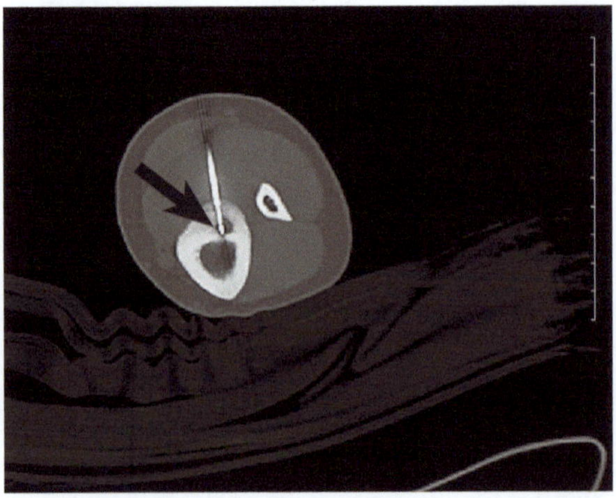

Fig. 6.5. A 17-year-old female patient with osteoid osteoma in the left tibia. Percutaneous and CT-guided approach. Note the exact positioning of the radiofrequency electrode in the center of the nidus

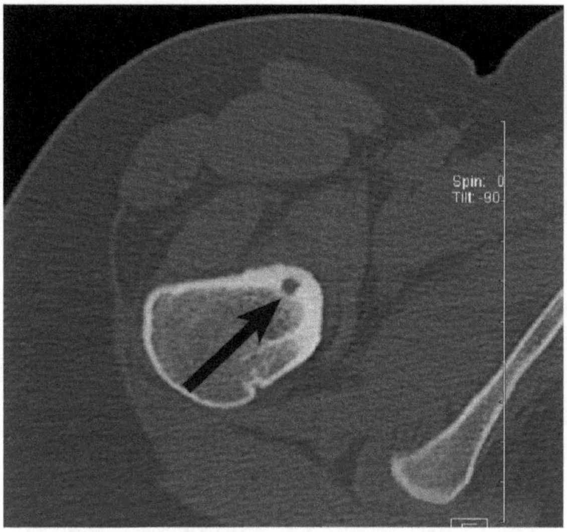

Fig. 6.6. A 19-year-old male patient with osteoid osteoma in the right femur. Note the nidus (*arrow*)

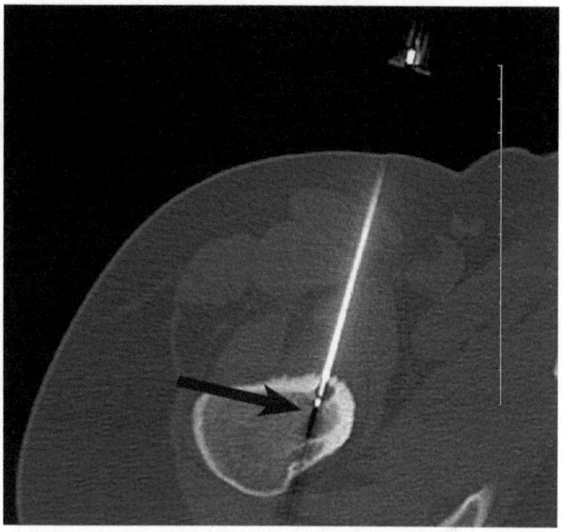

Fig. 6.8. A 19-year-old male patient with osteoid osteoma in the right femur. Percutaneous and CT-guided approach. Note the exact positioning of the radiofrequency electrode in the center of the nidus

the osteoid osteomas are observed in patients aged between 10 and 25 years. Half of the lesions occur in the femur and tibia. Pain can subside after several years of conservative treatment. Curative treatment of osteoid osteoma consists of completely removing the nidus (Woertler et al. 2001).

Percutaneous resection requires instruments of large caliber to ensure complete removal of the lesion. Consecutive structural weakness of the affected bone can lead to fracture, and therefore limitations of activity and weight-bearing. In the literature, the complication rate is reported to be >20% with the risk of bone fracture up to 5% (Ramseier and Exner 2006; Sans et al. 1999). RFA of osteoid osteoma requires the creation of only a small osseous access to the nidus to allow insertion of the electrode (Figs. 6.7, 6.8). Loss of bone substance is therefore minimal and does not result in significant structural weakening. The complication rate and the dimension of the therapy are much lower compared to surgical resection of the nidus (Ramseier and Exner 2006; Sans et al. 1999; Woertler et al. 2001).

Rosenthal et al. (1998) retrospectively compared outcomes for a series of patients treated by operative excision ($n=87$) or by RFA alone ($n=38$). The study reported no significant difference between the two approaches. The rates of recurrence showed no significant difference (11% RFA, 9% surgery) and no difference in complications (0% RFA, 2% surgery). The decreased need for hospitalization with RFA was significant in this study population.

Another recent case series reported primary success in 37 of 38 (97%) patients (25 males, 8 females, age range 5–43 years) who underwent CT-guided percutaneous RFA (Martel et al. 2005). All patients experienced sufficient pain relief to permit resumption of normal activities within 24 h of the procedure. During follow-up ranging 3–24 months, no major complications were reported.

There have been other studies showing good results with percutaneous RFA treatment. Reviewing the literature, the success rate is reported to be 94% (Table 6.1). Complications occurred in 2% of cases (Table 6.1).

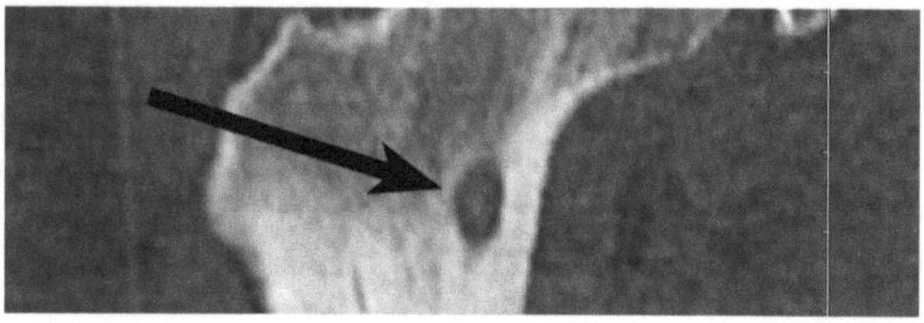

Fig. 6.7. A 19-year-old male patient with osteoid osteoma in the right femur. Reconstruction scan of the osteoid osteoma and the nidus

Table 6.1. Literature review. Different studies treating osteoid osteoma using radiofrequency ablation

Author	Year	Patients	Success rate (%)	Complications (%)
Barei et al.	2000	11	91	None
Lindner et al.	2001	58	100	1.7
Vanderschueren et al.	2002	97	92	2.1
Venbrux et al.	2003	9	89	22 (2/9)
Rosenthal et al.	2003	126	89	3.2
Cioni et al.	2004	38	92	5.3
Martel et al.	2005	38	100	5.3
Rimondi et al.	2005	97	98	2.1

Despite the weaknesses in the published clinical evidence, RFA of osteomas has become a standard of care based on the lower morbidity and quicker recovery time associated with the procedure compared to the standard alternative which is open surgery.

6.6.2 Bone Metastases

After lung and liver, bone is the third most common metastatic site and is relatively frequent among patients with primary malignancies of the breast, prostate, and lung. Bone metastases often cause osteolysis resulting in pain, fractures, decreased mobility, and reduced quality of life (Fig. 6.2). External beam irradiation often is the initial palliative therapy for osteolytic bone metastases (Fig. 6.3). However, pain from bone metastases is refractory to radiation therapy in 20%–30% of patients, while recurrent pain at previously irradiated sites may be ineligible for additional radiation due to risks of normal-tissue damage. RFA has been investigated as another alternative and upcoming technique for palliating pain from bone metastases (Jemal et al. 2004; Thomas et al. 1996).

Indications and contraindications for thermal ablation in the therapy of bone metastases are as follows:

Indications:

- Osteolytic bone metastases
- Painful bone metastases
- Not suitable or failed standard therapy

Contraindications:

- Hypervascular tumors
- Large lesion with impending fracture
- Tumors in contact with major neurovascular structures
- Internal fixation with metallic devices at the site of the tumor

Goetz et al. (2004a) reported a multicenter study in which 43 patients with painful osteolytic bone metastases were treated palliatively with RFA. Of the patients, 39 (91%) had previously received opioids to control pain from the lesion(s) treated with RFA, and 32 (74%) had prior radiation therapy to the same lesion. Mean pain score before therapy was 7.9 (range 4–10). At 4, 12, and 24 weeks after RFA, average pain scores decreased to 4.5, 3.0, and 1.4 respectively. Of the patients, 41 (95%) achieved a clinically significant improvement in pain scores.

Reviewing the literature, there are further retrospective trials available, which show a good success rate and only minor complications (Table 6.2) (Callstrom et al. 2002; Dupuy 1989; Goetz et al. 2004b).

6.7 Conclusion

RFA is a safe and minimally invasive tumor ablation therapy which rapidly reduces pain and improves quality of life in patients with bone metastases. Recent advances in different generator and applicator systems as well as in different guiding/monitoring technologies will overcome previous shortcomings. Particularly because of its ability to evaluate the results of the treatment immediately, RFA has the potential to be an effective option in the local treatment of bone tumors.

Table 6.2. Different retrospective trials treating painful bone metastases using radiofrequency ablation

Author	No. of patients	Reduction of pain (%)	Complications (%)
Dupuy (1989)	10	90	None
Callstrom et al. (2002)	12	92	None
Goetz et al. (2004a)	43	95	7

References

Albisinni U, Rimondi E, Bianchi G, Mercuri M (2004) Experience of the Rizzoli Institute in radiofrequency thermal ablation of musculoskeletal lesions. J Chemother 16 [Suppl 5]:75–78

Aronow S (1960) The use of radio-frequency power in making lesions in the brain. J Neurosurg 17:431–438

Barei DP, Moreau G, Scarborough MT, Neel MD (2000) Radiofrequency Ablation of Osteoid Osteoma. Clin Orthop Relat Res 373:115–124

Callstrom MRCJ, Goetz MP, Rubin J, Wong GY, Sloan JA, Novotny PJ, Lewis BD, Welch TJ, Farrell MA, Maus TP, Lee RA, Reading CC, Petersen IA, Pickett DD (2002) Painful metastases involving bone: feasibility of percutaneous CT- and US-guided radio-frequency ablation. Radiology 224:87–97

Cioni R, Armillotta N, Bargellini I, Zampa V, Cappelli C, Vagli P, Boni G, Marchetti S, Consoli V, Bartolozzi C (2004) CT-guided radiofrequency ablation of osteoid osteoma: long-term results. Eur Radiol 14(7):1203–1208

Dupuy D (1989) Radiofrequency ablation: an outpatient percutaneous treatment. Radiology 209:389

Dupuy D (1999) Radiofrequency ablation: an outpatient percutaneous treatment. Med Health RI 82:213–216

Goetz MP, Charboneau JW, Farrell MA, Maus TP, Welch TJ, Wong GY, Sloan JA, Novotny PJ, Petersen IA, Beres RA, Regge D, Capanna R, Saker MB, Gronemeyer DH, Gevargez A, Ahrar K, Choti MA, de Baere TJ, Rubin J (2004a) Percutaneous image-guided radiofrequency ablation of painful metastases involving bone: a multicenter study. J Clin Oncol 22:300–306

Goetz MP, Charboneau JW, Farrell MA, Maus TP, Welch TJ, Wong GY, Sloan JA, Novotny PJ, Petersen IA, Beres RA, Regge D, Capanna R, Saker MB, Gronemeyer DH, Gevargez A, Ahrar K, Choti MA, de Baere TJ, Rubin J (2004b) Percutaneous image-guided radiofrequency ablation of painful metastases involving bone: a multicenter study. J Clin Oncol 15:200–206

Haaga J (2005) Interventional CT: 30 years‘ experience. Eur Radiol 15:116–120

Hitchcock ERMT (1981) A comparison of results from center-median and basal thalamotomies for pain. Surg Neurol 15:341–351

Jakobs TFHR, Vick C, Reiser MF, Helmberger TK (2004) RFA in Tumoren des Knochens und der Weichteile. Radiologe 44:370–375

Jemal ATR, Murray T, Ghafoor A, Samuels A, Thun MJ (2004) Cancer statistics, 2004. CA Cancer J Clin 54:8–29

Kataoka MLRV, Lin PJ, Siewert B, Goldberg SN, Kruskal JB (2006) Multiple-image in-room CT imaging guidance for interventional procedures. Radiology 239(3):863–868

Laitinen LVAB, Hariz MI (1992) Leksell‘s posteroventral pallidotomy in the treatment of Parkinson‘s disease. J Neurosurg 76:53–61

Lindner NJ, Ozaki T, Roedl R, Gosheger G, Winkelmann W, Wortler K (2001) “Percutaneous radiofrequency ablation in osteoid osteoma”. J Bone Joint Surg Br 83(3):391–396

Livraghi TSL, Meloni MF, Gazelle GS, Halpern EF, Goldberg SN (2003) Treatment of focal liver tumors with percutaneous radio-frequency ablation: complications encountered in a multicenter study. Radiology 226:441–451

Martel J, Bueno A, Ortiz E (2005) Percutaneous radiofrequency treatment of osteoid osteoma using cool-tip electrodes. Eur Rad 56(3):403–408

Pinto CHTA, Vanderschueren GM, Hogendoorn PC, Bloem JL, Obermann WR (2002) Technical considerations in CT-guided radiofrequency thermal ablation of osteoid osteoma: tricks of the trade. AJR Am J Roentgenol 179:1633–1642

Ramseier LEDS, Exner GU (2006) Osteoid osteoma: CT guided drilling and radiofrequency ablation. Orthopade 19 Epub ahead

Rimondi E, Bianchi G, Malaguti MC, Ciminari R, Del Baldo A, Mercuri M, Albisinni U (2005) Radiofrequency thermoablation of primary non-spinal osteoid osteoma: optimization of the procedure. Eur Rad 15(7):1393–1399

Rosenthal DIHF, Wolfe MW, Jennings LC, Gebhardt MC, Mankin HJ (1998) Percutaneous radiofrequency coagulation of osteoid osteoma compared with operative treatment. J Bone Joint Surg Am 80:815–821

Rosenthal DI, Hornicek FJ, Torriani M, Gebhardt MC, Mankin HJ (2003) Osteoid osteoma: percutaneous treatment with radiofrequency energy. Radiology 229(1):171–175

Sans NG-FD, Assoun J, Jarlaud T, Chiavassa H, Bonnevialle P, Railhac N, Giron J, Morera-Maupome H, Railhac JJ (1999) Osteoid osteoma: CT-guided percutaneous resection and follow-up in 38 patients. Radiology 212:687–692

Silverman SGTK, Adams DF, Nawfel RD, Zou KH, Judy PF (1999) CT fluoroscopy-guided abdominal interventions: techniques, results, and radiation exposure. Radiology 212:673–681

Sweet VM, Hamlin H (1960) RF lesions in the central nervous system of man and cat. J Neurosurg 17:213–225

Teeuwisse WMGJ, Broerse JJ, Obermann WR, van Persijn van Meerten EL (2001) Patient and staff dose during CT guided biopsy, drainage and coagulation. Br J Radiol 74:720–726

Thomas CAC, Dienes HP, Emons B, Falk S, Gabbert H (1996) Spezielle Pathologie. Schattauer, Stuttgart,

Vanderschueren GM, Taminiau AH, Obermann WR, Bloem JL (2002) Osteoid osteoma: clinical results with thermocoagulation. Radiology 224(1):82–86

Venbrux AC, Montague BJ, Murphy KP, Bobonis LA, Washington SB, Soltes AP, Frassica FJ (2003) Image-guided percutaneous radiofrequency ablation for osteoid osteomas. J Vasc Interv Radiol 14(3):375–380

Woertler KVT, Boettner F, Winkelmann W, Heindel W, Lindner N (2001) Osteoid osteoma: CT-guided percutaneous radiofrequency ablation and follow-up in 47 patients. J Vasc Interv Radiol 12:717–722

Other

7

7.1 Head and Neck Lesions

MARTIN G. MACK and THOMAS J. VOGL

CONTENTS

7.1.1 Introduction

The head and neck area contains a multitude of small, complexly arranged anatomical structures; intimate knowledge of normal spatial relationships and variations is necessary to plan and implement appropriate therapy. Lesions often lie near vital structures, complicating diagnostic and therapeutic procedures. Improved visualization during such procedures can therefore provide the physician with critical information, permitting innovative procedures and improved outcomes.

Palliative treatment options for recurrent head and neck cancer are limited by the proximity of vital vascular and neural structures and the aggressive nature of most of these tumors. Laser-induced interstitial thermotherapy (LITT) is a recently developed minimally invasive treatment modality. It is a minimally invasive technique for local tumor destruction within solid organs.

M. G. MACK, MD, PD; T. J. VOGL, MD, Professor
Institute for Diagnostic and Interventional Radiology, University Hospital, Johann Wolfgang Goethe University, Theodor-Stern-Kai 7, 60590 Frankfurt, Germany

Experimental work has shown that a well-defined area of coagulative necrosis is obtained around the fiber tip, with minimal damage to surrounding structures.

MR-guided LITT offers a number of potential treatment benefits. First, MR imaging provides unparalleled topographic accuracy due to its excellent soft-tissue contrast and high spatial resolution. Secondly, the temperature sensitivity of specially designed MR sequences can be used to monitor the temperature elevation in the tumor and surrounding normal tissues. This enables the exact visualization of the growing coagulative necrosis. On-line MR imaging during LITT is essential for avoiding local complications due to laser treatment. Thirdly, recovery times, lengths of hospital stay, and the risk of infection and other complications can be reduced when compared with conventional palliative surgery. Finally, successful implementation of such minimal invasive procedures would significantly reduce costs in comparison to surgical procedures. A further, indirect advantage is the psychological effect due to avoidance of cosmetic deformities that can result from major reconstructive surgery.

A number of studies have already been performed to evaluate the potential of laser treatment for the local treatment of liver metastases, as well as other tumors.

7.1.2 Material and Methods

7.1.2.1 Laser System and Application Set

Laser coagulation was performed using a neodymium-YAG laser (Dornier MediLas 5060 or Dornier

MediLas 5100) with a specially developed flexible laser applicator. Furthermore an application kit for percutaneous treatment was developed and optimized for our purposes.

Laser light with a wavelength of 1046 nm was transmitted to tissue with a diffusing applicator. Laser light of this wavelength penetrates deeply into biological tissue, where photon absorption and heat conduction lead to hyperthermic and coagulative effects. The tissue destruction may be immediate or delayed.

The cooled power laser system (SOMATEX, Germany) for MR-guided minimally invasive percutaneous LITT of soft tissue tumors consists of an MR-compatible cannulation needle (length 20 cm, diameter 1.3 mm) with a tetragonally beveled tip and stylet; guide wire (length 100 cm); 9-Fr sheath with stylet; and a 7-Fr double-tube thermostable (up to 400°C) protective catheter (length 40 cm) also with a stylet, which enables internal cooling with saline solution (Fig. 7.1.1a). Cooling of the surface of the laser applicator modifies the radial temperature distribution so that the maximum temperature shifts into deeper tissue layers. The protective catheter prevents direct contact of the laser applicator with the patient and enables complete removal of the applicator even in the unlikely event of damage during treatment. This increases patient safety and simplifies the procedure. The catheter is transparent for laser radiation and resistant to heat (up to 400°C). Marks on the sheath and the protective catheter allow exact positioning of both in the lesion.

The system is fully compatible with MR imaging systems. Magnetite markers on the laser applicator allow an easier visualizing and positioning procedure.

The laser itself is installed outside of the examination unit. The laser light is transmitted via a 10-m-long optical fiber. The complete set-up used for LITT is shown in Figure 7.1.1.

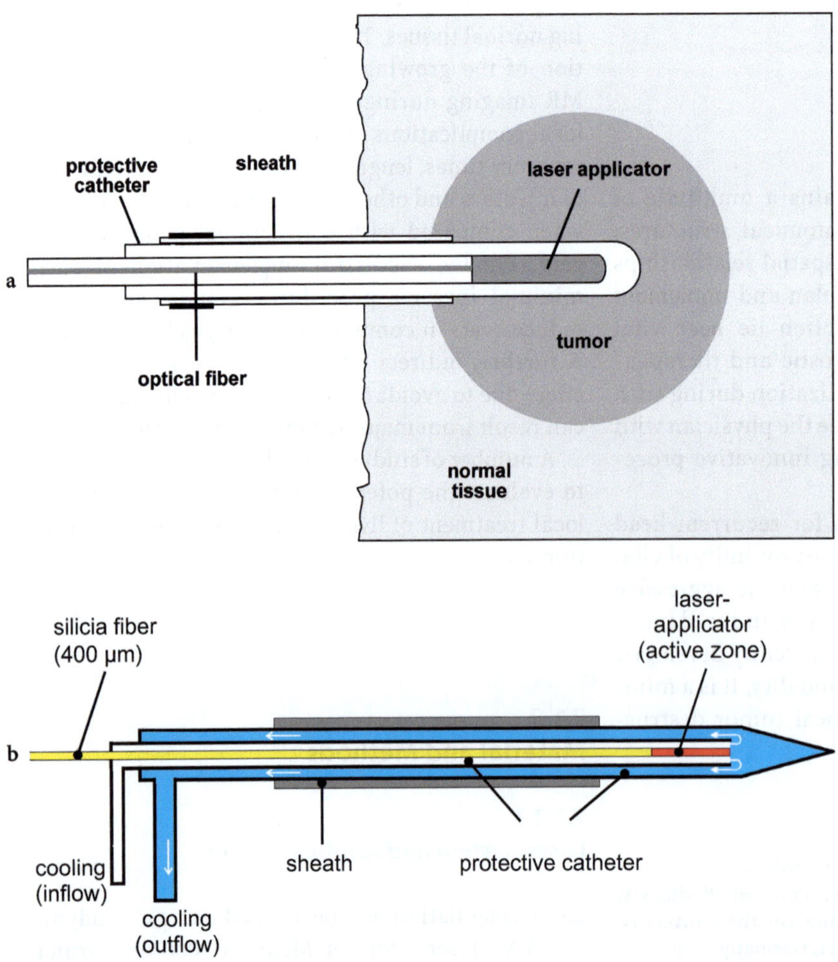

Fig. 7.1.1. **a** The drawing shows the set-up for laser-induced interstitial thermotherapy (*LITT*). **b** Internally cooled power laser application system with laser applicator

7.1.2.2
Technique of MR-Guided LITT

Informed consent is obtained from all patient. Prior to LITT treatment all patients undergo CT and a contrast-enhanced MRI study at least 2 days prior to the intervention. After localization of the tumor with CT local anesthesia was achieved with 20–30 ml of 1% mepivacaine (Scandicain, AstraZeneca, Wedel, Germany). Distance to the lesion and the puncture angle are calculated electronically. For targeting of both recurrent nasopharyngeal tumors and pleomorphic adenomas a subzygomatic approach to the lesion was chosen, which provided the best and safest access to the lesion. Lesions of the larynx and the floor of the mouth were punctured directly. After the procedure the needle track was closed with fibrin glue (Tissucol Duo S, Baxter, Vienna, Austria).

The LITT treatment was performed under MR guidance using a 0.5 tesla scanner (Privilig, Escint, Israel) by T_1-weighted GE sequences (TR/TE = 140/12, flip angle = 80°, matrix 128 × 256, 5 slices, slice thickness 8 mm, interslice gap 30%, acquisition time 15 s) in axial slice orientation and parallel to the laser applicators. These two sequences were repeated every minute. The entire LITT treatment was performed using local anesthesia and intravenously injected analgesics [pethidine 10–80 mg (Dolantin, Aventis Pharma, Frankfurt, Germany) and/or piritramid 5–15 mg (Dipidolor, Janssen-CILAG AG, Neuss, Germany)] and sedation (2–10 mg midazolam, Hoffmann-La Roche, Grenzach-Wyhlen, Germany).

7.1.2.3
MR Thermometry

MR thermometry is performed with a Turbo-FLASH sequence (TR/TE/TI = 7/3/400) as well as a Thermo-FLASH-2D sequence (TR/TE/Flip angle = 102/8/15), which was found to be more sensitive to thermal induced.

Before and after LITT treatment T_1-weighted (SE, GE), and T_2-weighted (SE) images are obtained. Of special importance is a dynamic Turbo-FLASH sequence protocol, which acquires images prior to as well as in short delays (6 s) following the intravenous administration of contrast over a length of 180 s. Follow-up studies including non-enhanced and contrast-enhanced sequences are performed 1, 4, 12, and 24 weeks following therapy. Qualitative and quantitative parameters including size, morphology, and contrast enhancement pattern at early and late follow-up are evaluated.

7.1.3
Results

All treated patients were suffering from recurrent benign or malignant tumors in the head and neck region. An interventional subzygomatic approach was used for recurrent tumors of the nasopharynx and parapharyngeal space. Tumors of the maxillary sinus were directly punctured from the anterior or lateral approach, and lesions of the neck and the floor of the mouth were punctured using either a anterior or lateral approach. The placement of the laser application systems was done under CT guidance in all cases.

Under CT guidance, optimal positioning of the cannula and mandrin was achieved in all patients (Figs. 7.1.2a, b, 7.1.3). All tolerated the puncture well on a moderate amount of systemic analgesics and local infiltrative anesthesia. After positioning of the protective catheter and insertion of the laser tip, the energy of the laser and the duration of the treatment were calculated individually, depending on the position of the laser tip in relation to the tumor borders, the homogeneity of the tumor, and its relationship to neighboring vascular structures, in particular the internal carotid artery and major branches of the external carotid artery, including the maxillary, lingual, and ascending pharyngeal arteries.

Pre-interventional scans were optimized individually to show the tumor as tissue with a signal intensity lower than that of fat and higher than that of muscle tissue. For each patient, these images were used as baseline for visualizing changes in signal loss during LITT.

Criteria for evaluating success of treatment included clinical data such as pain or other local symptoms as well as pre- and post-therapeutic changes in signal and tumor morphology. We were able to induce coagulative necrosis in all patients (volume range: 3 cm^3 to 25 cm^3) and to reduce clinical symptoms in most of the patients (Fig. 7.1.2b).

All LITT treatments were performed under local anesthesia on an outpatient basis. General anesthesia was not necessary for the procedure.

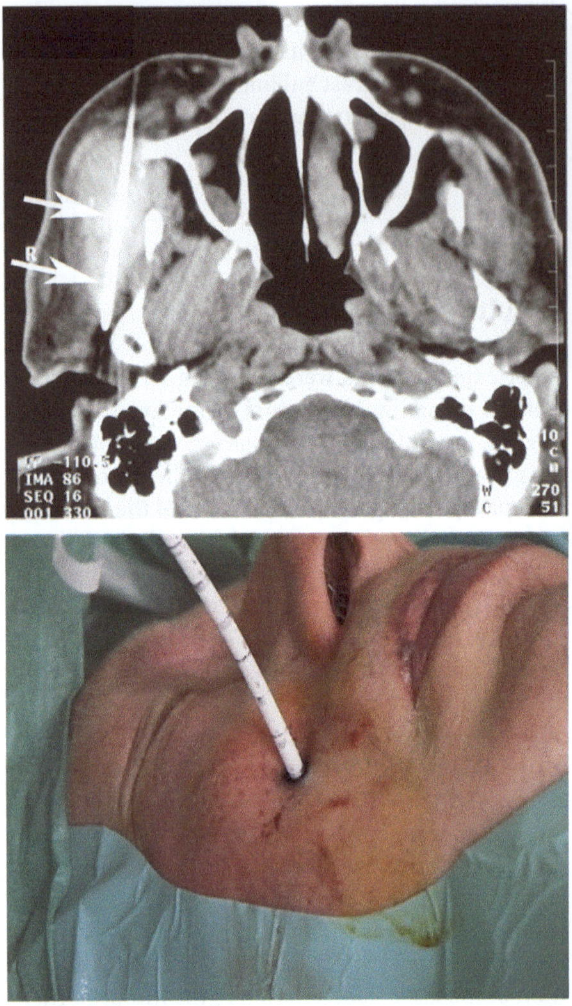

a

b

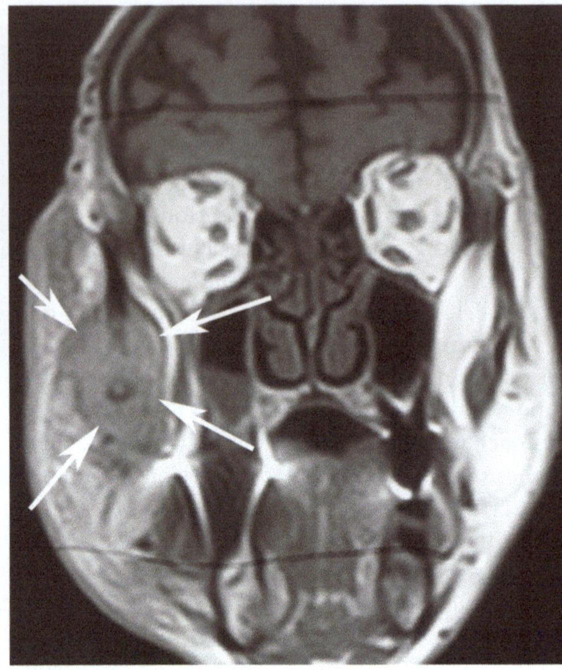

c

Fig. 7.1.2a–c. Metastases of a hepatocellular carcinoma in the masticator space. **a** CT-guided puncture of the lesion. Note the positioning of the needle (*arrows*). **b** The clinical image shows the laser application system in situ using a subzygomatic approach. **c** This contrast-enhanced T_1-weighted sequence after LITT (12 min, 22.8 W) shows a significant amount of necrosis (*arrows*)

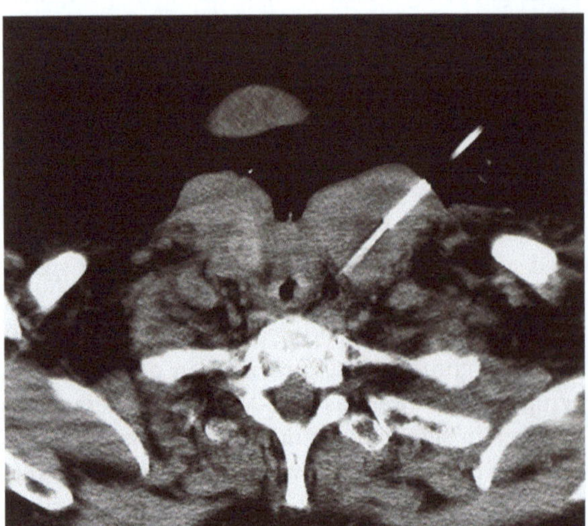

Fig. 7.1.3. CT-guided placement of a laser application system in parastomal recurrent tumors of a squamous cell carcinoma

7.1.4 Discussion

LITT is a widely used technique for minimally invasive tumor ablation throughout the body with a main focus on liver metastases. Palliative treatment options for recurrent head and neck cancer are limited by the proximity of vital vascular and neural structures and the aggressive nature of these tumors. A minimally invasive treatment modality such as interventional MR-guided LITT offers a number of potential treatment benefits. First, MR imaging provides unparalleled topographic accuracy due to its excellent soft-tissue contrast and high spatial resolution. Secondly, the temperature sensitivity of the Thermo-TurboFLASH and FLASH-2D sequences can be used to monitor the temperature elevation in the tumor and surrounding normal tissues, thus increasing safety. On-line MR imaging during LITT therefore allows early detection of local complications and treatment effects such as bleeding, hemorrhage, or necrosis. Thirdly, recovery times, lengths of hospital stay, and the risk of infection and other complications can be reduced when compared with conventional palliative surgery. Finally, successful implementation of such minimally invasive procedures would significantly reduce costs in comparison to surgical procedures. A further, indirect advantage is the psychological effect due to avoidance of cosmetic deformities that can result from major reconstructive surgery.

The clinical success of MR-guided LITT depends on three factors: the optimal localization of the laser applicator in the center of the lesion, controlled in all dimensions, an optimal "on-line monitoring" of the temperature and an exact documentation of the local tumor control rate.

The "on-line thermometry" with MRI allows an exact guidance of the thermotherapy. Contrast-enhanced MRI represents the superior parameter for the follow-up of the treated lesions.

Further Reading

Anzai Y, Lufkin RB, Saxton RE et al (1991) Nd:YAG interstitial laser phototherapy guided by magnetic resonance imaging in an ex vivo model: dosimetry of laser-MR-tissue interaction. Laryngoscope 101:755

Castro DJ, Saxton RE, Layfield LJ et al (1990) Interstitial laser phototherapy assisted by magnetic resonance imaging: a new technique for monitoring laser-tissue interaction. Laryngoscope 100:541

Chapman R (1998) Successful pregnancies following laser-induced interstitial thermotherapy (LITT) for treatment of large uterine leiomyomas by a minimally invasive method. Acta Obstet Gynecol Scand 77:1024

De Poorter J (1995) Noninvasive MRI thermometry with the proton resonance frequency method: study of susceptibility effects. Magn Reson Med 34:359

De Poorter J, De Wagter C, De Deene Y, Thomsen C, Stahlberg F, Achten E (1995) Noninvasive MRI thermometry with the proton resonance frequency (PRF) method: in vivo results in human muscle. Magn Reson Med 33:74

Eyrich GK, Bruder E, Hilfiker P et al (2000) Temperature mapping of magnetic resonance-guided laser interstitial thermal therapy (LITT) in lymphangiomas of the head and neck. Lasers Surg Med 26:467

Fiedler VU, Schwarzmaier HJ, Eickmeyer F et al (2001) Laser-induced interstitial thermotherapy of liver metastases in an interventional 0.5 Tesla MRI system: technique and first clinical experiences. J Magn Reson Imaging 13:729

Gewiese B, Beuthan J, Fobbe F, Stiller D, Muller G, Bose Landgraf J, Wolf KJ, Deimling M (1994) Magnetic resonance imaging-controlled laser-induced interstitial thermotherapy. Invest Radiol 29:345

Harth T, Kahn T, Rassek M, Schwabe B, Schwarzmaier HJ, Lewin JS, Modder U (1997) Determination of laser-induced temperature distributions using echo-shifted TurboFLASH. Magn Reson Med 38:238

Hynynen K, Darkazanli A, Damianou CA, Unger E, Schenck JF (1993) Tissue thermometry during ultrasound exposure. Eur Urol 1:12

Kahn T, Bettag M, Ulrich F et al (1994) MRI-guided laser-induced interstitial thermotherapy of cerebral neoplasms. J Comput Assist Tomogr 18:519

Le Bihan D, Delannoy J, Levin RL (1989) Temperature mapping with MR imaging of molecular diffusion: application to hyperthermia. Radiology 171:853

Mack MG, Straub R, Eichler K, Engelmann K, Roggan A, Woitaschek D, Böttger M, Vogl TJ (2001) Percutaneous MR imaging-guided laser-induced thermotherapy of hepatic metastases. Abdom Imaging 26:369

Matsumoto R, Oshio K, Jolesz FA (1992) Monitoring of laser and freezing-induced ablation in the liver with T1-weighted MR imaging. J Magn Reson Imaging 2:555

Orth K, Russ D, Duerr J et al (1997) Thermo-controlled device for inducing deep coagulation in the liver with the Nd:YAG laser. Lasers Surg Med 20:149

Panych LP, Hrovat MI, Bleier AR, Jolesz FA (1992) Effects related to temperature changes during MR imaging. J Magn Reson Imaging 2:69

Peters RD, Chan E, Trachtenberg J, Jothy S, Kapusta L, Kucharczyk W, Henkelman RM (2000) Magnetic resonance thermometry for predicting thermal damage: an application of interstitial laser coagulation in an in vivo canine prostate model [In Process Citation]. Magn Reson Med 44:873

Vogl TJ, Mack MG, Muller P, Phillip C et al (1995) Recurrent nasopharyngeal tumors: preliminary clinical results with interventional MR imaging-controlled laser-induced thermotherapy. Radiology 196:725

Vogl TJ, Mack MG, Hirsch HH, Müller P, Weinhold N, Wust P, Philipp C, Roggan R, Felix R (1997) In-vitro evaluation of MR-thermometry for laser-induced thermotherapy. Fortschr Röntgenstr 167:638

Vogl TJ, Mack MG, Straub R, Roggan A, Felix R (1997) Magnetic resonance imaging – guided abdominal interventional radiology: laser-induced thermotherapy of liver metastases. Endoscopy 29:577

Vogl TJ, Mack MG, Roggan A, Straub R, Eichler KC, Muller PK, Knappe V, Felix R (1998) Internally cooled power laser for MR-guided interstitial laser-induced thermotherapy of liver lesions: initial clinical results. Radiology 209:381

Vogl TJ, Muller PK, Mack MG, Straub R, Engelmann K, Neuhaus P (1999) Liver metastases: interventional therapeutic techniques and results, state of the art. Eur Radiol 9:675

Vogl TJ, Eichler K, Straub R, Engelmann K, Zangos S, Woitaschek D, Bottger M, Mack MG (2001) Laser-induced thermotherapy of malignant liver tumors: general principals, equipment(s), procedure(s) – side effects, complications and results. Eur J Ultrasound 13:117

Zhang Y, Samulski TV, Joines WT, Mattiello J, Levin RL, LeBihan D (1992) On the accuracy of noninvasive thermometry using molecular diffusion magnetic resonance imaging. Int J Hypertherm 8:263

Other

7.2 Breast

STEFAN O. R. PFLEIDERER and WERNER A. KAISER

CONTENTS

7.2.1 Epidemiology of Breast Cancer

Breast cancer is a major health problem and is the most common cancer in women in industrialized countries. Each year in Germany 55,100 new breast cancer cases are diagnosed. These cases represent 26.8% of all cancers which occur in women (ROBERT-KOCH INSTITUT 2004). Of these breast cancer patients, 40% are younger than 60 years. In North America one in eight women will develop breast cancer during her lifetime (GORDON et al. 2004).

After a follow-up period of more than 20 years it was reported that curative breast-conserving therapy (BCT) of breast cancer yields equivalent results compared to radical mastectomy (FISHER et al. 2002; VERONESI et al. 2002). Despite the fact that postoperative radiation therapy is necessary, most patients and surgeons prefer BCT, because the women want the superior cosmetic outcome and also the prognosis of breast cancer has basically improved over the years. Some 90% of patients with breast cancers in stage T1a present with a disease-free survival time of 20 years. Even for those with higher stages of cancer, radical mastectomy has become less important because patients can be referred to BCT after neoadjuvant chemotherapy and consecutive downstaging of the tumor (SINGLETARY 2001). Also important is the fact that breast cancers are being initially detected earlier, because of the rising sensitivity of imaging procedures, particularly MR mammography, which reaches a sensitivity of between 95% and 100% (KAISER and ZEITLER 1989). CADY (2000) estimated that the mean size of initially diagnosed breast cancers will be as small as 10 mm in 2010. Consequently breast cancer treatment shows a trend to less invasive methods and the evaluation of minimally invasive procedures is warranted. Thermal procedures play a key role in the minimally invasive ablation of tumors. Recently several reports dealing with the percutaneous, minimally invasive therapy of breast cancer have been published (KACHER and JOLESZ 2004). Procedures such as interstitial laser therapy (ILT) (DOWLATSHAHI et al. 2004; MUMTAZ et al. 1996; PFLEIDERER et al. 2003b), radiofrequency ablation (RFA) (BOEHM et al. 2001; BURAK et al. 2003; FORNAGE et al. 2004; HAYASHI et al. 2003) and high focused ultrasound (HIFU) (GIANFELICE et al. 2003a, b; HYHYHEN et al. 2001) destroy the tumor by heating it. In contrast, cryotherapy (HEWITT et al. 1997; PFLEIDERER et al. 2002, 2005) ablates tumor tissue by cooling a cryoprobe down to temperatures as low as –180°C. Until now cryotherapy has been used mainly in the ablation of liver tumors and prostate cancer (SEIFERT and MORRIS 1999). Recently a few reports about cryotherapy of breast cancer (MORIN et al. 2004;

S. O. R. PFLEIDERER, MD
W. A. KAISER, MD, Professor
Institute for Diagnostic and Interventional Radiology, Friedrich-Schiller-Universität Jena, Erlanger Allee 101, 07747 Jena, Germany

Pfleiderer et al. 2002, 2005) and of fibroadenomas (Kaufman et al. 2002, 2004; Littrup et al. 2005) were published.

Thermal destruction of the carcinoma makes adequate assessment of biological tumor markers and hormone receptor status impossible. Thus, minimally invasive breast biopsy, such as large-core breast biopsy or vacuum-assisted biopsy under sonographic, stereotactic or MR guidance for preablative histologic diagnosis, is necessary. Then determination of the presence of estrogen and progesterone receptors and HER-2/neu is performed to plan adjuvant therapies.

7.2.2 Interstitial Laser Therapy (ILT)

The effect of ILT is brought about through the interaction between the laser photons and the molecules of the tissue that is targeted by the laser beam. Three physical processes – absorption, diffusion, refraction – are responsible for the spread of the light in the tissue. Alterations of tissue structure during ILT, e.g., bleaching following coagulation or darkening after carbonization, lead to dynamic changes of these optical properties. The laser light is delivered directly to the target lesion by percutaneous optical fiber. The absorption of the laser light is responsible for the thermal effects of ILT after transformation of the laser energy to heat, which increases the temperature of the tissue and so creates a zone of thermal ablation.

ILT can be carried out directly after breast biopsy using a coaxial technique because the laser fiber is normally placed through a trocar. Afterwards the trocar is pulled back so that there is no danger of the outer cannula obscuring the light. Diffusing tips enable the treatment of larger volumes compared with bare fibers. An additional increase of the size of the necrotic zone can be achieved by cooling the laser fiber, avoiding carbonization of the tissue near the tip of the laser fiber (Vogl et al. 2002). An important advantage of ILT is that optical fibers are entirely MR compatible. MRI is possible during laser energy delivery, indeed MRI is not affected by light and the laser light delivery is not affected by MRI, while the laser device is located outside the scanner room. Furthermore MRI enables temperature mapping during ILT. It is reported that a focal increase of temperature can be visualized by a signal loss in T_1-weighted and diffusion-weighted images. The signal loss appears about 30 s after the onset of treatment and reaches its maximum after 270–400 s. Phase imaging can be used for temperature and dose monitoring as well (Fig. 7.2.1) (Fried et al. 1996; Hall-Craggs 2000; Mumtaz et al. 1996; Pfleiderer et al. 2003b; Steiner et al. 1998). A thermal ablation zone induced by ILT typically consists of a central cavity, which is surrounded by an area of pale tissue, and a hemorrhagic rim in the periphery beyond which viable tissue is found. In histology laser ablation zones are characterized by cells that are morphologically without abnormalities, showing hyperchromatic unsharp nuclei and hypereosinophilic cytoplasm reflecting protein coagulation in the pale zone. The hemorrhagic rim consists of cells that are less damaged and whose nuclei are only slightly hyperchromatic. In the neighborhood of these cells proliferating fibroblasts, blood vessels and red blood cells outside vessels in the interstitium are found. Dowlatshahi and coworkers (2002) reported on ILT of breast carcinomas in 56 patients with histologically proven invasive breast cancers of a diameter under 23 mm. They achieved total tumor destruction in 70% of the patients with early breast cancers. Of the 56 patients, 54 were operated on within 2 months after ILT; 16 of 54 patients (30%) showed residual tumor after ablation. The authors gave the following explanation for these therapeutic failures: four patients were treated during the learning phase and did not receive enough laser energy for effective treatment; two women were oversedated and moved during ILT, which was not realized; in four cases there were technical problems with the equipment, and in five women insufficient target visualization due to post-biopsy hematomas or excessive fluid infusion led to incomplete tumor destruction. The two patients who were not operated after ILT were followed up for 2 years. Initially the treated lesions shrank and were replaced by oil cysts. After resolution of the cysts, fibrosis was found in bioptic histology. No residual tumor was detected after 2 years (Dowlatshahi et al. 2002).

Harms (2001) performed ILT in 12 women with 22 breast lesions under magnetic resonance (MR) guidance. Using rotating delivery of excitation off-resonance (RODEO), breast MRI provides high contrast and improved resolution of breast cancers when localizing the tumor. General anesthetic was not required. After local anesthesia an MRI-com-

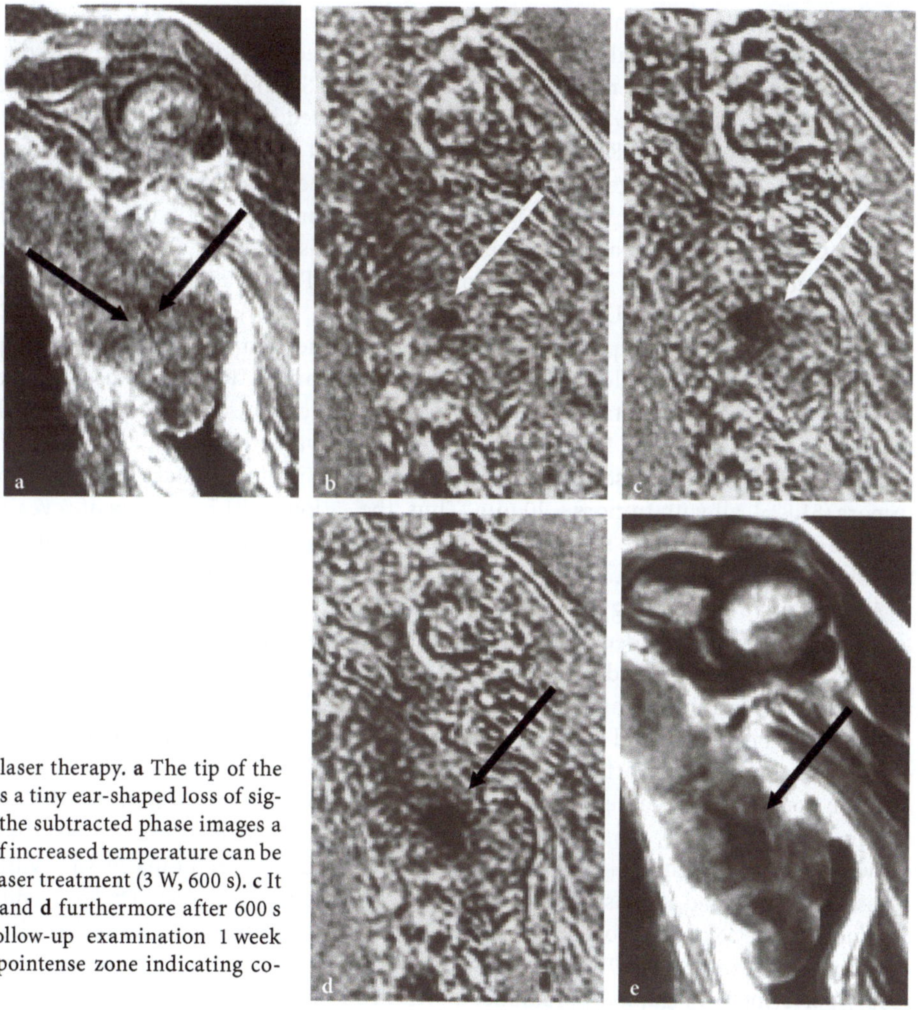

Fig. 7.2.1a–e. Interstitial laser therapy. **a** The tip of the laser fiber is visualized as a tiny ear-shaped loss of signal (*black arrows*). **b** On the subtracted phase images a small hypointense zone of increased temperature can be delineated after 120 s of laser treatment (3 W, 600 s). **c** It is expanding after 360 s and **d** furthermore after 600 s (*white arrows*). **e** The follow-up examination 1 week later shows an anlog hypointense zone indicating coagulation necrosis

patible needle was inserted into the cancer and ILT was controlled by MRI. The appearance of a hypointense zone indicated the heating area. Complete destruction was achieved in only three women who had tumors with diameters under 3 cm. In the other patients large tumors were destroyed incompletely (Harms 2001). Akimov et al. (1998) reported on 35 patients with primary breast cancer who were treated with ILT. In 28 patients, ILT was performed before radical resection, and in 7 patients it was the only invasive treatment. Of 7 patients treated without surgery, local tumor control was achieved in 5, and in 3 stage-I to stage-III patients disease-free survival was followed for 19–60 months. After ILT plus surgery, 3-year disease-free survival was 27% in premenopausal and 92% in menopausal patients.

7.2.3 Radiofrequency Ablation (RFA)

During radiofrequency ablation (RFA), alternating current is sent into the tissue through needle electrodes. The alternating current generates ionic movement and agitation as ions oscillate at the applied frequency. Localized friction results in tissue heating, which leads to cell death. Histologically tissue shows coagulation necrosis and protein denaturation after RFA. Macroscopically the ablation zone is characterized by a yellow-white center, which is surrounded by a hyperemic red rim reflecting hemorrhage (Mirza et al. 2001). Boehm and coworkers (2001) developed an experimental tumor model for RFA of breast tumors surrounded by fat to investigate the minimally invasive treatment of breast tumors with saline-enhanced RFA monitored by ultrasound (US). In total, 28 VX2 tumors were implanted into the retroperitoneum of 14 rabbits and monitored by B-mode US at regular intervals of 2–3 days. Saline-enhanced RFA (25 mm tip length) was performed 16 days after tumor implantation (10 min treatment time, 28 W, 15 ml/h infusion of 0.9% NaCl, which was increased to 30 ml/h in cases of an impedance increase). Thermal lesion growth was monitored by B-mode US. Treatment was considered complete if no relapse was detectable histopathologically after a follow-up period of up to 3 weeks. All tumor implantations were successful, reaching sizes of 5–38 mm 16 days after implantation. After RFA local relapses occurred in 14 of 27 tumors (51.8%), all with tumors > 20 mm. Thus, the method appears to be more successful with smaller tumors (Boehm et al. 2001).

All human studies dealing with percutaneous RFA to treat breast cancer included fewer than 30 patients. Jeffrey et al. (1999) treated 5 women with locally advanced breast cancer using RFA. The tumors had diameters of between 4 and 7 cm. Mastectomy was carried out immediately after RFA that generated ablation zones with a diameter of between 0.8 and 1.8 cm around the tip of the radiofrequency needle, showing cell death histologically in four of the five cases. One tumor had a focus of less than 1 mm with residual tumor. No periprocedural complications occurred (Jeffrey et al. 1999). Izzo and coworkers (2001) performed US-guided percutaneous RFA in 26 patients with biopsy-proven, invasive breast cancers which was followed by immediate resection. The size of the tumors ranged between 0.7 and 3 cm. Complete coagulation necrosis was achieved in 25 of the 26 patients (96%). One patient had a microscopic focus of viable tissue adjacent to the needle shaft which was interpreted to be rather unusual because viable tumors are seen at the periphery of the ablation zone and not in its center. In one case a complication occurred. After RFA a skin burn overlying the ablation zone was seen. Limitations of this study were that ultrasonographic monitoring of the treatment did not provide accurate measurement of the histopathologic zone of complete necrosis. The hyperechogenicity of the RF ablation zone and the dorsal acoustic shadowing made it impossible to monitor the deeper zones of treatment, resulting in a lack of real-time assessment of the adequacy of RFA (Izzo et al. 2001). Another group reported on US-guided RFA in 21 invasive breast cancers under 2 cm immediately prior to open surgical removal of the tumor. The prongs of an umbrella-shaped needle in the lesions were deployed with real-time US guidance. The effectiveness of RFA was evaluated by NADH staining of the operation specimen. In one woman who had neoadjuvant chemotherapy the target lesion was destroyed but residual invasive tumor occult in US and mammography was found in histology. In all, 20 woman were free of tumor after RFA. No adverse effects were observed (Fornage et al. 2004). MRI is not possible during RFA because of the high-frequency alternating current. On the other hand, MRI may be used for exact lesion and needle localization before, and reliable treatment response evaluation after, the onset of alternating current. With the highest sensitivity in breast cancer detection, MRI is capable of revealing multifocal disease by detecting lesions as small as 3 mm (Fischer et al. 2005). Hayashi and coworkers (2003) treated 22 postmenopausal women with core-biopsy-proven breast cancers measuring 3 cm or less. Resection took place between 1 and 2 weeks after US-guided RFA. Coagulative necrosis was complete in 19 of 22 patients. Disease at the ablation zone margin was found in 3 patients and 5 patients had disease distant to the ablation zone consisting of multifocal tumors (2 cases), in-transit metastasis (1 case), and extensive ductal carcinoma in situ with microinvasive carcinoma (2 cases). The procedure was well tolerated and cosmesis was excellent in all cases (Hayashi et al. 2003). The case report of Elliot et al. (2002) is the only example of stereotactically guided RFA of breast cancer. After mammographic-guided biopsy revealed an invasive ductal carcinoma with a size of 16 mm, a metallic clip was left to mark the lesion and it was treated using RFA. Then, 4 weeks later the ablation site was resected after wire localization. No viable tumor was detectable in the operation specimen. This was at least a proof-of-principle that RFA is feasible under stereotactic guidance.

7.2.4 High-Intensity Focused Ultrasound (HIFU)

High-intensity focused ultrasound (HIFU) has the same principle as conventional ultrasound. Many piezo elements emit US beams, which are brought to a tight focus. There, focal energy deposition by conversion of mechanical energy into heat causes protein denaturation and tissue necrosis. Arrest of cellular reproduction will take place if the temperature is maintained above 56°C for 1 s. Rapid thermo-induced irreversible cell death through coagulation necrosis occurs. During HIFU treatments, the temperature at the focus can rise rapidly above 80°C which, even for the shortest exposures, should lead to effective and complete cell damage. The high thermal gradient caused by reaching such high temperatures within seconds creates boundaries of the treatment area that are sharply demarcated without damage to the non-tumorous surrounding tissue. In other heating procedures the cooling effect of perfusion may inhibit the efficiency of treatment, whereas HIFU does not suffer from this limitation because the exposure times for a volume of a few cubic millimeters are below 3 s (Kennedy et al. 2003). The process is repeated in the entire tumor volume until the lesion is completely covered. MRI allows good anatomic resolution, and high sensitivity in tumor detection and temperature monitoring (Bohris et al. 1999). Thus, the combination of MRI and HIFU simultaneously enables the definition of tumor margins, noninvasive thermal therapy, and the control of the temperature at the current therapy site (Jolesz and Hynynen 2002). Huber and coworkers (2001) published an animal study and a case report about MRI-guided HIFU of breast cancer. The patient was in a prone position with her breast suspended in the water bath of the HIFU unit, which consisted of an ultrasound source, an MRI coil, and a hydraulically driven positioning system. When the US transducer was positioned exactly within a deviation of not more than 1 mm, HIFU sonications were sent to the tumor. The ultrasound focus was cigar shaped with a diameter of 1 mm and a length of 8.7 mm. The target volume was outlined by MRI. A close spacing of small foci resulted in overlapping treatment zones that covered the entire tumor volume. The passage of the surrounding tissue did not cause any damage. In contrast to other minimally invasive therapy procedures the focused ultrasound penetrated the skin without damaging it by the insertion of probes or needles. The published case was a patient with a 22-mm, invasive ductal carcinoma. Immediately after HIFU, MRI showed a non-enhancing area at the treated zoned. Open surgery was performed as a standard breast-conserving procedure 5 days after HIFU. In the operation specimen the treated zone presented as a white necrotic area with a hyperemic rim which corresponded well with the target outlined in the MR planning image. Chung et al. (1996) and Mulkern et al. (1998) treated 11 women using HIFU and achieved partial or total success in 73% of cases. They described problems due to patient motion, lesion undertreatment through inadequate power settings, and beam reflection caused by the formation of gas bubbles during treatment or local anesthetic.

Gianfelice and coworkers (2003a) reported on 17 patients who underwent MR-guided HIFU for treatment of breast cancer. Dynamic MR mammography was performed before and after the MRIgFUS treatment of small breast tumors (diameter <3.5 cm). The lesions were surgically resected and the presence of residual tumor was determined by histopathological analysis. A good correlation was found between parameters which were acquired by MR mammography and the percentage of residual viable tumor determined by histopathology. The amount of residual tumor ranged between 0% and 75%. Nine patients had residual tumor volumes of less than 10% and only four women did not show any viable tumor after HIFU. The parameters from MR mammography provided a reliable noninvasive method for assessing residual tumor following HIFU treatment of breast tumors. In a series of 12 women the same group reported (Gianfelice et al. 2003c) a treatment duration of between 35 and 133 min (median time 76.5 min). A mean of 46.7% of the tumor was within the targeted zone and a mean of 43.3% of the cancer tissue was destroyed. In the last nine patients who were treated with a more advanced HIFU system a mean of 95.6% of the tumor was within the target area and 88.3% of the cancer tissue was necrosed. Two patients did not show residual cancer (Fig. 7.2.2). Residual tumor was identified predominantly at the periphery of the tumor mass. The authors concluded that this fact indicated the need to increase the total targeted area by increasing the number of sonifications. Wu et al. (2003) published the largest trial on HIFU. They included 48 women and randomized them to undergo modified radical mastectomy (25 women) or HIFU and modified radical mastectomy 1–2 weeks later (23 women). After HIFU breast edema occurred and disappeared during a time interval of between 7 and 10 days after HIFU. Of 23 patients, 14 had minor symptoms such as heaviness of the treated breast or local pain but only 4 patients requested analgesics. The distance between tumor and nipple was at least 20 mm in all cases, and between tumor and skin, 5 mm. Histology revealed total cell death and coagulation necrosis inside the treated area proved by immunohistochemical methods.

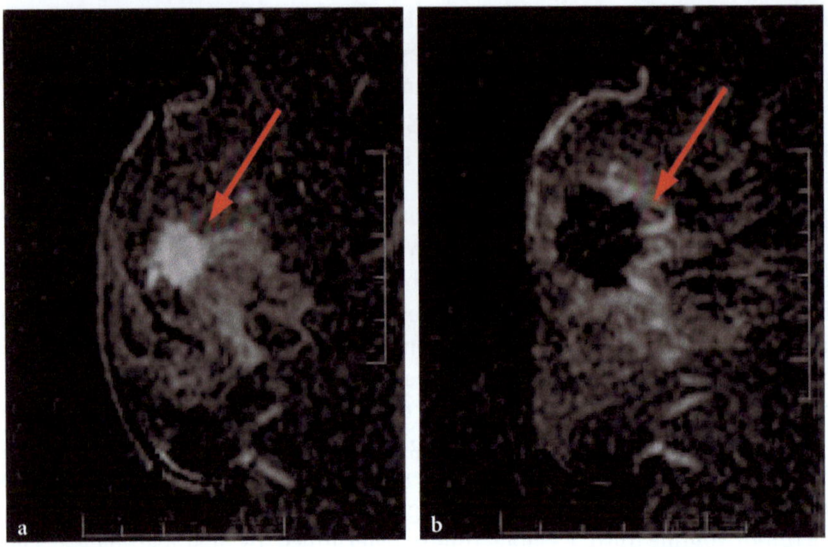

Fig. 7.2.2a,b. MRI-guided HIFU of breast cancer. **a** T_1-weighted subtracted MR image after gadolinium-DTPA application which shows a breast cancer (*arrow*) before HIFU. **b** After HIFU the lesion enhances no further, indicating effective ablation (with courtesy of Breastopia Namba Hospital, Miyazaki, Japan)

7.2.5 Microwave Ablation Therapy

Microwaves applied to living tissue produce dielectric heat by stimulation of the water molecules within the tissue and the cells. The rapid agitation of the water molecules results in frictional heating and thermo-induced coagulation necrosis. Using microwave ablation therapy in breast cancer two microwave phased array waveguide applicators compress the breast. The energy preferentially heats tissues with a high water content, such as breast cancer tissue, whereas the surrounding tissues, for instance adipose or connective tissue and breast parenchyma, with a lower water content absorb less thermal energy. Cooling of the overlying skin is necessary frequently. Gardner and colleagues (2002) performed microwave ablation in ten women with breast cancer. All tumors were surgically resected within 18 days after microwave ablation. A reduction of tumor size was found in 60% of the patients, using ultrasound. Histological evaluation of the operation specimens revealed tumor necrosis in 80% of cases. In another series 25 patients were treated using microwave ablation (Vargas et al. 2004). Histology revealed necrosis of the tumors, which had a mean diameter of 18 mm, in 68% of patients. Complete destruction of the invasive component of the tumor was achieved only in 2 of 25 women.

7.2.6 Cryotherapy

During cryotherapy three basic phenomena occur resulting in cell death:

- Rapid formation of intracellular and extracellular ice crystals, which leads to mechanical shear forces on cell membranes and organelles causing mechanical cell damage
- Cellular dehydration, which occurs due to shifting of water from intracellular to extracellular spaces by osmosis causing destruction of critical cellular components
- Ischemia as a result of vascular stasis and damage to the blood vessels, which prevents nutrients from reaching remnant viable cells

The faster low temperatures are reached, the more severe is the damage to the treated tissue. Compared to nitrogen-based systems, operating temperature is reached faster with argon-based systems, and cells are damaged more effectively. So Hewitt and coworkers (1997) compared nitrogen-based cryotherapy with cryoablation using argon gas. Three different 3-mm cryoprobes were used: an old liquid nitrogen probe (N-probe), a new N-probe featuring gas bypass, and an argon gas probe. Each probe was tested in two models:

- Fresh sheep liver at 20°C – the probe was inserted to a depth of 1.5 cm; the rate of ice-ball formation was monitored by recording radial temperatures every 15 s at 5, 10, 15, and 20 mm from the cryoprobe, and the ice-ball diameter was measured every 2.5 min. After 10 min, the probe was warmed and the time taken until it could be extracted from the liver was recorded.

- Warm water bath – the probe was immersed in warm water (42°C) for 15 min and the ice-ball diameter was measured at 5-min intervals.

Radial temperatures in liver declined more rapidly ($p < 0.001$) and the time to probe extraction was less ($p < 0.01$) when the argon gas system was used. The new N-probe performed better than its older counterpart, but was still slower than the argon gas system. In liver (20°C), ice-ball diameters were similar after 10 min, but in warm water, they were larger when the new N-probe was used ($p < 0.02$). It would appear that the argon gas system is initially faster, but it does not achieve as large an ice-ball in a warm environment as the liquid nitrogen system (Hewitt et al. 1997). The safety of cryotherapy has already been published: a world review about 5432 patients who underwent cryotherapy for prostate cancer mentioned 3 deaths (0.06%) after the intervention. Mortality after cryotherapy of liver tumors is reported to be 1.5%–1.6% due to cryoshock, which is uncommon in prostate therapy (Seifert and Morris 1999). The two minor complications in the study from our group in Jena (Pfleiderer et al. 2002) are most likely due to vessel damage during the insertion of the cryoprobe, which resulted in bleeding that was stopped after compression and the transformation of a hematoma to a seroma. While complications such as those that occur in cryoshock, for example fistulas that occurred in cryoablation of the liver or urethral strictures and incontinence with cryosurgery of the prostate, are unlikely to occur in breast therapy, skin or fatty tissue necrosis, hematoma, intercostals nerve damage and focal neuritis may occur. Our group (Pfleiderer et al. 2002, 2005) treated a total of 41 patients with biopsy-confirmed breast cancers using percutaneous cryotherapy. In all, 30 women had tumor diameters of 15 mm or smaller (Pfleiderer et al. 2005) (range 5–15 mm, median 12 mm) whereas 11 patients presented with cancers of 16 mm or more (Pfleiderer et al. 2002). After local anesthesia a 3-mm cryoprobe was placed into the tumor under ultrasound guidance (Fig. 7.2.3). All tumors were subjected to two freeze cycles with an interposing thawing cycle. The size of the ice-balls and the temperature at the tip of the probe (Fig. 7.2.4) were closely monitored during the procedure. The patients underwent surgery within 6 weeks and the specimens were evaluated histologically.

The median minimum temperature reached −146°C (range: −117°C to −167°C). In 5 of 29 patients who had tumors with a size of 15 mm or smaller, remnant ductal carcinoma in situ (DCIS) was histologically detectable after cryotherapy beyond the margin of the cryosite in the specimens after open surgery. In 24 women no viable tumor cells were found (Pfleiderer et al. 2005). No severe side-effects occurred. In one patient the cryo procedure was not performed completely due to technical problems.

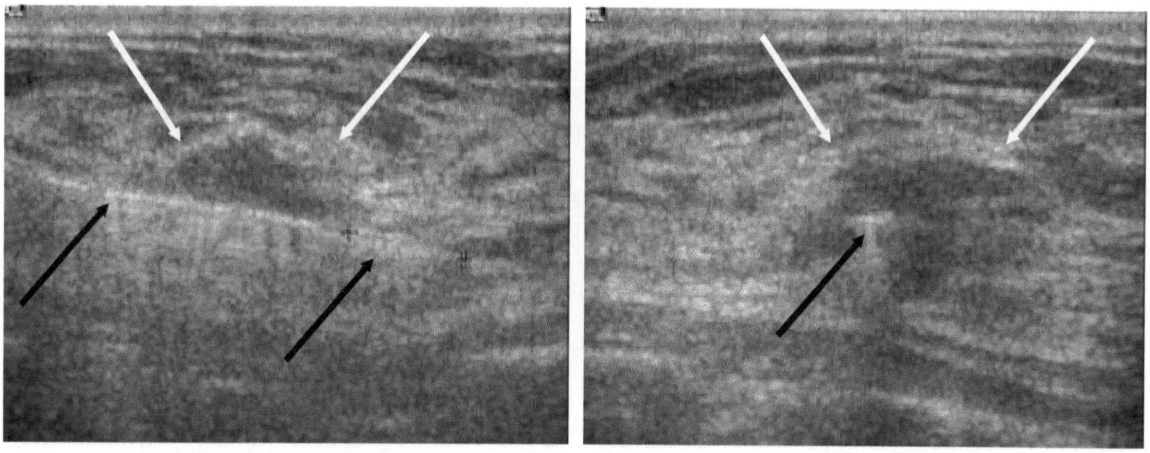
a b

Fig. 7.2.3a,b. Ultrasound image (B-mode) of the final position of the cryoprobe in a 70-year-old patient. **a, b** The cryoprobe (*black arrows*) passed the center of a histologically proven invasive ductal carcinoma (diameter 14 mm) (*white arrows*) in two planes. The patient was operated after cryotherapy. The histological evaluation of the specimens after open surgery did not reveal any residual viable tumor

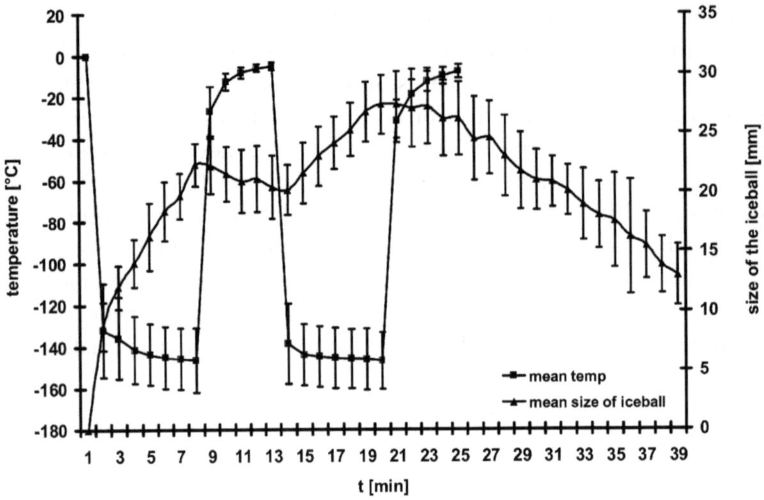

Fig. 7.2.4. Mean of temperature scores (*y*-axis, *left*) measured at the tip of the cryo probe and mean diameters of the ice-ball (*y*-axis, *right*) at each minute (*x*-axis) during the procedure in the first 16 patients

Incomplete destruction of the cancers was achieved in the 11 patients who presented with tumors that had a diameter of 16 mm or more (Pfleiderer et al. 2002). It has already been reported that clinical occult, remnant tumor is present even after breast-conserving surgery. Holland et al. (1985) found otherwise unsuspected foci of tumor in about 40% of mastectomy specimens that were sectioned serially. On the other hand, Karasawa et al. (2003) reported 102 of 348 patients with positive final pathological margin states, which means that cancer cells remained within 5 mm of the surgical margins after BCT. Only five patients had loco-regional tumor recurrence 5 years after radiation therapy, so residual viable tumor did not always result in tumor recurrence in this study. Preinterventional histological evaluation of the hormone receptor status is necessary after LCBB before the tumor cells are destroyed. In the current study the hormone receptor status of the cancers were all evaluated prior to cryotherapy and thus adjuvant therapy could be planned properly in all patients.

In contrast, many reports have shown that the pathologic margin status is one of the most important predictors for local recurrence and that it is still not clear whether obtaining a radical margin will decrease the rate of local recurrence after BCT (Chagpar et al. 2003; Singletary 2002). Nevertheless, residual tumor cells at the edge of the cryo zone should be avoided. Thus, sensitive imaging modalities such as MR mammography (Fischer et al. 2005) might be helpful and could be performed for therapy planning and preinterventional MR-guided breast biopsy (Pfleiderer et al. 2003a; Veltman et al. 2005). In addition, MR guidance may better monitor cryotherapy and seems adequate for delineating tumors from ice-balls, according to a recent paper of Morin et al. (2004). Using MR, frozen tissue may be very easily delineated from surrounding structures within all three dimensions. In contrast, only the surface of the ice-ball facing the transducer can be delineated using ultrasound. Due to acoustic shadowing the area behind the ice-ball cannot be detected completely (Fig. 7.2.5). Furthermore, ultrasound may underestimate the true microscopic extent of the tumor, which may result in the undertreatment of breast lesions. In the study of Morin et al. (2004) percutaneous cryosurgery was performed in 25 patients with operable invasive breast carcinoma, 4 weeks prior to their scheduled mastectomy under the guidance of near-real-time T_1-weighted FSE images of a 0.5-T open-configuration MR system. The cryo procedure resulted in no serious complications, either local or systemic. All tumoral tissues included in the cryogenic "ice-ball" were destroyed, with no viable histologic residues. Of the 25 patients, 13 presented with histologically detectable viable tumor residue after cryotherapy, indicating that the ice-ball did not cover the entire lesion. Roubidoux and colleagues (2004) treated nine patients with small solitary invasive breast cancers diagnosed at core biopsy using US-guided cryoablation and a 2.7-mm cryoprobe. Mean cancer size was 12 mm (range, 8–18 mm). A tabletop argon-gas-based cryoablation system with a double freeze-thaw protocol was used to treat cancers in an outpatient setting. Tumor sites were excised at lumpectomy 2–3 weeks after cryoablation. With US guidance, ice-balls (maximal mean size, 4.4 cm) were formed around cancers. Two of nine patients (22%) had residual cancer. One patient had a small focus of invasive cancer; one had extensive multifocal ductal carcinoma in situ (DCIS). No

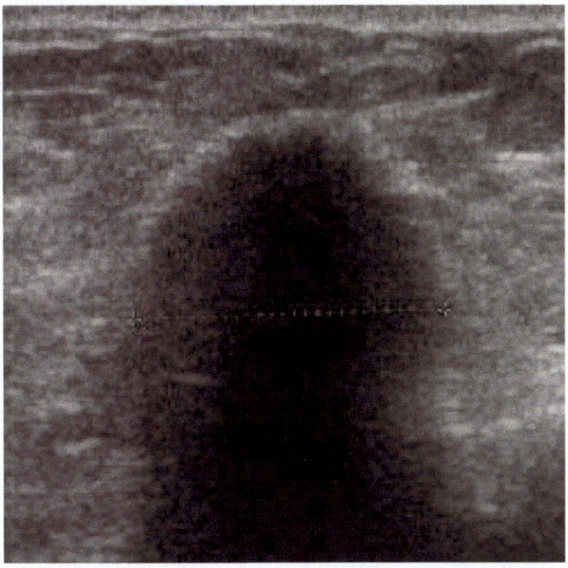

Fig. 7.2.5. The surface of the ice-ball could be well delineated in all cases on the ultrasound images showing the sickle-shaped hyperechoic surface of the ice-ball. The entire area behind the ice-ball is not visible because ice reflects ultrasound waves resulting in dorsal acoustic shadowing

residual invasive cancers occurred in tumors 17 mm or smaller or in cancers without spiculated margins at US. One tool to avoid remnant tumor as occurred in the study of Pfleiderer et al. (2002, 2005) or Roubidoux and coworkers (2004) may be preprocedural MR mammography. DCIS has a characteristic appearance in MR mammography, which has a rather good sensitivity of 92% in detecting high-grade DCIS (Neubauer et al. 2003). Thus, MR mammography may be helpful for excluding women with an extensive intraductal component from minimally invasive therapy.

Kaufman et al. (2004) performed percutaneous cryotherapy in women with fibroadenomas. US-guided cryoablation of core biopsy-proven benign fibroadenomas, other benign breast nodules, or nodular fibrocystic change was performed on 78 lesions in 63 patients. Then, 64 of 78 lesions (mean size 2.0 cm, range 0.8–4.2 cm) were followed-up for at least 12 months after cryoablation per protocol, which included 53 fibroadenomas. At 1 year, US tumor volume resorption was 88.3% overall (87.3% for fibroadenomas), and 73% of the entire group became nonpalpable to both clinician and patient (75% for fibroadenomas). Two of the fibroadenoma patients had their palpable residual nodule excised, both revealing necrotic debris and no viable tumor in the treated volume.

7.2.7 Summary

Numerous methods of image-guided percutaneous minimally invasive therapy for breast cancer are under investigation, while BCT is developing less invasive methods. All procedures destroy cancer tissue by depositing thermal energy within the tumorous lesion. All reports show partial destruction of the cancers to various extents. Limitations in local tumor control are still a limitation of almost all published studies. On the other hand, even after breast-conserving surgery, positive margins, which were not apparent from acute perioperative histology, occurred and may result in local cancer recurrence. Nevertheless the presence of tumor cells at the edge of the ablation zone after percutaneous treatment of breast cancer should be avoided. Up until now, breast-conserving surgery followed by irradiation and probably chemotherapy, depending on the lymph node status and the tumor extent, is still the gold standard in the treatment of breast cancer. However, to achieve wide acceptance, minimally invasive ablation therapies must lead to equivalent or even greater efficacy as surgical outcomes and, in the short-term, demonstrate total ablation with negative margins, while sparing normal tissue beyond the target volume. Furthermore long-term results after percutaneous ablation are not yet available. Thus, further studies with larger patient series have to be carried out, especially those without subsequent surgery but with adjuvant therapy regimens including state-of-the-art radiotherapy and chemotherapy.

References

Akimov AB, Seregin VE, Rusanov KV et al (1998) Nd:YAG interstitial laser thermotherapy in the treatment of breast cancer. Lasers Surg Med 22:257–267

Boehm T, Malich A, Reichenbach JR, Fleck M, Kaiser WA (2001) Percutaneous radiofrequency (RF) thermal ablation of rabbit tumors embedded in fat: a model for RF ablation of breast tumors. Invest Radiol 36:480–486

Bohris C, Schreiber WG, Jenne J et al (1999) Quantitative MR temperature monitoring of high-intensity focused ultrasound therapy. Magn Reson Imaging 17:603–610

Burak WE Jr, Agnese DM, Povoski SP et al (2003) Radiofrequency ablation of invasive breast carcinoma followed by delayed surgical excision. Cancer 98:1369–1376

Cady B (2000) Breast cancer in the third millennium. Breast J 6:280–287

Chagpar A, Yen T, Sahin A et al (2003) Intraoperative margin assessment reduces reexcision rates in patients with ductal carcinoma in situ treated with breast-conserving surgery. Am J Surg 186:371–377

Chung AH, Hynynen K, Colucci V, Oshio K, Cline HE, Jolesz FA (1996) Optimization of spoiled gradient-echo phase imaging for in vivo localization of a focused ultrasound beam. Magn Reson Med 36:745–752

Dowlatshahi K, Francescatti DS, Bloom KJ (2002) Laser therapy for small breast cancers. Am J Surg 184:359–363

Dowlatshahi K, Dieschbourg JJ, Bloom KJ (2004) Laser therapy of breast cancer with 3-year follow-up. Breast J 10:240–243

Elliott RL, Rice PB, Suits JA, Ostrowe AJ, Head JF (2002) Radiofrequency ablation of a stereotactically localized nonpalpable breast carcinoma. Am Surg 68:1–5

Fischer DR, Wurdinger S, Boettcher J, Malich A, Kaiser WA (2005) Further signs in the evaluation of magnetic resonance mammography: a retrospective study. Invest Radiol 40:430–435

Fisher B, Jeong JH, Anderson S et al (2002) Twenty-five-year follow-up of a randomized trial comparing radical mastectomy, total mastectomy, and total mastectomy followed by irradiation. N Engl J Med 347:567–575

Fornage BD, Sneige N, Ross MI et al (2004) Small (≤2-cm) breast cancer treated with US-guided radiofrequency ablation: feasibility study. Radiology 231:215–224

Fried MP, Morrison PR, Hushek SG, Kernahan GA, Jolesz FA (1996) Dynamic T1-weighted magnetic resonance imaging of interstitial laser photocoagulation in the liver: observations on in vivo temperature sensitivity. Lasers Surg Med 18:410–419

Gardner RA, Vargas HI, Block JB et al (2002) Focused microwave phased array thermotherapy for primary breast cancer. Ann Surg Oncol 9:326–332

Gianfelice D, Khiat A, Amara M, Belblidia A, Boulanger Y (2003a) MR imaging-guided focused ultrasound surgery of breast cancer: correlation of dynamic contrast-enhanced MRI with histopathologic findings. Breast Cancer Res Treat 82:93–101

Gianfelice D, Khiat A, Boulanger Y, Amara M, Belblidia A (2003b) Feasibility of magnetic resonance imaging-guided focused ultrasound surgery as an adjunct to tamoxifen therapy in high-risk surgical patients with breast carcinoma. J Vasc Interv Radiol 14:1275–1282

Gianfelice D, Khiat A, Amara M, Belblidia A, Boulanger Y (2003c) MR imaging-guided focused US ablation of breast cancer: histopathologic assessment of effectiveness – initial experience. Radiology 227:849–855

Gordon R, Wirth M, Schellenberg J, Sivaramakrishna R (2004) Workshop on alternatives to mammography. 18–20 September 2004

Hall-Craggs MA (2000) Interventional MRI of the breast: minimally invasive therapy. Eur Radiol 10:59–62

Harms SE (2001) Percutaneous ablation of breast lesions by radiologists and surgeons. Breast Dis 13:67–75

Hayashi AH, Silver SF, van der Westhuizen NG et al (2003) Treatment of invasive breast carcinoma with ultrasound-guided radiofrequency ablation. Am J Surg 185:429–435

Hewitt PM, Zhao J, Akhter J, Morris DL (1997) A comparative laboratory study of liquid nitrogen and argon gas cryosurgery systems. Cryobiology 35:303–308

Holland R, Veling SH, Mravunac M, Hendriks JH (1985) Histologic multifocality of Tis, T1-2 breast carcinomas. Implications for clinical trials of breast-conserving surgery. Cancer 56:979–990

Huber PE, Jenne JW, Rastert R et al (2001) A new noninvasive approach in breast cancer therapy using magnetic resonance imaging-guided focused ultrasound surgery. Cancer Res 61:8441–8447

Hynynen K, Pomeroy O, Smith DN et al (2001) MR imaging-guided focused ultrasound surgery of fibroadenomas in the breast: a feasibility study. Radiology 219:176–185

Izzo F, Thomas R, Delrio P et al (2001) Radiofrequency ablation in patients with primary breast carcinoma: a pilot study in 26 patients. Cancer 92:2036–2044

Jeffrey SS, Birdwell RL, Ikeda DM et al (1999) Radiofrequency ablation of breast cancer: first report of an emerging technology. Arch Surg 134:1064–1068

Jolesz FA, Hynynen K (2002) Magnetic resonance image-guided focused ultrasound surgery. Cancer J 8 [Suppl 1]: S100–S112

Kacher DF, Jolesz FA (2004) MR imaging-guided breast ablative therapy. Radiol Clin North Am 42:947–962, vii

Kaiser WA, Zeitler E (1989) MR imaging of the breast: fast imaging sequences with and without Gd-DTPA. Preliminary observations. Radiology 170:681–686

Karasawa K, Obara T, Shimizu T et al (2003) Outcome of breast-conserving therapy in the Tokyo Women's Medical University Breast Cancer Society experience. Breast Cancer 10:341–348

Kaufman CS, Bachman B, Littrup PJ et al (2002) Office-based ultrasound-guided cryoablation of breast fibroadenomas. Am J Surg 184:394–400

Kaufman CS, Bachman B, Littrup PJ et al (2004) Cryoablation treatment of benign breast lesions with 12-month follow-up. Am J Surg 188:340–348

Kennedy JE, Ter Haar GR, Cranston D (2003) High intensity focused ultrasound: surgery of the future? Br J Radiol 76:590–599

Littrup PJ, Freeman-Gibb L, Andea A et al (2005) Cryotherapy for breast fibroadenomas. Radiology 234:63–72

Mirza AN, Fornage BD, Sneige N et al (2001) Radiofrequency ablation of solid tumors. Cancer J 7:95–102

Morin J, Traore A, Dionne G et al (2004) Magnetic resonance-guided percutaneous cryosurgery of breast carcinoma: technique and early clinical results. Can J Surg 47:347–351

Mulkern RV, Panych LP, McDannold NJ et al (1998) Tissue temperature monitoring with multiple gradient-echo imaging sequences. J Magn Reson Imaging 8:493–502

Mumtaz H, Hall-Craggs MA, Wotherspoon A et al (1996) Laser therapy for breast cancer: MR imaging and histopathologic correlation. Radiology 200:651–658

Neubauer H, Li M, Kuehne-Heid R, Schneider A, Kaiser WA (2003) High grade and non-high grade ductal carcinoma in situ on dynamic MR mammography: characteristic findings for signal increase and morphological pattern of enhancement. Br J Radiol 76:3–12

Pfleiderer SO, Freesmeyer MG, Marx C, Kuhne-Heid R, Schneider A, Kaiser WA (2002) Cryotherapy of breast cancer under ultrasound guidance: initial results and limitations. Eur Radiol 12:3009–3014

Pfleiderer SO, Reichenbach JR, Azhari T, Marx C, Wurdinger S, Kaiser WA (2003a) Dedicated double breast coil for

magnetic resonance mammography imaging, biopsy, and preoperative localization. Invest Radiol 38:1–8
Pfleiderer SOR, Reichenbach JR, Wurdinger S et al (2003b) Interventional MR-mammography: manipulator-assisted large core biopsy and interstitial laser therapy of tumors of the female breast. Z Med Phys 13:198–202
Pfleiderer SO, Marx C, Camara O, Gajda M, Kaiser WA (2005) Ultrasound-guided, percutaneous cryotherapy of small (≤15 mm) breast cancers. Invest Radiol 40:472–477
Robert-Koch Institut (2004) Entwicklung der Überlebensraten von Krebspatienten in Deutschland, Brust. http://www.rki.de. In, 2004; 1–6
Roubidoux MA, Sabel MS, Bailey JE, Kleer CG, Klein KA, Helvie MA (2004) Small (<2.0 cm) breast cancers: mammographic and US findings at US-guided cryoablation-initial experience. Radiology 233:857–867
Seifert JK, Morris DL (1999) World survey on the complications of hepatic and prostate cryotherapy. World J Surg 23:109–113; discussion 113–104
Singletary SE (2001) Neoadjuvant chemotherapy in the treatment of stage II and III breast cancer. Am J Surg 182:341–346
Singletary SE (2002) Surgical margins in patients with early-stage breast cancer treated with breast conservation therapy. Am J Surg 184:383–393
Steiner P, Botnar R, Dubno B, Zimmermann GG, Gazelle GS, Debatin JF (1998) Radiofrequency-induced thermoablation: monitoring with T1-weighted and proton frequency-shift MR imaging in an interventional 0.5-T environment. Radiology 206:803–810
Vargas HI, Dooley WC, Gardner RA et al (2004) Focused microwave phased array thermotherapy for ablation of early-stage breast cancer: results of thermal dose escalation. Ann Surg Oncol 11:139–146
Veltman J, Boetes C, Wobbes T et al (2005) Magnetic resonance-guided biopsies and localizations of the breast: initial experiences using an open breast coil and compatible intervention device. Invest Radiol 40:379–384
Veronesi U, Cascinelli N, Mariani L et al (2002) Twenty-year follow-up of a randomized study comparing breast-conserving surgery with radical mastectomy for early breast cancer. N Engl J Med 347:1227–1232
Vogl TJ, Mack MG, Straub R et al (2002) MR-guided laser-induced thermotherapy with a cooled power laser system: a case report of a patient with a recurrent carcinoid metastasis in the breast. Eur Radiol 12 [Suppl 3]:S101–S104
Wu F, Wang ZB, Cao YD et al (2003) A randomised clinical trial of high-intensity focused ultrasound ablation for the treatment of patients with localised breast cancer. Br J Cancer 89:2227–2233

Treatment Strategies

(incl. Current Study Protocols and Flow-Charts)

Hepatocellular Carcinoma (HCC)

8

Thomas K. Helmberger

CONTENTS

8.1 Background

Hepatocellular carcinoma (HCC) is considered to be one of the most common malignancies worldwide, and the most common one in Africa and Asia. Over the last decade, a rising incidence of up to 10–15/100,000 per population has been seen in the Western world, with an estimate of 250,000 deaths and more than a million worldwide per year. By the year 2010, the World Health Organization expects that HCC will be the leading cause of cancer mortality surpassing lung cancer. This increasing incidence is most likely related to an increasing prevalence of chronic hepatitis C (HC) and B (HB) virus infections and other diseases inducing chronic inflammation (Befeler and Di Bisceglie 2002; Llovet et al. 2003).

For the US, an estimated ca. 4 million individuals carry the HC virus; similar figures might be true for Central Europe. Subsequently, 5%–10% of the infected HC virus carriers will develop HCC. In Africa and South East Asia aflatoxin B1 contamination and HB virus infection are the main causes of developing HCC. As in many other tumors, mutations or deletions of the tumor suppressor gene P53 seem to play an important role in HCC carcinogenesis, and this is especially true in aflatoxin B1 exposure.

Moreover, long-standing viral infection will result in the liver being chronically inflamed, which is linked to a permanent process of inflammation, necrosis, and regeneration, together with activation of proto-oncogenes and with potential mutations of the P53 tumor suppressor gene. Juengst et al. (2004) showed that the inflammatory-induced persistent oxidative damage enhances hepatocarcinogenesis.

This explains the high correlation between cirrhosis and HCC, in that cirrhosis will be present in up to 60% of patients with HCC. Additional factors supporting the development of cirrhosis are chronic alcohol abuse and metabolic diseases such as alpha-1 antitrypsin deficiency syndrome, hepatic porphyria, and hemochromatosis, which presents a risk of about 30% of developing HCC.

Taken together, hepatic cirrhosis of any etiology represents the major risk factor for HCC with additional increased incidence in viral hepatitis and idiopathic hemochromatosis (El-Serag and Mason 2000).

Unfortunately, the prognosis of untreated HCC is still poor. The mean survival time from diagnosis is only 3–8 months with a 5-year survival rate of less than 5% in patients with advanced disease when curative treatment is no longer possible. However, many patients will die due to liver failure in end-stage cirrhosis *with but not due to* their tumor (Llovet et al. 1999a, 2002a; Varela et al. 2003).

Therefore, given the facts of the high incidence of HCC in cirrhosis together with the dismal prognosis in late diagnosis, therapeutic strategies in HCC should incorporate concepts for early detection – screening in individuals at risk – and tailored therapy regimens.

T. K. Helmberger, MD
Professor, Department of Diagnostic and Interventional Radiology and Nuclear Medicine, Klinikum Bogenhausen, Engelschalkinger Strasse 77, 81925 Munich, Germany

8.2 Diagnosis of HCC

Usually, HCC is assessed by ultrasound, contrast-enhanced CT and MRI. Dependent on potential suspect findings in terms of nodules, the surveillance of a high-risk patient group can be adjusted according to the likelihood of malignancy. The European Association for the Study of the Liver (EASL; Bruix et al. 2001) makes the following recommendations:

- For nodules <1 cm in diameter, with a rather low HCC probability <50%, ultrasound should be performed every 3 months for follow-up
- For nodules between 1 and 2 cm in diameter, presenting a moderately high HCC probability, diagnosis should be established by biopsy; however, false-negative biopsies occur in 30%–40%
- For nodules between 2 and 3 cm in diameter, the high likelihood of malignancy can be established by concomitant findings of two imaging modalities confirming arterial hypervascularization in association with elevated alpha-fetoprotein over 400 ng/Ml
- For nodules >3 cm in diameter, with an almost 100% risk of malignancy, CT and MRI should be used for staging invasiveness.

A recent study comparing cross-sectional imaging and post liver transplantation specimens confirmed the superiority of contrast-enhanced MR angiography over contrast-enhanced CT, particularly in nodules between 1 and 2 cm (Burrel et al. 2003). Angiography and nuclear medicine studies no longer play a role in the primary diagnosis of HCC.

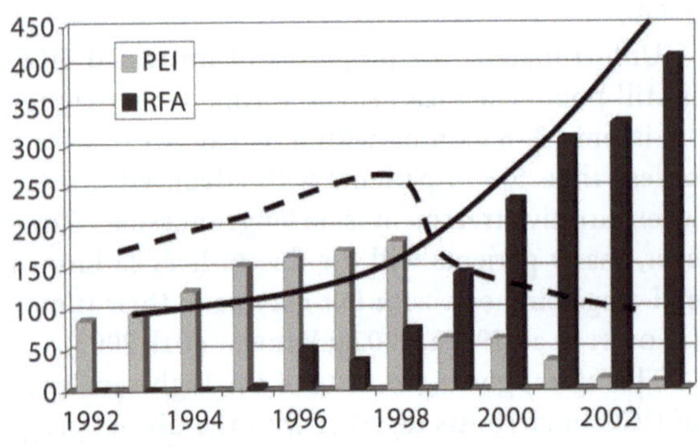

Fig. 8.1. Significant shift from percutanoeus ethanol injection to thermoablative therapy in hepatocellular carcinoma regarding published scientific papers over a period of 10 years (MedLine analysis)

Nevertheless, there is no general consensus on the best imaging method for the surveillance of patients at risk or for the most appropriate staging system. Most staging systems, for example Child-Turcotte-Pugh, TNM, and Okuda, the French staging classification, the Italian Cancer of the Liver Program (CLIP), or the Chinese University Prognostic Index (CUPI), assess only one key aspect of hepatic disease or are appropriate mainly in advanced tumoral stages. In contrast, the staging system proposed by the EASL group [the Barcelona-Clinic Liver Cancer (BCLC) staging system] incorporates four variables: tumor stage, degree of liver function impairment, patient's physical status, and cancer-related symptoms (Llovet et al. 2003). In contrast to all other staging systems the BCLC classification links the tumor stages defined by the variables to a treatment algorithm.

8.3 Implications for a Tailored Treatment Strategy

Treatment of HCC is based on four options: transplantation, resection, ablation, and embolization.

Liver transplantation is considered the only curative treatment because the tumor and the cause of the paraneoplastic disease, i.e., the cirrhotic liver, is removed. Patient selection is crucial for the success of transplantation. According to the Milan criteria the best long-term outcome rates can be achieved in patients with a single tumor <5 cm or with up to three tumors <3 cm in diameter (Fuster et al. 2005; Llovet et al. 2005; Mazzaferro et al. 2004). Applying these criteria, 5-year survival rates of 70%–80% with recurrence rates of less than 15% can be achieved. Nevertheless, the limitation of this procedure is still the worldwide shortage of organs together with tumor progression and/or deterioration of liver function during the waiting time, which causes a drop-out rate of 20%–50 % if the waiting time exceeds more than a year. Potential solutions to this problem might be adjuvant therapies to prevent tumor progression while the patient is on the transplant list, and living donor transplantation (Chui et al. 2004; Fuster et al. 2005; Llovet et al. 2005). While bridging procedures such as thermal ablation, transarterial chemoembolization, and chemotherapy can readily be performed, their impact

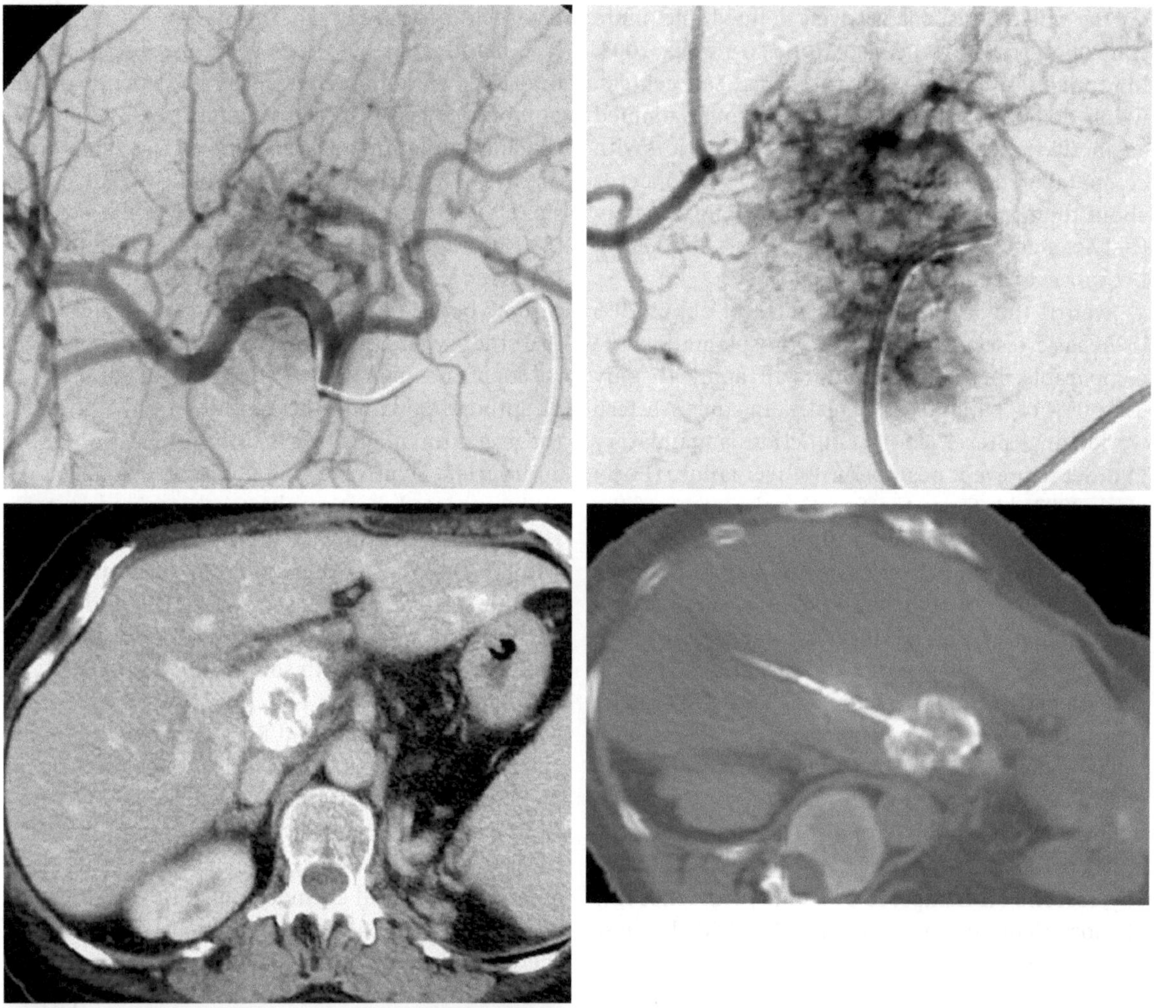

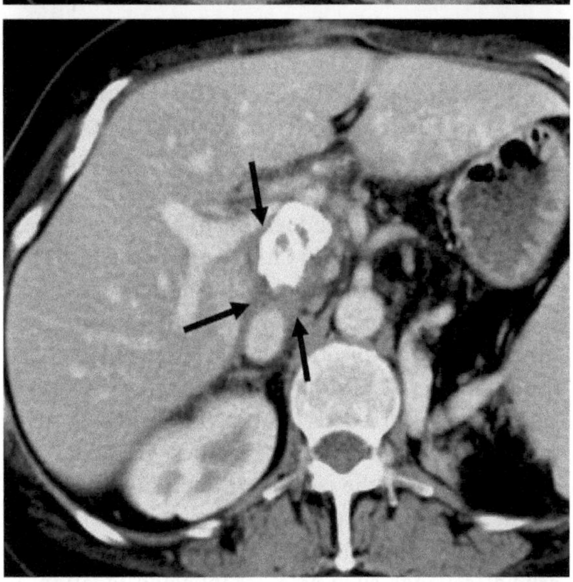

a b c d e

Fig. 8.2. **a** Hypervascularized HCC within the caudate lobe before transarterial chemoembolization (*TACE*). **b** Superselective placement of the catheter, initial phase of TACE. **c** Incomplete lipiodol storage of the tumor, but ideal demarcation for subsequent radiofrequency ablation (*RFA*). **d** Placement of an RFA electrode under CT-fluoroscopic guidance via a double oblique access route in the well visualized tumor. **e** Control scan 6 months after RFA; note the non-enhancing periphery of the tumor representing the safety margin of the former RFA and the shrinkage of the tumor (*arrows*). The lipiodol is still in place, confirming the complete devascularization of the tumor on the outcome is not yet well defined and more controlled trials are needed (Johnson et al. 2004; Mazzaferro et al. 2004). In specialized centers, living donor transplantation has become adopted as an alternative to cadaveric transplantation with comparable long-term survival rates, but concerns about the donors' morbidity and mortality remain (Befeler and Di Bisceglie 2002; Chui et al. 2004, Llovet et al. 2005).

Even if the 5-year survival rates of about 70% in hepatic resection and liver transplantation are comparable, hepatic resection will apply to only 5%–30% of patients, especially in the Western world, since preserved liver function is mandatory in order to prevent postoperative liver failure (Poon et al. 2002a,b). Since the functional reserve of the liver is one of the major limiting factors, patients with the following criteria are the best candidates for resection: no cirrhosis, a solitary, small (2 cm) HCC nodule, preserved liver function according to the BCLC criteria in terms of normal portal pressure (hepatic venous pressure gradient < 10 mmHg, no varices, no splenomegaly, normal platelet count < 100,000/mm^3), and normal bilirubin values. In contrast, patients with Child–Pugh A cirrhosis will tolerate liver resection of up to 50%; Child–Pough B and C cirrhosis, 20% and 5%, respectively. Additionally, resection is hampered by a high recurrence rate of more than 70% after 5 years. Most likely these high recurrence rates are triggered by the degree of differentiation, early microvascular invasion, and micro satellites of the primary tumor, as well as progression of the potentially underlying diffuse liver disease (Llovet et al. 1999b).

Unfortunately, the vast majority of patients with HCC are not suitable for any of the surgical treatment options; therefore, adjuvant, less invasive treatments have to be considered.

Percutaneous ethanol injection (PEI) has been widely used since the mid 1980s, with response rates of up to 100% and 5-year survival rates of about 60% in Child–Pugh A patients with tumors not larger than 2 cm. However, in larger tumors the complete response rates drop down to 60%–70% necessitating repeated procedures resulting in 5-year survival rates below 30% (Sala et al. 2004) (Table 8.1).

Recently a significant shift from PEI to radiofrequency ablation (RFA) procedures has been seen, reflected by the respective literature (Fig. 8.1). Fewer RFA treatment sessions are needed compared to PEI to obtain the same response, which, together with a superior local control rate, makes RFA the favorable procedure. The primary success rate of RFA mainly depends, in most studies, on the size of the HCC, while the recurrence rate depends on the number of lesions – reflecting most likely the multilocular inflammatory activity of the underlying disease – according to a recent multivariate analysis (Yamakado et al. 2004). However, Poon et al. (2004a) did not find a difference regarding the primary success rate between tumors < 3 cm (94%) and tumors between 3.1 cm and 8 cm in diameter (91%) in a study where they compared percutaneous, laparoscopic and open RFA procedures. The same group of authors explained these results by the effect of the users' learning curve and the application of the appropriate ablative technique (Poon et al. 2004b).

As expected, best results can be gained in early HCC in mild and moderate cirrhosis (Child A and B) (Table 8.2). Comparable to surgical results, Lencioni et al. (2005) showed 1-, 3-, and 5-year survival rates of 100%, 89%, and 61% respectively in Child A patients with solitary HCC after RFA. In this patient group, the 1-, 3-, and 5-year recurrence rates were 14%, 49%, and 81% respectively for the emergence of new tumors and 4%, 10%, and 10% for local tumor progression.

In patients with advanced tumor and/or liver disease not amenable to surgical and local ablative therapies, transarterial chemoembolization (TACE) is a widely accepted palliative treatment option. Even if there is no complete agreement on the optimal substances used for TACE, recent studies and pooled data from several randomized controlled trials have demonstrated that the survival rate after TACE is significantly superior than the natural course under best supportive care (Camma et al. 2002; Llovet et al. 2002b; Lo et al. 2002) (Table 8.3). Prognostic factors for an improved outcome after TACE are single- or multinodular, pseudoencapsulated tumors less than 8 cm in diameter in Child-Pugh A and B cirrhosis where a selective vascular approach to the tumor is achievable. On the other hand, patients with liver function decompensation should be excluded due to the potential risk of severe adverse events in terms of significant hepatic deterioration based on the TACE-induced ischemic insult (Huppert et al. 2004).

Furthermore, the combination of TACE and RFA might enhance the primary success rate and overcome the limitations of each single intervention in crucial settings such as a complicated location or when there is suspicion of satellite tumors (Fig. 8.2); however, sufficient study data supporting this concept are not yet available.

Table 8.1. HCC survival rates after *PEI* or a combination of PEI and TACE. (*HD* High density, *PEI* percutaneous ethanol injection, *RFA* radiofrequency ablation, *TACE* transarterial chemoembolization)

Author	No.	Method	HCC survival rates (%)		
			1 year	3 years	5 years
Tateishi et al. (1997)	61	OP (31)	89	73	64
		TAE + PEI (30)	93	73	42
Yamamoto et al. (1997)		TACE (50)	93	20	
		TACE+PEI (50)	95	50	
Lencioni et al. (1998)	CP A	TACE+PEI (48)		75	59
	CP B	TACE+PEI (38)		61	35
Tanaka et al. (1998)	CP A	TACE+PEI (22)		100	75
	all	TACE+PEI (83)		68	35
Livraghi (2001)	CP A	PEI (293)	98	79	47
	CP B	PEI (149)	93	63	29
	CP C	PEI (20)	64	12	0
Lencioni et al. (2003)	102	PEI (52)	96	88 (2 years)	–
		RFA (50)	100	98	–
Lin et al. (2004)	157	PEI (52)		50	
		HD PEI (53)		55	
		RFA (52)		74	
Sala et al. (2004)	282	PEI	87	51	27
Shiina et al. (2005)	232	PEI (114)		74 (4 years)	
		RFA (118)		57 (4 years)	

Table 8.2. HCC survival rates after thermoablative therapy

Author	No.	TU	Method	HCC survival rate (%)		
				1 year	3 years	5 years
Choi et al. (2004)	45	Rez. HCC	RFA	81	54	
Livraghi et al. (2004)	210	Early HCC	RFA	90	83	43
	164	Late HCC	RFA	68	49	28
Lencioni et al. (2004); Lencioni et al. (2005)	187	Early	RFA	97	71	48
Chen et al. (2005)	205	HCC	RFA	90	60	

Table 8.3. Meta-analysis of 13 studies/2140 patients treated by TACE. Survival figures related to tumor size and number, and Child-Pugh classification (Akashi et al. 1991; Alvarez et al. 2000; Hatanaka et al. 1995; Hsieh et al. 1992; Ikeda et al. 1991; Mondazzi et al. 1994; Poon et al. 2000; Savastano et al. 1999; Shijo et al. 1992; Takayasu et al. 2001; Yamamoto et al. 1992; Yamashita et al. 1991; Yoshioka et al. 1997)

	TU size, number		Child-Pugh	
	<5 cm, n=1	>5 cm, n>1	A	B
Survival at 1 year (%)	85–100	54–80	83-87	51-55
Survival at 3 years (%)	45–78	11–24	39–44	15-27
Survival at 5 years (%)	30–38	0–15	10–20	0–16

The treatment options for large, unresectable tumors are still very limited or not effective. In this scenario, yttrium-90 internal radiation, just recently approved by the Food and Drug Administration (FDA), is proving to be a new and promising method for the therapy of unresectable hepatic tumors. Technically yttrium-90 internal radiation therapy is comparable to TACE, while its effect is based on the combination of microembolization plus internal irradiation by beta-radiation. Yttrium-90 internal radiation in liver and pancreatic cancer was first described by Arial (1965). Since then a reasonable number of studies have been presented (Table 8.4).

Even if it is demonstrated that yttrium-90 is effective in terms of tumor response and improved survival in advanced primary hepatic malignancies, further validation of the method is necessary to define appropriate indications, dosage, and integration into a multimodal treatment concept.

In contrast to the variably invasive loco-regional ablative therapies, there are no valid data on systemic hormonal, chemotherapeutic, antiangiogenic, or receptor-directed therapies with 5-fluorouracil, doxorubicin, epirubicin, etoposide, cisplatin, and mitoxantrone, or with interferon, tamoxifen, capecitabine, thalidomide, and octreotide, in terms of their ability to improve patient survival or life quality in early or advanced HCC (Aguayo and Patt 2001).

8.4 Summary

Modern treatment of HCC should be directed by a multidisciplinary, individually customized therapy concept, since various therapeutic options are available. In spite of the lack of generally accepted

Table 8.4. Results of yttrium-90 internal radiation in advanced HCC. (*CR* Complete response, *PR* partial response)

Author	No.	Response	Survival
Lau et al. (1998)	71	26.7% PR by CT; 100% by AFP	–
Dancey et al. (2000)	22	20% PR + CR	1 year
Carr (2004)	65	38.4% by CT	649 days (Okuda I); 302 (Okuda II)
Geschwind et al. (2004)	80	–	628 days (Okuda I); 384 days (Okuda II)
Liu et al. (2004)	11	72% PR, 9% by CT, 75% by AFP	–
Goin et al. (2005)	121	–	466 days in low-risk group; 108 days in high-risk group

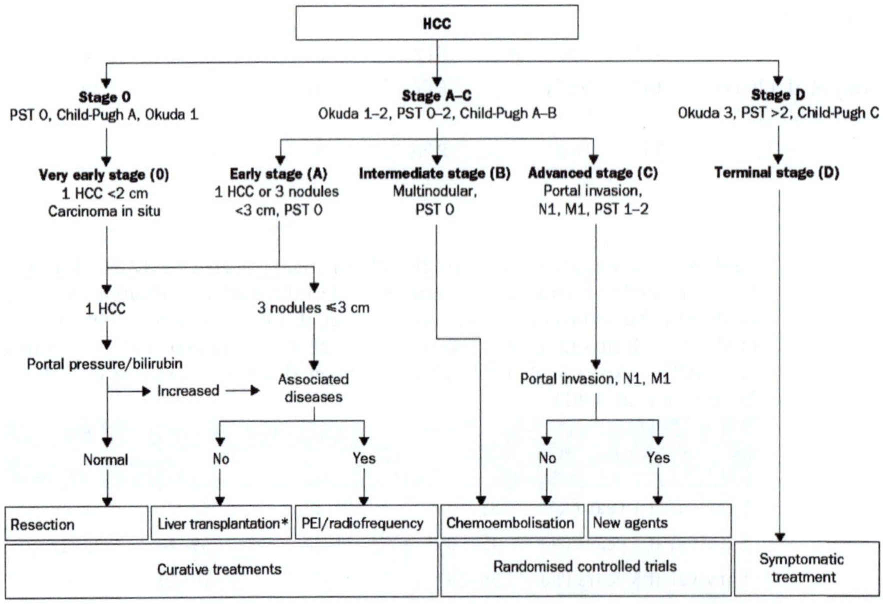

Fig. 8.3. Barcelona-Clinic Liver Cancer (*BCLC*) recommendation for a tailored stage-dependent treatment regimen directed by the performance status, severity of liver dysfunction, general condition of the patient, and treatment efficacy (according to Llovet et al. 2003)

guidelines on the therapy of HCC the BCLC recommendations provide a very practical and clinically effective staging and treatment classification in HCC, incorporating present valid data as much as possible (Fig. 8.3). Patients at an early stage are suitable for a surgical approach with resection in cases of single tumors and normal liver function, while liver transplantation is the method of choice for solitary tumors (<5 cm) in advanced cirrhosis or in multiple (≤3) small tumors (<3 cm). In non-surgical candidates percutaneous ablative therapies of small tumors are comparable to surgery in terms of 5-year survival. Multi-nodular, otherwise asymptomatic, tumors and compensated liver disease should be treated by TACE. Patients with advanced tumors and impaired liver function should be tested for new, experimental therapies, such as selective internal radiotherapy or antigenic and antiangiogenic therapies, under study conditions, while patients with end stage disease will be directed to symptomatic therapies.

References

Aguayo A, Patt YZ (2001) Nonsurgical treatment of hepatocellular carcinoma. Semin Oncol 28:503–513

Akashi Y, Koreeda C, Enomoto S et al (1991) Prognosis of unresectable hepatocellular carcinoma: an evaluation based on multivariate analysis of 90 cases. Hepatology 14:262–268

Alvarez R, Banares R, Echenagusia A et al (2000) [Prognostic factors for survival following transarterial chemoembolization in advanced hepatocellular carcinoma.] Gastroenterol Hepatol 23:153–158

Ariel I (1965) Treatment of inoperable primary pancreatic and liver cancer by the intra-arterial administration of radioactive isotopes (Y90 radiating microspheres). Ann Surg 162:267–278

Befeler AS, Di Bisceglie AM (2002) Hepatocellular carcinoma: diagnosis and treatment. Gastroenterology 122:1609–1619

Bruix J, Sherman M, Llovet JM et al (2001) Clinical management of hepatocellular carcinoma. Conclusions of the Barcelona-2000 EASL conference. European Association for the Study of the Liver. J Hepatol 35:421–430

Burrel M, Llovet JM, Ayuso C et al (2003) MRI angiography is superior to helical CT for detection of HCC prior to liver transplantation: an explant correlation. Hepatology 38:1034–1042

Camma C, Schepis F, Orlando A et al (2002) Transarterial chemoembolization for unresectable hepatocellular carcinoma: meta-analysis of randomized controlled trials. Radiology 224:47–54

Carr B (2004) Hepatic arterial 90Yttrium glass microspheres (Therasphere) for unresectable hepatocellular carcinoma: interim safety and survival data on 65 patients. Liver Transpl 10(2) [Suppl. 1]:107–110

Chen MH, Yang W, Yan K et al (2005) Treatment efficacy of radiofrequency ablation of 338 patients with hepatic malignant tumor and the relevant complications. World J Gastroenterol 11:6395–6401

Choi D, Lim HK, Kim MJ et al (2004) Recurrent hepatocellular carcinoma: percutaneous radiofrequency ablation after hepatectomy. Radiology 230:135–141

Chui AK, Rao AR, Island ER et al (2004) Multimodality tumor control and living donor transplantation for unresectable hepatocellular carcinoma. Transplant Proc 36:2287–2288

Dancey JE, Shepherd FA, Paul K et al (2000) Treatment of nonresectable hepatocellular carcinoma with intrahepatic 90Y-microspheres [In Process Citation]. J Nucl Med 41:1673–1681

El-Serag HB, Mason AC (2000) Risk factors for the rising rates of primary liver cancer in the United States. Arch Intern Med 160:3227–3230

Fuster J, Charco R, Llovet JM et al (2005) Liver transplantation in hepatocellular carcinoma. Transpl Int 18:278–282

Geschwind JF, Salem R, Carr BI et al (2004) Yttrium-90 microspheres for the treatment of hepatocellular carcinoma. Gastroenterology 127:S194–S205

Goin JE, Salem R, Carr BI et al (2005) Treatment of unresectable hepatocellular carcinoma with intrahepatic yttrium 90 microspheres: a risk-stratification analysis. J Vasc Interv Radiol 16:195–203

Hatanaka Y, Yamashita Y, Takahashi M et al (1995) Unresectable hepatocellular carcinoma: analysis of prognostic factors in transcatheter management. Radiology 195:747–752

Hsieh MY, Chang WY, Wang LY et al (1992) Treatment of hepatocellular carcinoma by transcatheter arterial chemoembolization and analysis of prognostic factors. Cancer Chemother Pharmacol Suppl 31:S82–S85

Huppert PE, Lauchart W, Duda SH et al (2004) Chemoembolization of hepatocellular carcinomas: which factors determine therapeutic response and survival? Rofo 176:375–385

Ikeda K, Kumada H, Saitoh S et al (1991) Effect of repeated transcatheter arterial embolization on the survival time in patients with hepatocellular carcinoma. An analysis by the Cox proportional hazard model. Cancer 68:2150–2154

Johnson EW, Holck PS, Levy AE et al (2004) The role of tumor ablation in bridging patients to liver transplantation. Arch Surg 139:825–829; discussion 829–830

Jungst C, Cheng B, Gehrke R et al (2004) Oxidative damage is increased in human liver tissue adjacent to hepatocellular carcinoma. Hepatology 39:1663–1672

Lau WY, Ho S, Leung TW et al (1998) Selective internal radiation therapy for nonresectable hepatocellular carcinoma with intraarterial infusion of 90yttrium microspheres. Int J Radiat Oncol Biol Phys 40:583–592

Lencioni R, Paolicchi A, Moretti M et al (1998) Combined transcatheter arterial chemoembolization and percutaneous ethanol injection for the treatment of large hepatocellular carcinoma: local therapeutic effect and long-term survival rate. Eur Radiol 8:439–444

Lencioni RA, Allgaier HP, Cioni D et al (2003) Small hepatocellular carcinoma in cirrhosis: randomized comparison of radio-frequency thermal ablation versus percutaneous ethanol injection. Radiology 228:235–240

Lencioni R, Crocetti L, Cioni D et al (2004) Percutaneous radiofrequency ablation of hepatic colorectal metastases:

technique, indications, results, and new promises. Invest Radiol 39:689–697
Lencioni R, Cioni D, Crocetti L et al (2005) Early-stage hepatocellular carcinoma in patients with cirrhosis: long-term results of percutaneous image-guided radiofrequency ablation. Radiology 234:961–967
Lin SM, Lin CJ, Lin CC et al (2004) Radiofrequency ablation improves prognosis compared with ethanol injection for hepatocellular carcinoma ≤4 cm. Gastroenterology 127:1714–1723
Liu MD, Uaje MB, Al-Ghazi MS et al (2004) Use of Yttrium-90 TheraSphere for the treatment of unresectable hepatocellular carcinoma. Am Surg 70:947–953
Livraghi T (2001) Percutaneous ethanol injection in the treatment of hepatocellular carcinoma in cirrhosis. Hepatogastroenterology 48:20–24
Livraghi T, Meloni F, Morabito A et al (2004) Multimodal image-guided tailored therapy of early and intermediate hepatocellular carcinoma: long-term survival in the experience of a single radiologic referral center. Liver Transpl 10:S98–S106
Llovet JM, Bru C, Bruix J (1999a) Prognosis of hepatocellular carcinoma: the BCLC staging classification. Semin Liver Dis 19:329–338
Llovet JM, Fuster J, Bruix J (1999b) Intention-to-treat analysis of surgical treatment for early hepatocellular carcinoma: resection versus transplantation. Hepatology 30:1434–1440
Llovet JM, Fuster J, Bruix J (2002a) Prognosis of hepatocellular carcinoma. Hepatogastroenterology 49:7–11
Llovet JM, Real MI, Montana X et al (2002b) Arterial embolisation or chemoembolisation versus symptomatic treatment in patients with unresectable hepatocellular carcinoma: a randomised controlled trial. Lancet 359:1734–1739
Llovet JM, Burroughs A, Bruix J (2003) Hepatocellular carcinoma. Lancet 362:1907–1917
Llovet JM, Schwartz M, Mazzaferro V (2005) Resection and liver transplantation for hepatocellular carcinoma. Semin Liver Dis 25:181–200
Lo CM, Ngan H, Tso WK et al (2002) Randomized controlled trial of transarterial lipiodol chemoembolization for unresectable hepatocellular carcinoma. Hepatology 35:1164–1171
Mazzaferro V, Battiston C, Perrone S et al (2004) Radiofrequency ablation of small hepatocellular carcinoma in cirrhotic patients awaiting liver transplantation: a prospective study. Ann Surg 240:900–909
Mondazzi L, Bottelli R, Brambilla G et al (1994) Transarterial oily chemoembolization for the treatment of hepatocellular carcinoma: a multivariate analysis of prognostic factors. Hepatology 19:1115–1123
Poon RT, Ngan H, Lo CM et al (2000) Transarterial chemoembolization for inoperable hepatocellular carcinoma and postresection intrahepatic recurrence. J Surg Oncol 73:109–114
Poon RT, Fan ST, Lo CM et al (2002a) Long-term survival and pattern of recurrence after resection of small hepatocellular carcinoma in patients with preserved liver function: implications for a strategy of salvage transplantation. Ann Surg 235:373–382
Poon RT, Fan ST, Tsang FH et al (2002b) Locoregional therapies for hepatocellular carcinoma: a critical review from the surgeon's perspective. Ann Surg 235:466–486
Poon RT, Ng KK, Lam CM et al (2004a) Effectiveness of radiofrequency ablation for hepatocellular carcinomas larger than 3 cm in diameter. Arch Surg 139:281–287
Poon RT, Ng KK, Lam CM et al (2004b) Learning curve for radiofrequency ablation of liver tumors: prospective analysis of initial 100 patients in a tertiary institution. Ann Surg 239:441–449
Sala M, Llovet JM, Vilana R et al (2004) Initial response to percutaneous ablation predicts survival in patients with hepatocellular carcinoma. Hepatology 40:1352–1360
Savastano S, Miotto D, Casarrubea G et al (1999) Transcatheter arterial chemoembolization for hepatocellular carcinoma in patients with Child's grade A or B cirrhosis: a multivariate analysis of prognostic factors. J Clin Gastroenterol 28:334–340
Shiina S, Teratani T, Obi S et al (2005) A randomized controlled trial of radiofrequency ablation with ethanol injection for small hepatocellular carcinoma. Gastroenterology 129:122–130
Shijo H, Okazaki M, Higashihara H et al (1992) Hepatocellular carcinoma: a multivariate analysis of prognostic features in patients treated with hepatic arterial embolization. Am J Gastroenterol 87:1154–1159
Takayasu K, Muramatsu Y, Maeda T et al (2001) Targeted transarterial oily chemoembolization for small foci of hepatocellular carcinoma using a unified helical CT and angiography system: analysis of factors affecting local recurrence and survival rates. AJR Am J Roentgenol 176:681–688
Tanaka K, Nakamura S, Numata K et al (1998) The long term efficacy of combined transcatheter arterial embolization and percutaneous ethanol injection in the treatment of patients with large hepatocellular carcinoma and cirrhosis. Cancer 82:78–85
Tateishi H, Oi H, Masuda N et al (1997) Appraisal of combination treatment for hepatocellular carcinoma: long-term follow-up and lipiodol-percutaneous ethanol injection therapy. Semin Oncol 24:S6-81–S86-90
Varela M, Sala M, Llovet JM et al (2003) Review article: natural history and prognostic prediction of patients with hepatocellular carcinoma. Aliment Pharmacol Ther 17 [Suppl 2]:98–102
Yamakado K, Nakatsuka A, Akeboshi M et al (2004) Combination therapy with radiofrequency ablation and transcatheter chemoembolization for the treatment of hepatocellular carcinoma: short-term recurrences and survival. Oncol Rep 11:105–109
Yamamoto K, Masuzawa M, Kato M et al (1992) Analysis of prognostic factors in patients with hepatocellular carcinoma treated by transcatheter arterial embolization. Cancer Chemother Pharmacol Suppl 31:S77–S81
Yamamoto K, Masuzawa M, Kato M et al (1997) Evaluation of combined therapy with chemoembolization and ethanol injection for advanced hepatocellular carcinoma. Semin Oncol 24:S6-50–S56-55
Yamashita Y, Takahashi M, Koga Y et al (1991) Prognostic factors in the treatment of hepatocellular carcinoma with transcatheter arterial embolization and arterial infusion. Cancer 67:385–391
Yoshioka H, Sato M, Sonomura T et al (1997) Factors associated with survival exceeding 5 years after transcatheter arterial embolization for hepatocellular carcinoma. Semin Oncol 24:S6-29–S26-37

Bone

9

Thomas K. Helmberger and Ralf-Thorsten Hoffmann

CONTENTS

9.1 Background

The typical clinical signs in bone tumours are pain, destruction and destabilization, immobilization, neurologic deficits, and finally functional impairment. Primary malignant bone tumours are a rare entity, accounting for about 0.2% of all malignancies. Also benign primary bone tumours are in total rare and mostly asymptomatic. The most common symptomatic benign bone tumour is osteoid osteoma with an incidence of 1:2000.

In contrast, secondary osseous malignancies may occur in about 30%–70% of all malignant diseases. For example, in breast and prostate cancer bone metastases can be found in about 70% and 60%, respectively. Metastatic disease to the bones is strongly correlated to the presence of red bone marrow. Therefore, bone metastasis is mostly found within the spine (69%), in the pelvis (41%), in the femoral (25%), and in the skull (14%) bones.

Pain relief and stabilization are the primary goals of every therapy for bone tumours. Surgery is the classic therapy providing different levels of cure: in the best case resection together with full functional reconstruction is possible; nevertheless, in most cases only resection (amputation) and/or palliative stabilization is achievable. Therefore, in most cases where surgery is no longer applicable radiotherapy and/or chemotherapy including hormonal therapy, depending on the primary tumour, will be administered. Unfortunately, the response to these therapies is limited and has a high risk of recurrence. This problem stimulated the utilization of more target-oriented, less invasive and minimally invasive techniques such as local thermal ablation, which has excellent results in the treatment of solid organ tumours.

9.2 Indication

The major indication for thermal ablation in bone tumours is pain. Secondarily, local tumour destruction may support destruction of the tumoral matrix, which may enhance repair processes and consequently prolong the process of functional preservation.

In this setting, thermal ablation will be mainly a symptomatic, supportive (palliative) therapy, which can also be applied in conjunction with other therapies such as resection, radiotherapy or chemotherapy. In contrast to the treatment of malignant tumours, local thermal ablation is considered the method of choice in treatment of symptomatic benign bone tumours such as osteoid osteomas.

T. K. Helmberger, MD
Professor, Department of Diagnostic and Interventional Radiology and Nuclear Medicine, Klinikum Bogenhausen, Englschalkinger Strasse 77, 81925 Munich, Germany
R.-T. Hoffmann, MD
Department of Clinical Radiology, University Hospitals – Grosshadern, Ludwig-Maximilians-University of Munich, Marchioninistrasse 15, 81377 Munich, Germany

9.3 Thermal Ablation in Osteoid Osteomas

Osteoid osteoma is a benign lesion of unknown origin. Typically, the lesion is formed by a central, vascularized nidus surrounded by a reactive sclerosis with a diameter of less than 2 cm, in contrast to the larger osteoblastoma. Because of the central nidus, a vascular malformation is discussed as being the origin of these lesions. Most of the tumours occur in the first three decades of life, with a male predominance (male:female = 2:1). Osteoid osteomas can be found in any bone of the body; however, the spine is the preferred localization, where 50% of all osteoid osteomas occur in the lumbar spine, and 75% of the tumours in the pedicles of the vertebrae. Other typical localizations are femur, radius, knee and ankle.

Clinically, the leading sign is a well-circumscribed sharp pain, mainly during the night, which responds well to acetylsalicylic acid intake. Unfortunately, the salicylate test is positive only in about two-thirds of the cases. After 5–6 years the pain and discomfort may be relieved spontaneously (Klein et al. 1992; Shankman et al. 1997).

In plain radiograms osteoid osteoma is often not identifiable at all or only cortical thickening can be appreciated. In CT the ivory-like, dense ossification surrounding the nidus is the key sign of osteoid osteoma. Bone scintigraphy may be helpful to identify an osteoid osteoma per se but the hot spot typically reflects the zone of intensified osteoblastic activity rather than the nidus. In MRI the nidus presents typically as a hyperintense small nodular area on T_2-weighted imaging within an area of low or no signal due to the dense surrounding bone.

The typical radiographic appearance of an osteoid osteoma together with the clinical symptoms and a positive aspirin test (i.e. pain relief) confirms the diagnosis (Klein and Shankman 1992; Shankman et al. 1997; Pinto et al. 2002) (Figs. 9.1a, 9.2a).

In general, osteoid osteoma is cured when the nidus is destroyed. This can be achieved by complete removal of the lesion or by just destroying the nidus, which is thought responsible for the symptoms.

In surgery – which used to be considered the treatment of choice – the osteoid osteoma is removed en bloc since the enostal nidus is, in general, not visible. In open surgery the hypersclerosed tumour is often not identifiable precisely; therefore, a substantial amount of bone has to be resected, which may cause complications such as fractures due to the subsequent weakening of the bone. Moreover, ineffective surgery with a high recurrence rate or residual tumour is not uncommon. Also C-arm fluoroscopic-guided drilling of the nidus/lesion is often not successful because the quality afforded by the available imaging systems is generally not sufficient to identify the nidus. Furthermore, the size of the drilling devices, ranging 3–10 mm of internal diameter, may also cause complications, such as incomplete removal with subsequent recurrence, skin burns at the entry site, haematoma, dysaesthesia, infections and fractures.

These restrictions and disadvantages of open and percutaneous resection stimulated the utilization of minimally invasive techniques such as image-guided drilling, alcohol injection, radiofrequency and laser ablation. Radiofrequency and laser ablation have become clinically well accepted due to their easy handling and high success rate, whereas percutaneous drilling and alcohol injection are significantly limited by the imprecise control of the size and morphology of lesion damage and a high recurrence rate (Rosenthal et al. 1998, 2003).

In contrast, the nidus can easily be identified by CT, which can guide a minimally invasive device into the nidus. In some cases the nidus is "encapsulated" by the surrounding reactive sclerosis. Then, it can be impossible to penetrate the bone with the ablation device directly. In such cases the access route to the nidus must be prepared by drilling a hole. For this purpose generally a bone biopsy cannula with a crown cut is suitable. Nevertheless, the sclerosis surrounding the nidus can be so hard that a mechanical drilling device is necessary to create the access route (Fig. 9.1). When the access is established the tip of the probe can be placed directly into the nidus.

Creating the access route to the nidus and placing a radiofrequency electrode or laser probe into it can be quite painful, which necessitates adequate pain management. In the authors' experience, in adults conscious sedation together with systemic and local anaesthesia is sufficient in most cases; in children general anaesthesia is usually mandatory. Other groups perform laser or radiofrequency ablation under general anaesthesia or regional nerve block only (Gangi et al. 2007).

The usually small volume of the nidus must be accommodated by the size of the active tip of any ablative device. If the active tip – either a radiofrequency or a laser device – is inappropriately large unwanted ablation of adjacent soft tissue as far as the skin may occur.

Generally, only small amounts of energy are needed to destroy the nidus. Typically, a power of 3–10 W over 4–10 min, i.e. energy of 500–6000 J will be sufficient. Higher energies, especially if used at the start, will result in immediate charring around the probe tip ending the process of ablation prematurely.

To avoid secondary harm to structures near to an osteoid osteoma, special attention must be paid to lesions close to joints, neuroforamina, and neurovascular bundles, and also in cases where a bone lamella between the nidus and adjacent structures is missing. Cooling with saline or a glucose bath may prevent thermal damage to adjacent nervous structures (Fig. 9.2). Therefore, a transarticular approach and immediate vicinity to joint spaces and neuroforamina must be avoided. To protect the skin in cases where only a thin soft-tissue layer is between the lesion and the skin, as in tibial osteoid osteomas, an ice pack around the shaft of the probe is recommended (Venbrux et al. 2003; Cantwell et al. 2004; Cioni et al. 2004; Rimondi et al. 2005; Gebauer et al. 2006; Ghanem 2006; Albisinni and Malaguti 2007; Gangi et al. 2007).

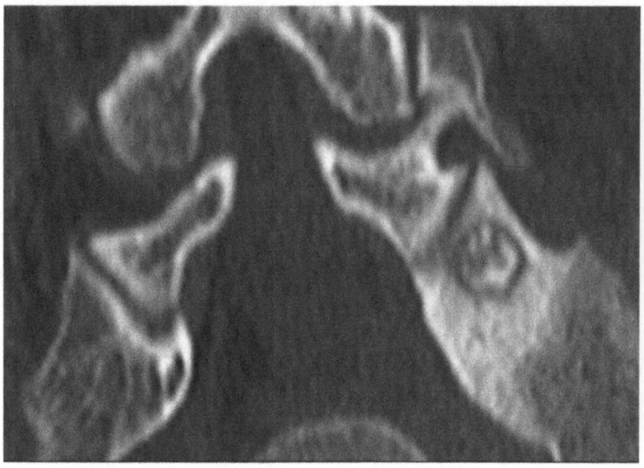

a

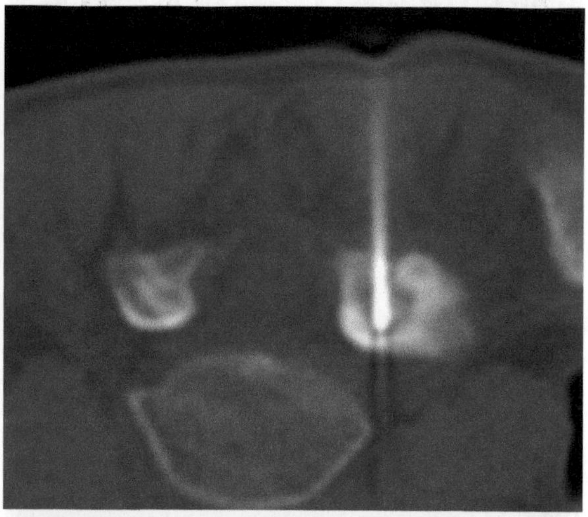

b

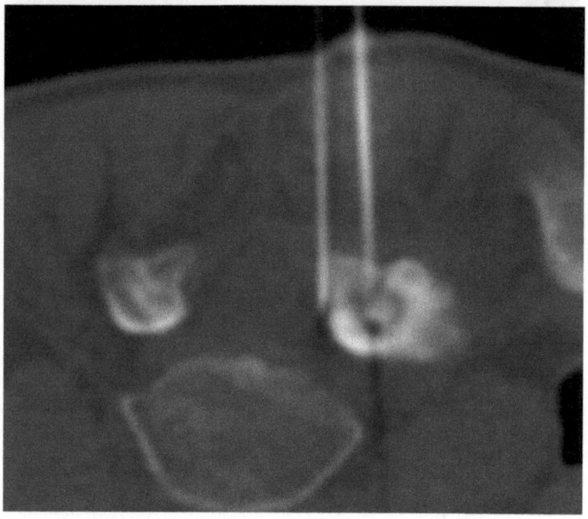

c

Fig. 9.1. **a** An 11-year-old girl with an osteoid osteoma of the left pedicle of the sixth vertebra of the thoracic spine. Note the partially sclerosed nidus together with the dense surrounding hyperostosis. **b** The dense cortical lamella was perforated by a biopsy cannula with a crown cut. **c** Subsequently, a radiofrequency single electrode with an active tip of 1 cm was placed into the nidus. To protect adjacent myelin structures a 21-gauge needle was placed into the epidural space for saline flushing

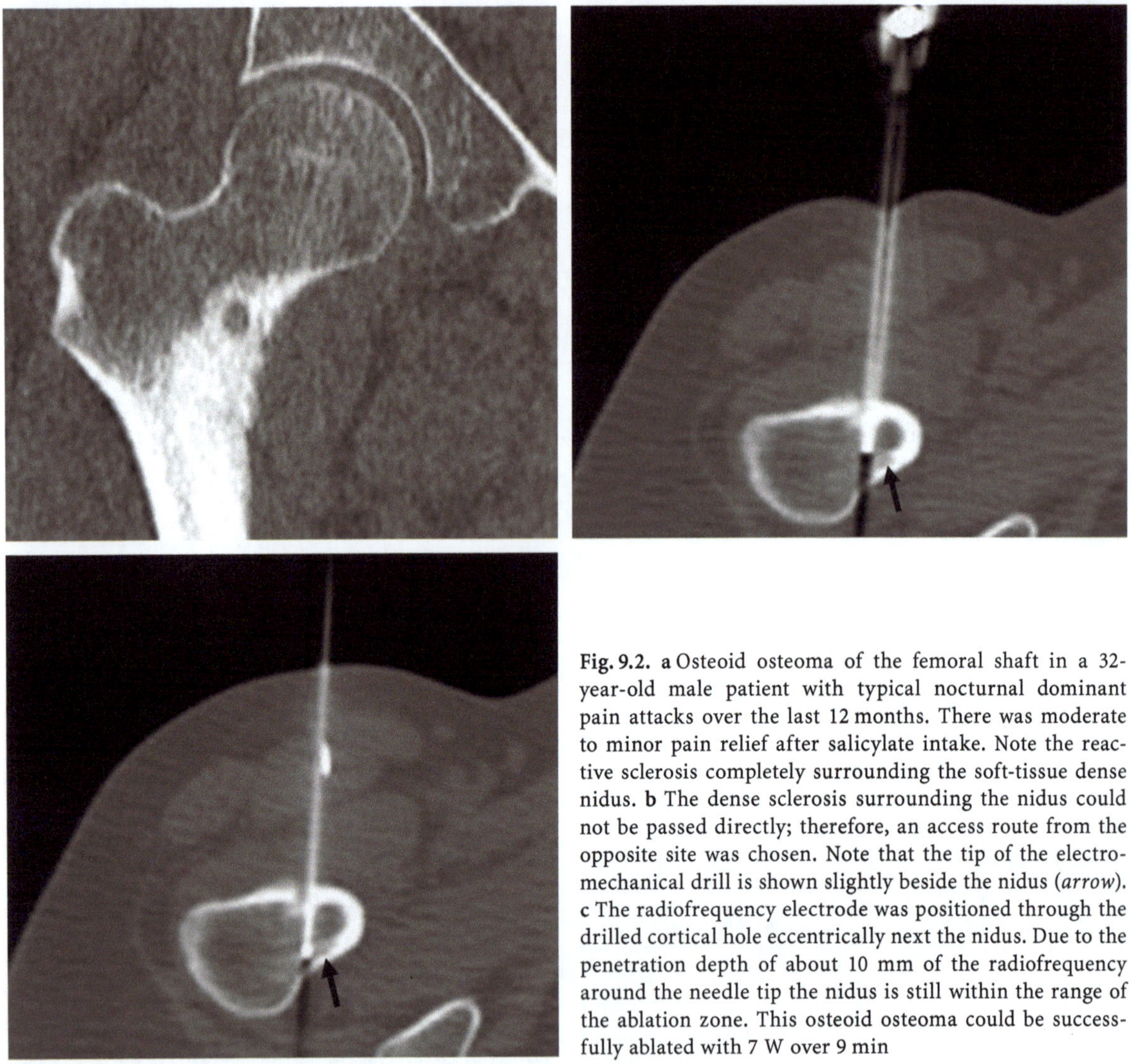

a b c

Fig. 9.2. **a** Osteoid osteoma of the femoral shaft in a 32-year-old male patient with typical nocturnal dominant pain attacks over the last 12 months. There was moderate to minor pain relief after salicylate intake. Note the reactive sclerosis completely surrounding the soft-tissue dense nidus. **b** The dense sclerosis surrounding the nidus could not be passed directly; therefore, an access route from the opposite site was chosen. Note that the tip of the electromechanical drill is shown slightly beside the nidus (*arrow*). **c** The radiofrequency electrode was positioned through the drilled cortical hole eccentrically next the nidus. Due to the penetration depth of about 10 mm of the radiofrequency around the needle tip the nidus is still within the range of the ablation zone. This osteoid osteoma could be successfully ablated with 7 W over 9 min

9.4 Results of Thermal Ablation in Osteoid Osteomas

The primary success in terms of pain relief ranges from 60% to 85% and reaches 90%–100% after a second treatment (Woertler et al. 2001; Ghanem 2006; Simon and Dupuy 2006; Gangi et al. 2007) (Table 9.1). These results compare very well or are even superior to the results from classic, surgical therapy. Ronkainen et al. (2006) showed that the non-invasive procedure of MRI-guided laser ablation is cheaper than surgery, especially regarding the number and mean cost of sick days taken and days of restricted weight-bearing for both superficial and deep lesions (Ronkainen et al. 2006).

9.5 Thermal Ablation in Malignant Bone Tumours

While primary malignant bone tumours are rare, bone metastases are a common finding among all malignancies. More than 50% of all patients with metastatic disease to the musculoskeletal system will present with symptoms – mainly pain – and will have severe constraints regarding quality of life for their remaining lifetime.

The classic oncological therapies, such as surgery, chemotherapy, radiation therapy and administration of analgesics, also target bone metastases and their clinical symptoms. In this setting, the time and effort of any therapy and its direct consequences, e.g. recovery periods, morbidity and mortality, must be correlated to the short- and mid-term benefits regarding overall life expectancy and quality. More and more patients are encountering multi-modality, sequential therapies, in which tumours may lose their sensitivity to chemotherapy, the number of radiation treatments is limited by the maximum suitable radiation dose, and where supportive analgesic therapy becomes intolerable because of increasing side-effects. Nevertheless, these "prolonged" therapies will result in "prolonged" survival times in many cases, even though intensified supportive care is often necessary. Regarding supportive care in particular, local ablative therapies such as radiofrequency and laser ablation as well as osteoplasty with local cement injection (Kelekis et al. 2005) (see Chap. 2.10) have become increasingly accepted as techniques for palliation of pain caused by soft-tissue and osseous tumours (Goetz et al. 2004; Callstrom and Charboneau 2005; Gangi et al. 2005), despite the fact that thermal ablation and osteoplastic augmentation are quite different regarding their mode of action.

9.6 Results of Thermal Ablation in Malignant Bone Tumours

In recent years several minimally invasive treatment approaches for pain management in malignant bone tumours have been presented. Most data exist on osteo- or cementoplasty for osseous augmentation, followed by radiofrequency ablation. There are a few studies on combination therapies, such as osteoplasty together with radiation therapy or radiofrequency ablation (Table 9.2). With a success rate of almost 90% of immediate post-procedural pain relief there seems as yet to be no significant difference between the various single techniques and combination methods. Nevertheless, the mode of action of pain relief may differ substantially between the treatment modalities – and is probably not yet completely understood. In thermal ablation, periosteal nociceptors may be destroyed by direct impact of heat, while in cementoplasty the cytotoxic effects and development

Table 9.1. Primary and secondary success rate of thermoablation in osteoid osteoma

Author	No. of patients/ procedures	First-time success.	Second-time success	Total success	Complications	Follow-up (months)
Barei et al. (2000)	11/11	10/11	–	10/11 (90.9%)	–	18.7
Lindner et al. (2001)	58/61	55/58 (94.8%)	3/3 (100%)	58/58 (100%)	Burns (n=1)	23 (6–41)
Vanderschueren et al. (2002)	97/121	74/97 (76%)	15/23 (65%)	89/97 (92%)	Burns (n=1) broken needle (n=1)	41 (5–81)
Rosenthal et al. (2003)	263/271	107/117) 91%	–	112/126 (89%)	Anesthesia (n=1), sympathic dystrophy (n=1), cellulitis (n=1)	24
Cioni et al. (2004)	38/44	30/38 (78.9%)	5/6 (83.3%)	35/38 (92.1%)	Burns (n=1), osteomyelitis (n=1)	35.5 (12–66)
Martel et al. (2005)	38/39	37/38 (97.4%)	1/1 (100%)	38/38 (100%)	Burns (n=1), tendinitis (n=11)	3–24
Rimondi et al. (2005)	97/114	82/97 (84.5%)	13/15 (86.7%)	95/97 (98%)	Burns (n=1), phlebitis (n=1)	3–12
Gangi et al. (2007)	114/114	112/114 (99.1%)		113/114 (99.1%)	Reflex sympathetic dystrophy (n=1), hyperalgesia (n=1), hyperesthesia (n=1), vasomotor disturbances (n=1)	58.5 (13–130)
Total	**717/775**	**88.8%**	**87.0%**	**95.1%**	**3.4% (26/775)**	**33.5 (3–130)**

of heat by polymerization of the cement components will affect neuronal structures. Furthermore, stabilization by cement reduces or eliminates the macro- and micro-destabilization of the affected osseous structure and in consequence reduces the mechanical stress on the periosteal nerve plexus. It remains to be elucidated whether and to what extent the release of necrosis factors and interleukins as well as osteclast inhibition enhance the process of pain relief.

It remains unclear whether the combination therapy of thermal ablation together with cementoplasty, for example, is superior to a single therapy (Fig. 9.3). Nevertheless, there are a few cases of painful bone tumours with a dense stroma that hinders cement injection. In cases such as these, thermal ablation may soften the tumour's stroma allowing subsequent cement instillation (Schaefer et al. 2002; Fourney et al. 2003; Hierholzer et al. 2003; Masala et al. 2003; Wenger 2003; Halpin et al. 2004; Masala et al. 2004; Halpin et al. 2005; Mont'Alverne et al. 2005; Cheung et al. 2006; Brodano et al. 2007; Calmels et al. 2007; Jakobs et al. 2007).

9.7 Complications

The overall complication rate for all minimally invasive treatment options for benign and malignant bone tumours is less than 4%, with no reports of major complications according to the SIR classification (Tables 9.1, 9.2). Typical and usually self-limiting complication or side-effects include: bleeding at the entry site of the puncture device, skin burns in thermal ablation systems, and neurological symptoms due to direct thermal (e.g. close vicinity to nerve or joint structures in osteoid osteomas) or mechanical (e.g. cement leakage) damage. Specific complications relate to specific methods, such as cement-induced pulmonary embolism, and depend mainly on the technical procedure rather than the indication for the intervention.

Incomplete treatment with residual or recurrent complaints should also be considered to be complications, since further action is needed (Cioni et al. 2004; Cribb et al. 2005; Guglielmi et al. 2005; Barragan-Campos et al. 2006; Weber et al. 2006; Gangi et al. 2007).

Table 9.2. Primary and secondary success rate of different ablation therapies in malignant bone tumours in terms of pain relief. (*Cryo* Cryoplasty, *KP* kyphoplasty, *OP* osteoplasty, *R* radiation therapy, *RFA* radiofrequency ablation)

Author	No. of patients/ procedures	Method	Primary success (%0	Long-term success	Complications	Follow-up (months)
Weill et al. (1996)	37/52	OP	94	73%	Neurologic (*n*=3)	13
Alvarez et al. (2003)	21	OP + R (15), surgery (3)	81	–	Neuritis (*n*=1)	5.6 (1–18)
Fourney et al. (2003)	56/97	OP/KP	84	–	0	4.5 (1–19.7)
Goetz et al. (2004)	43	RFA	95	–	Burns (*n*=1), transient incontinence (*n*=1), fracture (*n*=1)	16
Jagas et al. (2005)	21/21	OP + R	100		0	1–8
Jang and Lee 2005	28/72	OP + R	89	–	0	1–9
Kelekis et al. (2005)	14/23	OP	92	–	Leakage (*n*=1)	9 (1–24)
Mont'Alverne et al. (2005)	12/12 (axis)	OP	80		Neurologic (*n*=2)	6.9
Toyota et al. (2005)	17/23	RFA + OP	100	82.4%	Haematoma (*n*=1)	1–30
Callstrom et al. (2006)	14/22	Cryo	67	86%	0	3–24
Calmels et al. (2007)	52/59	OP	86	92%	Neurologic (*n*=4) Haematothorax (*n*=1), pulmonary embolism (*n*=2)	17
Hoffmann et al. (2007)	22/28	RFA + OP	90.9	100%	0	7.7 (3–15)
Total	**337/428**		**88.2**	**86.7%**	**17/428 (4.0%)**	**8.5 (1–30)**

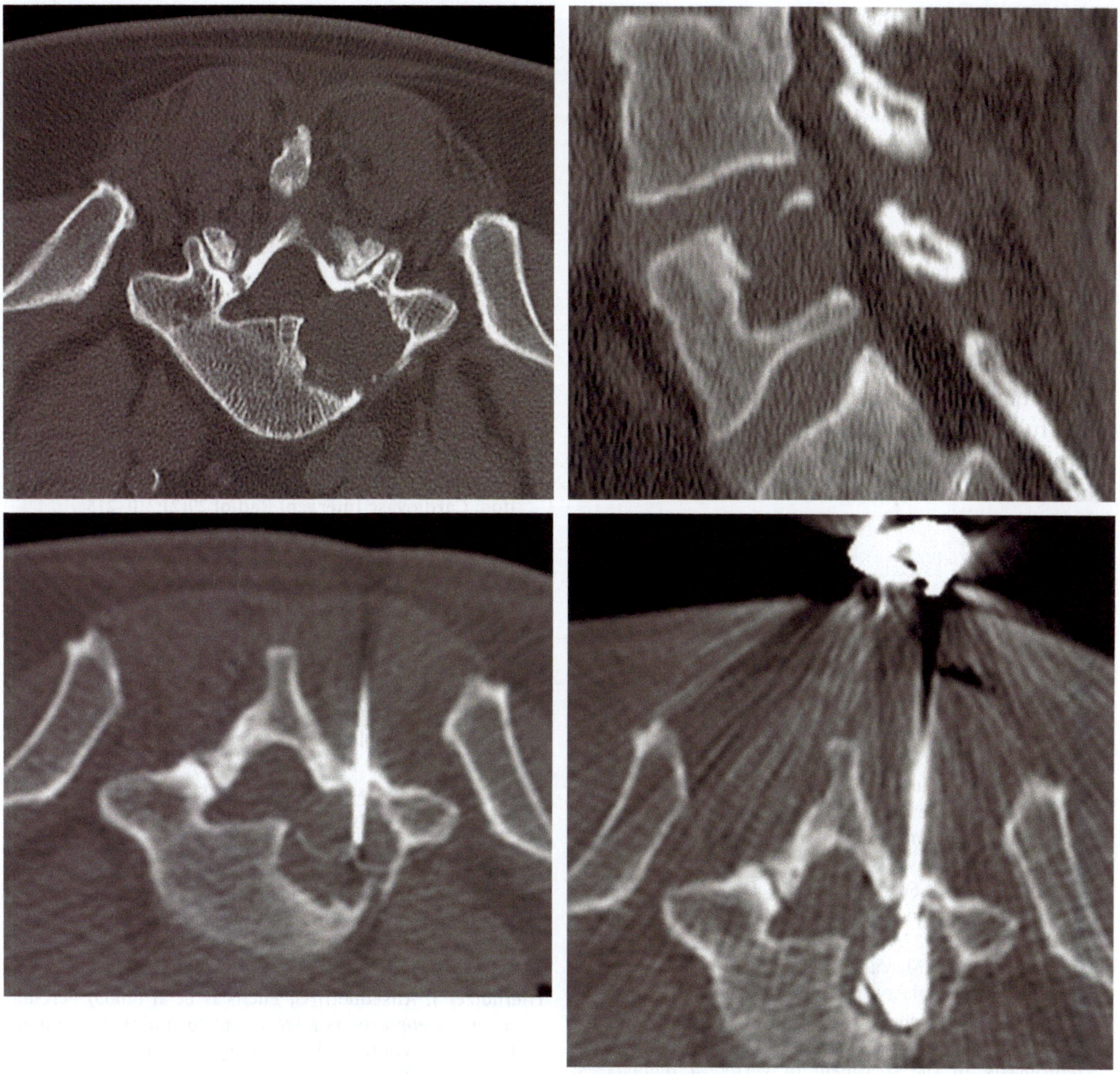

Fig. 9.3a–d. **a** A 58-year-old male patient with renal cell cancer and a symptomatic metastasis to the fifth lumbar vertebra. Note that the posterior lamina of the vertebra is already penetrated. **b** The coronal re-formation displays the total cranio-caudal extent. **c** The lamina of the pedicle could be passed by the umbrella-like electrode and the tines could be deployed within the tumoral cavity. Under conscious sedation without any neurological sensations the ablation procedure was performed with 10 W over 10 min until the impedance rose significantly, aborting the energy delivery. **d** Subsequently, in the same session, a vertebroplasty needle was placed into the tumor cavity and 2.5 ml of PMMA cement were injected under CT-fluoroscopic guidance. Within 24 h the patient was free of pain and presented during the follow-up period of 30 months with no tumor or pain recurrence

9.8 Summary

At present, the experience with local thermal ablation and/or augmentation for adjuvant thermal ablation is very limited. Nevertheless, it seems that there is high potential for synergistic and complementary therapeutic concepts to both enhance the efficacy of established therapies and be used as an alternative therapeutic option in cases where established options are no longer applicable (Poggi et al. 2003; Goetz et al. 2004; Kelekis et al. 2005; Simon and Dupuy 2006).

The benefits of thermal ablation and cement augmentation are their ease of use, their high success rate and their low complication rate. There are no major contraindications to these therapies; moreover, they can easily be repeated and combined with other treatment options such as radiotherapy or surgery.

The excellent results achieved using thermal ablation to treat osteoid osteomas mean that it must be considered to be the method of first choice, superior to surgical resection.

Furthermore, in malignant bone tumours, when surgery and/or radiotherapy are no longer applicable, these methods offer a new, very effective therapeutic option for pain management. The exact role of minimally invasive ablative therapies among the huge armamentarium of different treatment options is not fully defined; therefore, additional study evidence must be obtained to appreciate the high potential of these therapies.

References

Albisinni U,,Malaguti C (2007) An unusual complication of radiofrequency ablation treatment of osteoid osteoma. Clin Orthop Relat Res [Epub ahead of print]

Alvarez L, Perez-Higueras A, Quinones D et al (2003) Vertebroplasty in the treatment of vertebral tumors: postprocedural outcome and quality of life. Eur Spine J 12(4):356–360

Barei DP, Moreau G, Scarborough MT et al (2000) Percutaneous radiofrequency ablation of osteoid osteoma. Clin Orthop Relat Res 373:115–124

Barragan-Campos HM, Vallee JN, Lo D et al (2006) Percutaneous vertebroplasty for spinal metastases: complications. Radiology 238(1):354–362

Brodano GB, Cappuccio M, Gasbarrini A et al (2007) Vertebroplasty in the treatment of vertebral metastases: clinical cases and review of the literature. Eur Rev Med Pharmacol Sci 11(2):91–100

Callstrom MR, Charboneau JW (2005) Percutaneous ablation: safe, effective treatment of bone tumors. Oncology (Williston Park) 19 [11 Suppl. 4]:22–26

Callstrom MR, Atwell TD, Charboneau JW et al (2006) Painful metastases involving bone: percutaneous image-guided cryoablation – prospective trial interim analysis. Radiology 241(2):572–580

Calmels V, Vallee JN, Rose M et al (2007) Osteoblastic and mixed spinal metastases: evaluation of the analgesic efficacy of percutaneous vertebroplasty. AJNR Am J Neuroradiol 28(3):570–574

Cantwell CP, Obyrne J, Eustace S (2004) Current trends in treatment of osteoid osteoma with an emphasis on radiofrequency ablation. Eur Radiol 14(4):607–617

Cheung G, Chow E, Holden L et al (2006) Percutaneous vertebroplasty in patients with intractable pain from osteoporotic or metastatic fractures: a prospective study using quality-of-life assessment. Can Assoc Radiol J 57(1):13–21

Cioni R, Armillotta N, Bargellini I et al (2004) CT-guided radiofrequency ablation of osteoid osteoma: long-term results. Eur Radiol 14(7):1203–1208

Cribb GL, Goude WH, Cool P et al (2005) Percutaneous radiofrequency thermocoagulation of osteoid osteomas: factors affecting therapeutic outcome. Skeletal Radiol 34(11):702–706

Fourney DR, Schomer DF, Nader R et al (2003) Percutaneous vertebroplasty and kyphoplasty for painful vertebral body fractures in cancer patients. J Neurosurg 98 [1 Suppl.]:21–30

Gangi A, Basile A, Buy X et al (2005) Radiofrequency and laser ablation of spinal lesions. Semin Ultrasound CT MR 26(2):89–97

Gangi A, Alizadeh H, Wong L et al (2007) Osteoid osteoma: percutaneous laser ablation and follow-up in 114 patients. Radiology 242(1):293–301

Gebauer B, Tunn PU, Gaffke G et al (2006) Osteoid osteoma: experience with laser- and radiofrequency-induced ablation. Cardiovasc Intervent Radiol 29(2):210–215

Ghanem I (2006) The management of osteoid osteoma: updates and controversies. Curr Opin Pediatr 18(1):36–41

Goetz MP, Callstrom MR, Charboneau JW et al (2004) Percutaneous image-guided radiofrequency ablation of painful metastases involving bone: a multicenter study. J Clin Oncol 22(2):300–306

Guglielmi G, Andreula C, Muto M et al (2005) Percutaneous vertebroplasty: indications, contraindications, technique, and complications. Acta Radiol 46(3):256–268

Halpin RJ, Bendok BR, Liu JC (2004) Minimally invasive treatments for spinal metastases: vertebroplasty, kyphoplasty, and radiofrequency ablation. J Support Oncol 2(4):339–351; discussion 352–355

Halpin RJ, Bendok BR, Sato KT et al (2005) Combination treatment of vertebral metastases using image-guided percutaneous radiofrequency ablation and vertebroplasty: a case report. Surg Neurol 63(5):469–474; discussion 474–475

Hierholzer J, Anselmetti G, Fuchs H et al (2003) Percutaneous osteoplasty as a treatment for painful malignant bone lesions of the pelvis and femur. J Vasc Interv Radiol 14(6):773–777

Hoffmann RT, Jakobs TF, Trumm C et al (2007) Radiofrequency ablation in combination with osteoplasty for the treatment of bone malignancies. J Vasc Interv Radiol (in press)

Jagas M, Patrzyk R, Zwolinski J et al (2005) Vertebroplasty with methacrylate bone cement and radiotherapy in the treatment of spinal metastases with epidural spinal cord compression. Preliminary report. Ortop Traumatol Rehabil 7(5):491–498

Jakobs TF, Trumm C, Reiser M et al (2007) Percutaneous vertebroplasty in tumoral osteolysis. Eur Radiol 17(8):2166–2175

Jang JS, Lee SH (2005) Efficacy of percutaneous vertebroplasty combined with radiotherapy in osteolytic metastatic spinal tumors. J Neurosurg Spine 2(3):243–248

Kelekis A, Lovblad KO, Mehdizade A et al (2005) Pelvic osteoplasty in osteolytic metastases: technical approach under fluoroscopic guidance and early clinical results. J Vasc Interv Radiol 16(1):81–88

Klein MH, Shankman S (1992) Osteoid osteoma: radiologic and pathologic correlation. Skeletal Radiol 21(1):23–31

Lindner NJ, Ozaki T, Roedl R et al (2001) Percutaneous radiofrequency ablation in osteoid osteoma. J Bone Joint Surg Br 83(3):391–396

Llovet JM, Burroughs A, Bruix J (2003) Hepatocellular carcinoma. Lancet 362(9399):1907–1917

Martel J, Bueno A, Ortiz E (2005) Percutaneous radiofrequency treatment of osteoid osteoma using cool-tip electrodes. Eur J Radiol 56(3):403–408

Masala S, Fiori R,Massari F et al (2003) Vertebroplasty and kyphoplasty: new equipment for malignant vertebral fractures treatment. J Exp Clin Cancer Res 22 [4 Suppl.]:75–79

Masala S, Lunardi P, Fiori R et al (2004) Vertebroplasty and kyphoplasty in the treatment of malignant vertebral fractures. J Chemother 16 [Suppl. 5]:30–33

Mont'Alverne F, Vallee JN, Cormier E et al (2005) Percutaneous vertebroplasty for metastatic involvement of the axis. AJNR Am J Neuroradiol 26(7):1641–1645

Pinto CH, Taminiau AH, Vanderschueren GM et al (2002) Technical considerations in CT-guided radiofrequency thermal ablation of osteoid osteoma: tricks of the trade. AJR Am J Roentgenol 179(6):1633–1642

Poggi G, Gatti C, Melazzini M et al (2003) Percutaneous ultrasound-guided radiofrequency thermal ablation of malignant osteolyses. Anticancer Res 23(6D):4977–4983

Rimondi E, Bianchi G, Malaguti MC et al (2005) Radiofrequency thermoablation of primary non-spinal osteoid osteoma: optimization of the procedure. Eur Radiol 15(7):1393–1399

Ronkainen J, Blanco Sequeiros R, Tervonen O (2006) Cost comparison of low-field (0.23 T) MRI-guided laser ablation and surgery in the treatment of osteoid osteoma. Eur Radiol 16(12):2858–2865

Rosenthal DI, Hornicek FJ, Wolfe MW et al (1998) Percutaneous radiofrequency coagulation of osteoid osteoma compared with operative treatment. J Bone Joint Surg Am 80(6):815–821

Rosenthal DI, Hornicek FJ, Torriani M et al (2003) Osteoid osteoma: percutaneous treatment with radiofrequency energy. Radiology 229(1):171–175

Schaefer O, Lohrmann C, Herling M et al (2002) Combined radiofrequency thermal ablation and percutaneous cementoplasty treatment of a pathologic fracture. J Vasc Interv Radiol 13(10):1047–1050

Shankman S, Desai P, Beltran J (1997) Subperiosteal osteoid osteoma: radiographic and pathologic manifestations. Skeletal Radiol 26(8):457–462

Simon CJ, Dupuy DE (2006) Percutaneous minimally invasive therapies in the treatment of bone tumors: thermal ablation. Semin Musculoskelet Radiol 10(2):137–144

Toyota N, Naito A, Kakizawa H et al (2005) Radiofrequency ablation therapy combined with cementoplasty for painful bone metastases: initial experience. Cardiovasc Interv Radiol 28(5):578–583

Vanderschueren GM, Taminiau AH, Obermann WR et al (2002) Osteoid osteoma: clinical results with thermocoagulation. Radiology 224(1):82–86

Venbrux AC, Montague BJ, Murphy KP et al (2003) Image-guided percutaneous radiofrequency ablation for osteoid osteomas. J Vasc Interv Radiol 14(3):375–380

Weber CH, Krotz M, Hoffmann RT et al (2006) [CT-guided vertebroplasty and kyphoplasty: comparing technical success rate and complications in 101 cases.] Rofo 178(6):610–617

Weill A, Chiras J, Simon JM et al (1996) Spinal metastases: indications for and results of percutaneous injection of acrylic surgical cement. Radiology 199(1):241–247

Wenger M (2003) Vertebroplasty for metastasis. Med Oncol 20(3):203–209

Woertler K, Vestring T, Boettner F et al (2001) Osteoid osteoma: CT-guided percutaneous radiofrequency ablation and follow-up in 47 patients. J Vasc Interv Radiol 12(6):717–22

Subject Index

O

P

R

S

T

U

V

W

List of Contributors

Andreas Boss, MD
Institute for Diagnostic Radiology
University Clinics
Eberhards-Karls-University
Hoppe-Seyler-Strasse 3
72076 Tübingen
Germany

Damian Dupuy, MD
Diagnostic Radiology
Rhode Island Hospital
Warren Alpert Medical School of Brown University
593 Eddy Street
Providence, RI 02903
USA

Katrin Eichler, MD
Institute for Diagnostic and Interventional Radiology
University Hospital
Johann Wolfgang Goethe University
Theodor-Stern-Kai 7
60590 Frankfurt am Main
Germany

Thomas K. Helmberger, MD
Professor, Department of Diagnostic and
Interventional Radiology and Nuclear Medicine
Klinikum Bogenhausen, Academic Teaching
Hospital of the Technical University Munich
Engelschalkinger Strasse 77
81925 Munich
Germany

Ralf-Thorsten Hoffmann, MD
Department of Cinical Radiology
University Hospitals – Grosshadern
Ludwig-Maximilians-University of Munich
Marchioninistrasse 15
81377 Munich
Germany

Norbert Hosten, MD
Professor, Department of Diagnostic Radiology
and Neuroradiology
University Hospital
Sauerbruchstrasse
17475 Greifswald
Germany

Tobias F. Jakobs, MD
Department of Clinical Radiology
University Hospitals – Grosshadern
Ludwig-Maximilians-University of Munich
Marchioninistrasse 15
81377 Munich
Germany

Werner A. Kaiser, MD
Professor, Institute for Diagnostic and
Interventional Radiology
Friedrich-Schiller-University
Erlanger Allee 101
07747 Jena
Germany

Gerhard Kirsch, MD
Nuclear Medicine Department
University Hospital
Fleischmannstrasse 42
17475 Greifswald
Germany

Michael Kirsch, MD
Professor, Department of Diagnostic Radiology and
Neuroradiology
University Hospital
Sauerbruchstrasse
17475 Greifswald
Germany

Andreas Lubienski, MD
Institut für Radiologie der Universität Lübeck
Ratzeburger Allee 160
23538 Lübeck
Germany

Martin G. Mack, MD
PD, Institute for Diagnostic and
Interventional Radiology
University Hospital
Johann Wolfgang Goethe University
Theodor-Stern-Kai 7
60590 Frankfurt am Main
Germany

ANDREAS H. MAHNKEN, MD, MBA
Department of Diagnostic Radiology
University Hospital, RWTH Aachen University
Pauwelsstrasse 30
52074 Aachen
Germany

KONRAD MOHNIKE, MD
Klinik für Radiologie und Nuklearmedizin
Universitätsklinikum Magdeburg AöR
Leipziger Strasse 44
39120 Magdeburg
Germany

HERWART MÜLLER, MD
Oncological Surgery
Hammelburg Hospitals
Ofenthaler Weg 20
97762 Hammelburg
Germany

MOHAMMED NABIL, MD
Institute for Diagnostic and Interventional Radiology
University Hospital
Johann Wolfgang Goethe University
Theodor-Stern-Kai 7
60590 Frankfurt am Main
Germany

PHILIPPE L. PEREIRA, MD
Institute for Diagnostic Radiology
University Clinics
Eberhards-Karls-University
Hoppe-Seyler-Strasse 3
72076 Tübingen
Germany

STEFAN O. R. PFLEIDERER, MD
Institute for Diagnostic and Interventional Radiology
Friedrich-Schiller-University
Erlanger Allee 101
07747 Jena
Germany

DIRK PROSCHEK, MD
Orthopedic University Hospital
Johann Wolfgang Goethe University
Marienburgstrasse 2
60528 Frankfurt am Main
Germany

MAXIMILIAN F. REISER, MD
Professor and Chairman
Department of Clinical Radiology
University Hospitals - Grosshadern and Innenstadt
Ludwig-Maximilians-University of Munich
Marchioninistrasse 15
81377 Munich
Germany

JENS RICKE, MD
Professor, Klinik für Radiologie und Nuklearmedizin
Universitätsklinikum Magdeburg AöR
Leipziger Strasse 44
39120 Magdeburg
Germany

MARTIN SIMON, MD
Institut für Radiologie der Universität Lübeck
Ratzeburger Allee 160
23538 Lübeck
Germany

KARIN STEINKE, MD
Associate Professor, Medical Imaging
Royal Brisbane and Womens Hospital
Herston, 4029 QLD
Australia

CHRISTOPH TRUMM, MD
Department of Cinical Radiology
University Hospitals - Grosshadern
Ludwig-Maximilians-University of Munich
Marchioninistrasse 15
81377 Munich
Germany

THOMAS J. VOGL, MD
Professor, Institute for Diagnostic and
Interventional Radiology, University Hospital
Johann-Wolfgang-Goethe-University
Theodor-Stern-Kai 7
60590 Frankfurt am Main
Germany

STEPHAN ZANGOS, MD
Institute for Diagnostic and Interventional Radiology
University Hospital
Johann-Wolfgang-Goethe-University
Theodor-Stern-Kai 7
60590 Frankfurt am Main
Germany

ANDREAS ZINKE, MD
Professor, Nuclear Medicine Department
University Hospital
Fleischmannstrasse 42
17475 Greifswald
Germany

MEDICAL RADIOLOGY Diagnostic Imaging and Radiation Oncology

Titles in the series already published

DIAGNOSTIC IMAGING

Innovations in Diagnostic Imaging
Edited by J. H. Anderson

Radiology of the Upper Urinary Tract
Edited by E. K. Lang

The Thymus - Diagnostic Imaging, Functions, and Pathologic Anatomy
Edited by E. Walter, E. Willich, and W. R. Webb

Interventional Neuroradiology
Edited by A. Valavanis

Radiology of the Pancreas
Edited by A. L. Baert, co-edited by G. Delorme

Radiology of the Lower Urinary Tract
Edited by E. K. Lang

Magnetic Resonance Angiography
Edited by I. P. Arlart, G. M. Bongartz, and G. Marchal

Contrast-Enhanced MRI of the Breast
S. Heywang-Köbrunner and R. Beck

Spiral CT of the Chest
Edited by M. Rémy-Jardin and J. Rémy

Radiological Diagnosis of Breast Diseases
Edited by M. Friedrich and E.A. Sickles

Radiology of the Trauma
Edited by M. Heller and A. Fink

Biliary Tract Radiology
Edited by P. Rossi, co-edited by M. Brezi

Radiological Imaging of Sports Injuries
Edited by C. Masciocchi

Modern Imaging of the Alimentary Tube
Edited by A. R. Margulis

Diagnosis and Therapy of Spinal Tumors
Edited by P. R. Algra, J. Valk, and J. J. Heimans

Interventional Magnetic Resonance Imaging
Edited by J. F. Debatin and G. Adam

Abdominal and Pelvic MRI
Edited by A. Heuck and M. Reiser

Orthopedic Imaging
Techniques and Applications
Edited by A. M. Davies and H. Pettersson

Radiology of the Female Pelvic Organs
Edited by E. K.Lang

Magnetic Resonance of the Heart and Great Vessels
Clinical Applications
Edited by J. Bogaert, A.J. Duerinckx, and F. E. Rademakers

Modern Head and Neck Imaging
Edited by S. K. Mukherji and J. A. Castelijns

Radiological Imaging of Endocrine Diseases
Edited by J. N. Bruneton in collaboration with B. Padovani and M.-Y. Mourou

Trends in Contrast Media
Edited by H. S. Thomsen, R. N. Muller, and R. F. Mattrey

Functional MRI
Edited by C. T. W. Moonen and P. A. Bandettini

Radiology of the Pancreas
2nd Revised Edition
Edited by A. L. Baert. Co-edited by G. Delorme and L. Van Hoe

Emergency Pediatric Radiology
Edited by H. Carty

Spiral CT of the Abdomen
Edited by F. Terrier, M. Grossholz, and C. D. Becker

Liver Malignancies
Diagnostic and Interventional Radiology
Edited by C. Bartolozzi and R. Lencioni

Medical Imaging of the Spleen
Edited by A. M. De Schepper and F. Vanhoenacker

Radiology of Peripheral Vascular Diseases
Edited by E. Zeitler

Diagnostic Nuclear Medicine
Edited by C. Schiepers

Radiology of Blunt Trauma of the Chest
P. Schnyder and M. Wintermark

Portal Hypertension
Diagnostic Imaging-Guided Therapy
Edited by P. Rossi
Co-edited by P. Ricci and L. Broglia

Recent Advances in Diagnostic Neuroradiology
Edited by Ph. Demaerel

Virtual Endoscopy and Related 3D Techniques
Edited by P. Rogalla, J. Terwisscha Van Scheltinga, and B. Hamm

Multislice CT
Edited by M. F. Reiser, M. Takahashi, M. Modic, and R. Bruening

Pediatric Uroradiology
Edited by R. Fotter

Transfontanellar Doppler Imaging in Neonates
A. Couture and C. Veyrac

Radiology of AIDS
A Practical Approach
Edited by J.W.A.J. Reeders and P.C. Goodman

CT of the Peritoneum
Armando Rossi and Giorgio Rossi

Magnetic Resonance Angiography
2nd Revised Edition
Edited by I. P. Arlart, G. M. Bongratz, and G. Marchal

Pediatric Chest Imaging
Edited by Javier Lucaya and Janet L. Strife

Applications of Sonography in Head and Neck Pathology
Edited by J. N. Bruneton in collaboration with C. Raffaelli and O. Dassonville

Imaging of the Larynx
Edited by R. Hermans

3D Image Processing
Techniques and Clinical Applications
Edited by D. Caramella and C. Bartolozzi

Imaging of Orbital and Visual Pathway Pathology
Edited by W. S. Müller-Forell

Pediatric ENT Radiology
Edited by S. J. King and A. E. Boothroyd

Radiological Imaging of the Small Intestine
Edited by N. C. Gourtsoyiannis

Imaging of the Knee
Techniques and Applications
Edited by A. M. Davies and V. N. Cassar-Pullicino

Perinatal Imaging
From Ultrasound to MR Imaging
Edited by Fred E. Avni

Radiological Imaging of the Neonatal Chest
Edited by V. Donoghue

Diagnostic and Interventional Radiology in Liver Transplantation
Edited by E. Bücheler, V. Nicolas, C. E. Broelsch, X. Rogiers, and G. Krupski

Radiology of Osteoporosis
Edited by S. Grampp

Imaging Pelvic Floor Disorders
Edited by C. I. Bartram and J. O. L. DeLancey
Associate Editors: S. Halligan, F. M. Kelvin, and J. Stoker

Imaging of the Pancreas
Cystic and Rare Tumors
Edited by C. Procacci and A. J. Megibow

High Resolution Sonography of the Peripheral Nervous System
Edited by S. Peer and G. Bodner

Medical Radiology Diagnostic Imaging and Radiation Oncology

Titles in the series already published

Radiation Oncology

Lung Cancer
Edited by C.W. Scarantino

Innovations in Radiation Oncology
Edited by H. R. Withers and L. J. Peters

Radiation Therapy of Head and Neck Cancer
Edited by G. E. Laramore

Gastrointestinal Cancer – Radiation Therapy
Edited by R.R. Dobelbower, Jr.

Radiation Exposure and Occupational Risks
Edited by E. Scherer, C. Streffer, and K.-R. Trott

Radiation Therapy of Benign Diseases
A Clinical Guide
S. E. Order and S. S. Donaldson

Interventional Radiation Therapy Techniques – Brachytherapy
Edited by R. Sauer

Radiopathology of Organs and Tissues
Edited by E. Scherer, C. Streffer, and K.-R. Trott

Concomitant Continuous Infusion Chemotherapy and Radiation
Edited by M. Rotman and C. J. Rosenthal

Intraoperative Radiotherapy – Clinical Experiences and Results
Edited by F. A. Calvo, M. Santos, and L.W. Brady

Radiotherapy of Intraocular and Orbital Tumors
Edited by W. E. Alberti and R. H. Sagerman

Interstitial and Intracavitary Thermoradiotherapy
Edited by M. H. Seegenschmiedt and R. Sauer

Non-Disseminated Breast Cancer
Controversial Issues in Management
Edited by G. H. Fletcher and S.H. Levitt

Current Topics in Clinical Radiobiology of Tumors
Edited by H.-P. Beck-Bornholdt

Practical Approaches to Cancer Invasion and Metastases
A Compendium of Radiation Oncologists' Responses to 40 Histories
Edited by A. R. Kagan with the Assistance of R. J. Steckel

Radiation Therapy in Pediatric Oncology
Edited by J. R. Cassady

Radiation Therapy Physics
Edited by A. R. Smith

Late Sequelae in Oncology
Edited by J. Dunst and R. Sauer

Mediastinal Tumors. Update 1995
Edited by D. E. Wood and C. R. Thomas, Jr.

Thermoradiotherapy and Thermochemotherapy
Volume 1:
Biology, Physiology, and Physics
Volume 2:
Clinical Applications
Edited by M.H. Seegenschmiedt, P. Fessenden, and C.C. Vernon

Carcinoma of the Prostate
Innovations in Management
Edited by Z. Petrovich, L. Baert, and L.W. Brady

Radiation Oncology of Gynecological Cancers
Edited by H.W. Vahrson

Carcinoma of the Bladder
Innovations in Management
Edited by Z. Petrovich, L. Baert, and L.W. Brady

Blood Perfusion and Microenvironment of Human Tumors
Implications for Clinical Radiooncology
Edited by M. Molls and P. Vaupel

Radiation Therapy of Benign Diseases
A Clinical Guide
2nd Revised Edition
S. E. Order and S. S. Donaldson

Carcinoma of the Kidney and Testis, and Rare Urologic Malignancies
Innovations in Management
Edited by Z. Petrovich, L. Baert, and L.W. Brady

Progress and Perspectives in the Treatment of Lung Cancer
Edited by P. Van Houtte, J. Klastersky, and P. Rocmans

Combined Modality Therapy of Central Nervous System Tumors
Edited by Z. Petrovich, L. W. Brady, M. L. Apuzzo, and M. Bamberg

Age-Related Macular Degeneration
Current Treatment Concepts
Edited by W. A. Alberti, G. Richard, and R. H. Sagerman

Radiotherapy of Intraocular and Orbital Tumors
2nd Revised Edition
Edited by R. H. Sagerman, and W. E. Alberti

Modification of Radiation Response
Cytokines, Growth Factors, and Other Biolgical Targets
Edited by C. Nieder, L. Milas, and K. K. Ang

Radiation Oncology for Cure and Palliation
R. G. Parker, N. A. Janjan, and M. T. Selch

Clinical Target Volumes in Conformal and Intensity Modulated Radiation Therapy
A Clinical Guide to Cancer Treatment
Edited by V. Grégoire, P. Scalliet, and K. K. Ang

Advances in Radiation Oncology in Lung Cancer
Edited by Branislav Jeremić

New Technologies in Radiation Oncology
Edited by W. Schlegel, T. Bortfeld, and A.-L. Grosu

Technical Basis of Radiation Therapy
4th Revised Edition
Edited by S. H. Levitt, J. A. Purdy, C. A. Perez, and S. Vijayakumar

CURED I • LENT
Late Effects of Cancer Treatment on Normal Tissues
Edited by P. Rubin, L. S. Constine, L. B. Marks, and P. Okunieff

Clinical Practice of Radiation Therapy for Benign Diseases
Contemporary Concepts and Clinical Results
Edited by M. H. Seegenschmiedt, H.-B. Makoski, K.-R. Trott, and L. W. Brady

Springer

MIX
Papier aus verantwortungsvollen Quellen
Paper from responsible sources
FSC® C105338

If you have any concerns about our products,
you can contact us on
ProductSafety@springernature.com

In case Publisher is established outside the EU,
the EU authorized representative is:
Springer Nature Customer Service Center GmbH
Europaplatz 3, 69115 Heidelberg, Germany

Printed by Libri Plureos GmbH
in Hamburg, Germany